Farm Animals: A Veterinary Science Perspective

Farm Animals: A Veterinary Science Perspective

Edited by Ryan Jaxon

MURPHY & MOORE
www.murphy-moorepublishing.com

Published by Murphy & Moore Publishing,
1 Rockefeller Plaza,
New York City, NY 10020, USA
www.murphy-moorepublishing.com

Farm Animals: A Veterinary Science Perspective
Edited by Ryan Jaxon

International Standard Book Number: 978-1-63987-223-7 (Hardback)

Cataloging-in-Publication Data

Farm animals : a veterinary science perspective / edited by Ryan Jaxon.
p. cm.
Includes bibliographical references and index.
ISBN 978-1-63987-223-7
1. Domestic animals. 2. Veterinary medicine. 3. Zoology, Economic. 4. Domestic animals--Diseases.
5. Animal health. I. Jaxon, Ryan.
SF745 .F37 2022
636.089--dc23

TABLE OF CONTENTS

PREFACE

Farm animals or livestock are animals that are raised in an agricultural setting for the production of meat, milk, eggs, fur, wool or leather. This includes animals such as sheep, cattle, swine, poultry, goats, etc. Traditionally, farm animals were not confined within enclosures, allowing them the freedom to forage for food. Such practices have now mostly been replaced by intensive animal farming. Poultry are kept in cages or barns under controlled conditions, while dairy cows and beef cattle are kept in high density feedlots or in zero-grazing conditions. This leads to an increased susceptibility to developing internal and external parasites, and other diseases. To avoid such circumstances from arising and for optimal production, proper feeding, hygiene, good husbandry and veterinary care are essential. Routine vaccinations and use of antibiotics when necessary can prevent many diseases from occurring. Such measures can prevent the spread of contagious diseases between animals, and between animals and humans. The topics included in this book on farm animals are of utmost significance and bound to provide incredible insights to readers. While understanding the long-term perspectives of the topics, the book makes an effort in highlighting their impacts as a modern tool in the sustenance of animal health and welfare in the farm. With state-of-the-art inputs by acclaimed experts of this field, this book targets students and professionals.

This book is the end result of constructive efforts and intensive research done by experts in this field. The aim of this book is to enlighten the readers with recent information in this area of research. The information provided in this profound book would serve as a valuable reference to students and researchers in this field.

At the end, I would like to thank all the authors for devoting their precious time and providing their valuable contribution to this book. I would also like to express my gratitude to my fellow colleagues who encouraged me throughout the process.

Editor

1

Plasma pharmacokinetics and muscle disposition of marbofloxacin in chickens

Urzúa, N.[1], Errecalde, C.[1], Prieto, G.[1*], Lüders, C.[2], Picco, E.[3], Paula Tonini, M.[1]

[1]Department of Pharmacology, Faculty of Agriculture and Veterinary, National University of Río Cuarto, Río Cuarto, Argentina

[2]School of Veterinary Medicine, Catholic University of Temuco, Temuco, Chile

[3]Department of Pharmacology, Faculty of Veterinary Sciences, National University of the Litoral, Esperanza, Argentina

Key words:
chickens, HPLC, marbofloxacin, pharmacokinetics

Correspondence
Prieto, G.
Department of Pharmacology, Faculty of Agriculture and Veterinary, National University of Río Cuarto, Río Cuarto, Argentina

Email: gprieto@ayv.unrc.edu.ar

Abstract:

BACKGROUND: Reports on the pharmacokinetics of marbofloxacin in birds are scarce, even when it is a useful tool in poultry production. **OBJECTIVES:** Determining marbofloxacin kinetic parameters in plasma and muscle arrangement after intravenous and oral administrations and establishing its withdrawal period. **METHODS:** Clinical healthy chickens (1.08±0.22 kg) were used as experimental subjects, formed in groups of 5. In Group A (n= 45) birds received 2 mg/kg of marbofloxacin intravenously while group B (n= 65) was given the same oral dose after fasting for 12 hours. Blood samples in the groups and 5 g of muscle were obtained at different times, in A group up to 24 hours and in B group until 120 hours after application. Once the samples were obtained and treated, marbofloxacin was quantified by HPLC. **RESULTS:** Marbofloxacin in fasted chickens is almost completely absorbed (F= 97%), mean residence time is moderate (6.9 hours), with a high volume of distribution. Orally, mean residence time is less in plasma (4.9 hours) and the withdrawal time was calculated 2.5 days. **CONCLUSIONS:** The kinetic results are consistent with those presented by other fluoroquinolones in poultry and are in line with short production cycles in chickens.

Introduction

Marbofloxacin (MBFX) is a second generation fluoroquinolone marketed exclusively for veterinary medicine (Spreng et al., 1995; Martinez et al., 2006). Like other fluoroquinolones, it inhibits DNA gyrase (topoisomerase II) and topoisomerase IV creating complexes with the enzyme, which result in conformational changes, exerting antimicrobial activity against Gram negative bacteria, some Gram positive and Mycoplasma spp (García et al., 1999; Sidhu et al., 2010; Shan et al., 2013). MBFX is an organic acid, with good tissue penetration, high volume of distribution, and weak binding to plasma proteins (Anadón et al., 2002; Goudah and Hasabelnaby, 2010; Yang et al., 2014), being active at low concentrations (Ding et al., 2013). It differs from other fluoroquinolones, in the presence of an oxadiazine ring, conferring a long elimination half-life ($t_{1/2}\beta$) and high bioavailability (Goudah and Hasabelnaby, 2010; Yuan et al., 2010). These characteristics demonstrate that marbofloxacin presents a great potential for the treatment of bacterial infections in Veterinary Medicine (Thomas et al., 2001).

Investigations on MBFX pharmacokinetics in comestible birds are scarce, counting those of Anadón et al. (2002), Huang et al. (2003), and Ding et al. (2010) in chickens, Goudah and Hasabelnaby (2010) and Yuan et al. (2010) in ducks and Haritova et al. (2006, 2013) in turkeys and quail. Demonstrating short to moderate mean residence time in these species, ranging from 2.99 to 5.96 hours, the latter registered in chickens (Anadón et al., 2002), bioavailability ranges in chickens varies from 56.2% (Anadón et al., 2002) to 95.7% (Huang et al., 2003). Half-life elimination is fast in quails 2.01 (h) (Haritova et al., 2013), but slower in chickens being 5.6 and 6.5 hours after intravenous application, reported by Anadón et al. (2002) and Huang et al. (2003), respectively. The objective of this study was to describe the pharmacokinetic variables of MBFX in plasma and muscle disposition after intravenous and oral administrations, estimating MBFX withdrawal time in chickens.

Materials and Methods

Animals: 110 Ross line chickens from a farm near Río Cuarto city (Argentina) were used; these 30-day-old birds were clinically healthy, with a weight of 1.08±0.22 kg. The birds were transferred to the Veterinary Medicine Faculty at the National University of Río Cuarto and housed in a conditioned box for an acclimatization period of seven days before the study, at a temperature of 18°C, with food and water ad libitum

Experimental design (Broiler management): 110 chickens were randomly divided into two groups of 45 (A) and 65 (B) chickens respectively, with five replicates each one. Both were given a single dose of MBFX of 2 mg/kg, intravenously for group A and orally for B, after 12 hours of fasting. Following MBFX administration, according to the techniques approved by the Bioethics Committee of the National University of Río Cuarto, batches of five animals per time were slaughtered at different times, A (0.25, 0.5, 1, 2, 4, 6, 8, 12, 24 hours) and B (0.25, 0.5, 1, 2, 4, 6, 8, 12, 24, 48, 72, 96, 120 hours). Blood samples from each bird (5 ml) were centrifuged at 2500 rpm x 10 minutes and the plasma obtained was saved in sterile vials. Furthermore, samples of 5 grams of pectoral muscle were obtained and stored at -20 °C along with plasma until processing. Determination of plasma and muscle concentrations of MBFX was taken out by HPLC, using the modified technique of Bottcher et al. (2001).

HPLC conditions: MBFX and internal standard (enrofloxacin 2.5 μg/ml) were eluted isocratically with a flow rate of 0.8 ml/min using a mobile phase consisting of deionized water, acetonitrile, and triethylamine (790:200:10 V/V/V) adjusted to pH 3 with phosphoric acid. Calibrating the wavelength of fluorescence detector at 295 nm (excitation) and 490 nm (emission), respectively.

Sample preparation: The modified method of Böttcher et al. (2001) was used for the quantification of MBFX in plasma and tissue samples. Plasma samples were prepared by placing them in an Eppendorf tube 150 μL of plasma, 600 μL of extraction solution (ES) consisting of deionized water, methanol and perchloric acid in a ratio (500: 500: 1 v/ v/ v), 40 μL of internal standard, and 150 μL of deionized water. underwent agitation by vortex for 30 seconds, and then they were/it was centrifuged at 13,500 rpm for 25 min at 4°C. The obtained supernatant was filtered on nylon membrane 0.22 μm. A similar process/procedure was used for muscle samples, taking 150 mg of muscle to which 600 μL of ES, 40 μL of internal standard, and 150 μL of deionized water were added; the samples were mechanically homogenized for 1 minute and kept in refrigeration at 4°C for 12 hours for subsequent centrifugation for 25 min at 13,500 rpm at 4°C, filtering the supernatant through 0.22

µm nylon membrane.

Calibration of the chromatographic method: For testing, plasma and muscle samples were used, added with known MBFX concentrations from 0.009 to 2.5 µg/ml for plasma and 0.004 to 1.25 µg/mg for muscle. Determining the degree of adjustment of the area values index and their respective calibration by linear regression.

Data analysis: MBFX average concentrations, obtained in plasma at different times and routes, were processed by means of PK Solution 2.0 kinetic software (Farrier, 1999), in order to obtain plasma pharmacokinetic parameters. Oral bioavailability (F) was determined using the equation F = (AUCoral) / (AUCiv) (Baggot, 2002; Bousquet-Melou and Toutain, 2004).

Withdrawal period in muscle was performed by analysis of muscle residues, using the EMEA WT 1.4 Software (Hekman and Hoogland, 1996), with a confidence interval of 95%. Maximum residue limit (MRL) was established in 150 µg/kg, according to FDA and EMEA directives for MBFX.

Results

Calibration method: The method proved to be linear in the examined interval (r2 > 0.99). Intra and interassay coefficients of variation were < 1.73%. 50 µl of plasma and muscle injection provides the quantitation limits of 0,006 µg/ml and 0.07 µg/mg, respectability. Recovery tests performed to establish the precision of the extractive method in plasma samples showed a percentage of 86%, whereas in muscle it was 87%.

Intravenous and oral administrations of marbofloxacin: Figure 1 shows mean (±SD) plasma and muscle marbofloxacin concentrations versus time, whereas in Table 1 mean (±SD) values for intravenous and oral plasma pharmacokinetics parameters are shown. After a 2 mg/kg single oral dose, marbofloxacin was quickly absorbed, resulting in 0.8 µg/mlCmax, evidenced by Tmax and t½abs values of 1 and 0.126 hours respectively in plasma. It was also rapidly and widely distributed after intravenous administration, reflected by a 0.9 hour t½α and a 3.88 L/kg Vdárea, suggesting good tissue penetration; removal was slow (t½β 6.45 hours) and the plasma clearance (Clt) was 6.94 ml/min/kg.

Marbofloxacin analysis in muscle: Orally, MBFX residues were detected in muscle

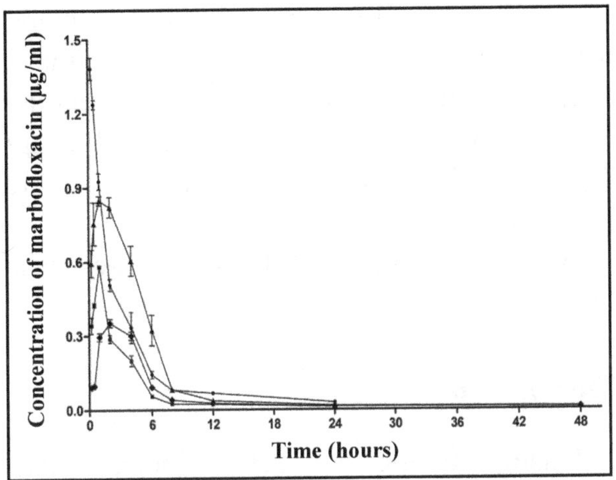

Figure 1. Marbofloxacin plasma and muscle concentration vs. time profiles, after intravenous and oral 2 mg/kg single dose in chickens (data as mean ± SD). i.v plasma —■— oral plusma —●— i.v muscle —◆— oral plusma —▲—

Table 1. Mean ± SD marbofloxacina pharmacokinetics parameters, after intravenous and oral 2 mg/kg single dose in chickens. Abbreviations: Cmax, maximum plasma concentration; Tmáx time to peak concentration; t½abs, absorption half-life; t½α distribution half-life; t½α elimination half-life; AUC, area under the curve; F (%), bioavailability; Vd area, volume of distribution; MRT, mean residence time and Cl, plasma clearance.

Pharmacokinetic parameters	IV	Oral
Cmax(µg/ml)	-	0.8
T*max* (h)	-	1.0
t½abs (h)	-	0.12
t½α (h)	0.9	2.88
t½α (h)	6.45	4.71
AUC (µg-h/ml)	4.8	4.7
F%	-	98
Vdarea L/kg	3.88	2.83
MRT (h)	6.9	4.9
Clt (L/h/kg)	0.416	0.417

up to 48 hours after administration, reaching a maximum concentration of 0.351 µg/mg 2 hours post-administration, while intravenously, the maximum concentration was 0.342 µg/mg, and residues were detected until 24 hours post-application (Fig. 1).

Withdrawal time for MBFX in muscle was estimated to be 2.5 days.

Discussion

Plasma kinetic parameters indicate that marbofloxacin oral administration has rapid absorption, reflected by a Cmax of 0.8 µg/ml, 1 hour post-administration, similar to 1.05 µg/ml obtained by Anadón et al. (2002), but less than 1.84 µg/ml obtained by Huang et al. (2003) at higher doses (2.5 mg/kg). Yuan et al., 2011 showed a Cmax of 1.13 µg/ml in ducks with a of 2.5 mg/g dose, meanwhile Haritova et al. (2003) reported 0.67 µg/ml in turkeys with a dose of 2 mg/kg, reaching Tmax 1 hour post-administration, similar to Anadón et al., 2002, Huang et al., 2003, and Ding et al., 2013 in chickens. The volume of distribution indicates a high tissue passage after intravenous application, greater than that obtained by Anadón et al. (2002) and Huang et al. (2003).

Under the rapid dissolution in intestinal media of fluoroquinolones (Kim & Nightingale, 2000; Scholar, 2002), marbofloxacin plasma concentrations could be measured from 15 minutes to 48 hours after oral administration, and these data were consistent with other studies conducted with these drugs in chickens (Anadón et al., 2002; Huang et al., 2003).

The AUCárea obtained in the study, 4.8 mg-h/ml, is lower than in chickens. Anadón et al. (2002) observed values of 10.5 mg-h/ml, giving 2 mg/kg repeated for three days, whereas Ding et al. (2013) obtained 9.8 g-h/ml, in infected animals at 5 mg/kg in repeated doses. Since fluoroquinolones are dose-dependent antimicrobials, treatments with high and repeated doses may increase the AUC.

Oral bioavailability (F= 98%) is similar to 95% reported by Huang et al. (2003), but higher than 56.8% cited by Anadón et al. (2002); this difference is attributable to the 12 hour fasting.

The high dissolution in the intestinal environment and the amphoteric character of marbofloxacin must be considered.

Plasma t½β was 6.4 hours, similar to that presented in other studies with MBFX in chickens by Anadón et al. (2002), Huang et al. (2003), and Ding et al. (2013), in which the time periods were 5.26, 6.48, and 6.8 hours, respectively. An oxadiazinic ring in MBFX structure determinates the pharmacokinetic characteristics associated with elimination half-life and bioavailability (Haritova et al., 2006), showing a moderate plasma permanence reflected by t½β and TMR. These data are consistent with the history of fluoroquinolones in poultry (Anadón et al., 2002; Ding et al., 2013) with greater tissue retention.

Marbofloxacin kinetic profile after oral and intravenous administration is consistent with that described by Anadón et al. (2002), Huang et al. (2003), Haritova et al. (2006), Yuan et al. (2011), and Ding et al. (2013) for this drug in birds.

After oral administration, muscle disposition occurs quickly detecting levels at 15 minutes and after 72 hours post-application (Anadón et al., 2002; Huang et al., 2003; Ding et al., 2013). The disposition curve versus time in muscle shows the most significant levels between 1 and 4 hours; considerable tissue levels are attributable to reduced plasma proteins binding, lipid solubility, and amphoteric characteristics determining poor ionization of the drug in blood thus facilitating passage through membranes, and slower elimination compared to the plasma (Thomas et al., 2000; Anadón et al., 2002; Baggot, 2002; Guiguére et al., 2013.)

The withdrawal period of 2.5 days agrees with that calculated by Anadón et al. (2002), but is less than that presented by Yang et al.

(2014), estimated in four days but not calculated with the software used here. The withdrawal period of this experience, which influences when choosing an antimicrobial in poultry, is reasonable and consistent with the brevity of broiler production cycles.

References

1. Anadón, A., Martinez-Larrañaga, M.R., Díaz, M.J., Martinez, M.A., Frejo, M.T., Martínez, M., Tafur, M., Castellano, V.J. (2002) Pharmacokinetic characteristics and tissue residues for marbofloxacin and its metabolite N-desmethyl marbofloxacin in broiler chickens. Am J Vet Res. 63: 927-93.
2. Baggot, J.D. (2002) En: Terapéutica Antimicrobiana Veterinanria: Principios de BiodiSponibilidad Y Disposición De Los Fármacos Antimicrobianos. Prescott J. (ed.). (3rd ed.) Buenos Aires, Argentina p. 43-76.
3. Böttcher, S., Baum, H., Hoppe-Tychy, T., Benz, C. (2001) An HPLC assay as a microbiological assay to determine levofloxacin in soft tissue, bone, bile and serum. J Pharm Biomed Anal. 25: 197-203.
4. Ding, H., Wang, L., Shen, X., G.U, X., Zeng, D., Zeng, Z. (2013) Plasma and tissue pharmacokinetics of marbofloxacin in experimentally infected chickens with Mycoplasma gallisepticum and *Escherichia coli*. J Vet Pharmacol Therap. 36: 511-515.
5. Farrier, D.S. (1999) PK Solutions 2.0, Non-compartmental Pharmacokinetics. Data Analysis. Ashland, USA.
6. García, M.A., Solansa, C., Aramayonab, J.J., Ruedab, S., Breganteb, M.A. (1999) Determination of marbofloxacin in plasma samples by high-performance liquid chromatography using fluorescence detection. J Chromatogr B. 729: 157-161.
7. Giguére, S., Prescott, J., Dowling, P., (2013) Antimicrobial Therapy in Veterinary Medicine. John Wiley and Sons. (eds.). (5th ed.) Wiley Blackwell. Iowa, USA.
8. Goudah, A., Hasabelnaby, S. (2010) The disposition of marbofloxacin after single dose intravenous, intramuscular and oral administration to Muscovy duck. J Vet Pharmacol Therap. 34: 197-201.
9. Haritova, A.M., Dimitrova, D., Dinev, T., Moutafchieva, R., Lashev, L. (2013) Comparative pharmacokinetics of enrofloxacin, danofloxacin and marbofloxacin after intravenous and oral administration in Japanese Quail (*Conturnix conturnix japónica*). J avian Med Surg. 1: 23-31.
10. Haritova, A.M., Rusenova, N.V., Parvanov, P.R., Lashev, L.D., Fink- Gremmels, J. (2006) Integration of pharmacokinetic and pharmacodynamic indices of marbofloxacin in turkeys. Antimicrob Agents Chemother. 50: 3779-3785.
11. Hekman, P. (1996) WT1.4 Withdrawal time calculation program. Freeware, distributed by the European Agency for the Evaluation of Medicinal Products (EMEA), London, UK.
12. Huang, X.H., Chen, Z.L., Zhang, S.T., Zeng, Z.L. (2003) Influence of experimentally *Pasteurella multocida* Infection on the pharmacokinetics of marbofloxacin in broiler chickens. Acta Veterinaria et Zootechnica Sinica. 34: 98-102.
13. Kim, M., Nightingale, C. (2000) The Quinolones:Pharmacokinect and pharmacodynamic of the fluoroquinolones. Andriole, V. (ed.) (3rd ed.) California, USA. p. 169-193.
14. Martinez, M., McDermott, P., Walker, R. (2006) Pharmacology of the fluoroquinolones: a perspective for the use in domestic animals. Vet J. 172: 10-28.
15. Shan, Q., Wang, J., Yang, F., Ding, H., Liang, C., Lv, Z., Li, Z., Zen, Z. (2013) Pharmacokinetic/pharmacodynamic relationship of marbofloxacin against *Pasteurella multocida* in a tissue-cage model in yellow cattle. J Vet Pharmacol Therap. 37: 222-230.
16. Sidhu, P.K., Landoni, M.F., AliAbadi F.S., Lees, P. (2010) Pharmacokinetic and phar-

macodynamic modelling of marbofloxacin administered alone and in combination with tolfenamic acid in goats. Vet J. 184: 219-229.

17. Spreng, M., Deleforge, J., Thomas, V., Boisram_e, B., Drugeon, H. (1995) Antibacterial activity of marbofloxacin. A new fluoroquinolone for veterinary use against canine and feline isolates. J Vet Pharmacol Therap. 18: 284-289.
18. Thomas, E., Caldow G.L., Borell, D., Davot J.L (2001) A field comparison of the efficacy and tolerance of marbofloxacin in the treatment of bovine respiratory disease. J Ve Pharmacol Therap. 24: 353-358.
19. Thomas, E., Grandemange, E., Pommier, P., Wessel-Robert, S., Davot, J.L (2000) Field evaluation of efficacy and tolerance of a 2% marbofloxacin injectable solution for the treatment of respiratory disease in fattening pigs. Vet Q. 22: 131-135.
20. Toutain, P., Bousquet-Mélou, A. (2004) Bioavailability and its assessment. J Vet Pharmacol Therap. 27: 455-466.
21. Yang, F., Yang, Y.R., Wang, L., Huang, X.H., Qiao, G., Zeng, Z.L. (2014) Estimating marbofloxacin withdrawal time in broiler chickens using a population physiologically based pharmacokinetics model. J Vet Pharmacol Therap. 37: 579-588.
22. Yuan, L.G., Wang, R., Sun, L.H., Luo, X.Y., Sun, J., Fang, B.H., Liu, Y.H. (2011) Pharmacokinetics of marbofloxacin in Muscovy ducks (*Carina moschata*). J Vet Pharmacol Therap. 30: 10-15.

2

Relationship between ghrelin and estrogen in the ovary of pregnant sheep

Sookhtehzari, A.[1*], **Alirezaei, M.**[2]

[1]*Department of Clinical Sciences, School of Veterinary Medicine, Lorestan University, Khorramabad, Iran*
[2]*Division of Biochemistry, School of Veterinary Medicine, Lorestan University, Khorramabad, Iran*

Key words:
corpora lutea, estrogen, follicle, ghrelin, sheep

Correspondence
Sookhtehzari, A.
Department of Clinical Sciences, School of Veterinary Medicine, Lorestan University, Khorramabad, Iran

Email: asookhthezary@yahoo.com

Abstract:

BACKGROUND: Ghrelin, an endogenous ligand for the growth secretagogue receptor is predominantly produced in the stomach and an expression of ghrelin has recently been identified in placenta and ovary. **OBJECTIVES:** Therefore, we decited to measure ovarian ghrelin as quantitative and evaluate the correlation between ghrelin and estrogen during second half of ovine pregnancy. **METHODS:** The ovarian samples were collected from 40 pregnant sheep in 3, 3.5, 4, 4.5 and 5 months of pregnancy in a local abattoir. Follicles and active corpora lutea (CL) were dissected from surrounding tissues, separately. The samples were homogenized with phosphate buffer (0.1 M, pH=7.4) on liquid nitrogen to provide fluid samples. Ghrelin and estrogen concentrations were measured by ELISA method and expressed as milligram (mg) and picogram (pg) per mg of tissue protein, respectively. **RESULTS:** There was a linear correlation between ghrelin and estrogen in ovarian follicles ($r=0.97$ and $p=0.004$), but not in CL. Follicular ghrelin significantly increased in 4, 4.5 and 5 months ($p<0.001$) but CL ghrelin significantly decreased in the 4.5 month of ovine pregnancy ($p<0.01$). Estrogen concentration was also significantly higher in 4-5 months of pregnancy in ovarian follicles ($p<0.001$) but potent CL indicated higher estrogen level only in the 5th month of pregnancy ($p<0.001$). **CONCLUSIONS:** These results emphasize the role of ghrelin in the reproductive system and open a new window to future studies.

Introduction

In recent years, there has been increasingly more evidence to support the biological actions of ghrelin than those originally anticipated (Alirezaei et al., 2015; Du et al., 2010; Dupont et al., 2010; Du et al., 2009; Rak and Gregoraszczuk 2008; Caminos et al., 2003). Ghrelin has been identified as an endogenous ligand for growth hormone secretagogue receptor (GHSR) that regulates growth hormone (GH) secretion, regulates food intake, increases appetite and contributes to insulin release and energy homeostasis as well as acingt as an antioxidant peptide (Alirezaei et al., 2015; Kheradmand et al. 2010, 2011; Neamati et al. 2011; Kojima and Kangawa 2005; Obay et al. 2008). Expression of ghrelin has been identified in an array of tissues and cell types including the stomach, small intestine, pancreas, lymphocytes, placenta, kidney, lung, pituitary and brain (Gualillo et al., 2003, Du et al., 2009).

This ubiquitous distribution suggests that locally produced ghrelin might exert paracrine/autocrine effects in different tissues (Du et al., 2010).So, this may be the case in various reproductive organs such as endometrium, placenta, testis and ovary (Du et al., 2010; Garcia et al., 2007; Harrison et al., 2007). Recently, new evidence strongly indicated that the ghrelin and ghrelin receptors (GHS-R1a, GHS-R1b) are present in the mammalian and non-mammalian ovary (Dupont et al., 2010) and expression of ghrelin mRNA in ovarian tissue has been reported (Rak and Gregoraszczuk 2008; Caminos et al., 2003; Gnanapavan et al., 2002). In this regard, ghrelin is found in human, rat, pig and sheep ovary (Dupont et al., 2010; Zhang et al., 2008; Sirotkin et al., 2006; Miller et al., 2005; Caminos et al., 2003; Gaytan et al., 2003). Ghrelin is expressed during the estrous cycle and pregnancy and the relative mRNA levels depend on the stage of the cycle with the highest expression during the development the corpora lutea in sheep ovary (Dupont et al., 2010). Likewise, strong ghrelin immunostaining was observed in ovarian follicles at all development stages (Miller et al., 2005; Du et al., 2009). These results encouraged the researchers to provide further evidence regarding the role of this hormone in reproduction of domestic animals.

It is well known that the ovary is a complex organ in which different endocrine and locally produced steroidal and non-steroidal regulators cooperate to ensure complete ovarian function (Rak and Gregoraszczuk 2008). It has been recently shown that a factor that directly regulates ghrelin gene expression in the stomach of rats is estrogen, which plays a critical role in ghrelin expression and production (Sakata et al., 2006). This finding confirmed that the produced estrogen in the stomach regulates ghrelin gene expression and the published data have demonstrated that ghrelin is produced by the ovarian follicle, increases estradiol secretion and influences aromatase activity in prepubertal pig ovaries (Rak and Gregoraszczuk 2008). Our previous report also demonstrated changes of aromatase activity (a key enzyme for estrogen synthesis) in follicles and corpora lutea during the second half of ovine pregnancy (Sokhtehzari et al., 2011). In order to better understand the potential relationship between ghrelin and estrogen, the concentrations were measured in follicles and corpora lutea per milligram of tissue protein. Hence, the aim of the present study was to evaluate the relationship between ghrelin and estrogen during the second half of ovine pregnancy.

Materials and Methods

Animals and tissue collection: A total of 120 pregnant sheep (24-48 months of age) were used in this study from November 2014 to January 2015 at the abattoir in Lorestan province, Khorram Abad, Iran. The stage (month) of pregnancy was estimated by measuring foetal size, based on the crown-rump length of the fetus (Sivachelvan et al., 1996). The ovarian samples were collected from the pregnant sheep using a pair of surgical scissors for 3, 3.5, 4, 4.5 and 5 months of pregnancy, immediately after slaughter at the local abattoir. The ovaries were transported at ice-cold temperature to the biochemical laboratory. All follicles were collected from the surface with a surgical blade and functional corpora lutea (CL) was dissected from the 40 ovarian samples in order to provide 8 samples for each stage of pregnancy (5 stage × 8 samples=40). The samples were stored at -70 °C for a maximum of up to 2 months prior to biochemical analysis.

Tissue preparation and biochemical analysis: The tissues were thawed and manually homogenized in cold phosphate buffer (0.1 M, pH=7.4) on liquid nitrogen as described previously (Alirezaei et al. 2015) and debris were removed by centrifugation at 2000 RPM for 20 min (Centrifuge 5415 R; Rotofix 32A, Germany). Supernatants were recovered and used for protein measurement, ghrelin content and estrogen concentration. Protein content of tissue homogenates was determined using a colorimetric method of Lowry with bovine serum albumin as a standard (Lowry et al., 1951).

Ghrelin measurement: Ghrelin content was measured by an enzyme-linked immunosorbent assay (ELISA) kit (Bioassay Technology Laboratory, Shanghi, China) based on the biotin double antibody sandwich technology via an ELISA reader (STAT FAX, 2100, USA) at 450 nm. This kit was prepared to assay the ghrelin in the sample of sheep's serum, blood samples and other related biological fluids. The detectable level of this kit was 20 to 320 ng/l and the coefficients of inter-and intra-assay precision were <12 % and <10 %, respectively. The ghrelin concentration was expressed as mg/mg protein of tissue homogenates (mg/mg of tissue protein).

Estrogen measurement: Estrogen concentration was assayed by the competitive ELISA method according to the manufacturer's instructions kit (Dia Metra, Foligno (PN), Italy), as described previously in our laboratory (Sokhtehzari et al., 2011). In brief, 25 µl of the each E2 standard (0, to 2000 pg/ml in duplicate, for standard curve preparation) and 25 µl of tissue homogenates were transferred to the anti-E2 IgG-coated wells of the plate. The immunoreaction was initiated by adding 200 µl of the E2-HRP conjugate solution to each well, followed by incubation at 37 °C for 2 h. The content from each well was removed and washed with 300 µl of distilled water, 5-6 times. The water was completely drained out from each well. Next, 100 µl of TMB substrate was dispensed into each well and incubated at 25 °C for 30 min in dark condition. Color development was stopped with 100 µl of stop solution. Absorbance was taken at 450 nm using an ELISA reader. Calculation from the measured absorbance of the samples was interpolated from the standard curve to obtain the values. The cross reactivity of the antibody used, calculated according to manufacturer's instructions kit were: estradiol 100%, estrone 2%, estriol 0.39%, and testosterone 0.02%. Estrogen concentration was expressed as pg/mg of tissue homogenates (pg/mg of tissue protein).

Statistical analysis: Statistical analysis was performed using the statistical package GraphPad PRISM version 5 (GraphPad Software Inc., San Diego, CA, USA). All variables were tested for normal and homogeneous variances by Leven's statistic test. All results are presented as mean± (S.E.M.). The statistical differences were applied among all stages of pregnancy by one-way analysis of variance (ANOVA) with Tukey's post hoc analysis. Pearson's correlation and linear regression tests were also used between ghrelin and estrogen concentrations in follicles and corpora lutea. A calculated P value of less than 0.01 was considered statistically significant.

Results

Values represent Mean ± SEM of estrogen and ghrelin concentrations in follicles and corpora lutea during second half of ovine pregnancy. Figure 1 indicates that estrogen concentration in follicles significantly increased in the months 4, 4.5 and 5 in comparison with 3 and 3.5 months of ovine pregnancy ($p<0.001$) and there was a tendency to increase follicular estrogen from 4 to 5 months in pregnant sheep. There was also a significant increase of follicular ghrelin in 4, 4.5 and 5 months of pregnancy when compared to both 3 and 3.5 months in pregnant sheep ($p<0.001$, Figure 2). The estrogen concentration of active CL significantly increased in 5th month when compared to other months ($p<0.001$; Figure 3). In contrast, there was a significant decrease in ghrelin concentration for the 4.5 month of pregnancy as compared to the 5th month in functional CL ($p<0.0$; Figure 4).

Regarding correlation between ghrelin and

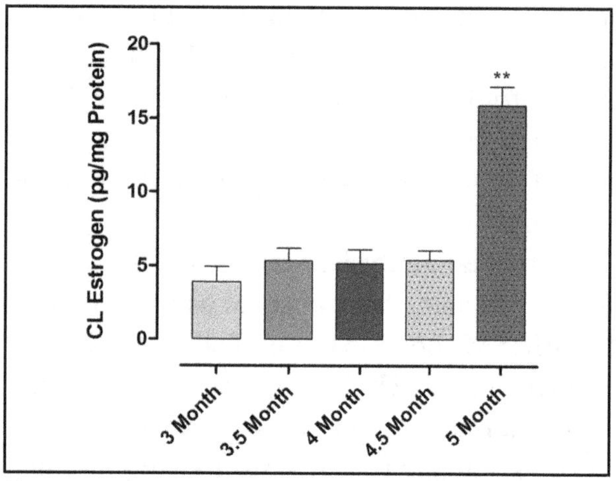

Figure 1. Estrogen concentration in follicles during second half of ovine pregnancy. Values represent mean± SEM of estrogen (pg/mg protein of follicle). **Asterisk indicates statistical difference versus 4, 4.5 and 5months of pregnancy ($p<0.001$).

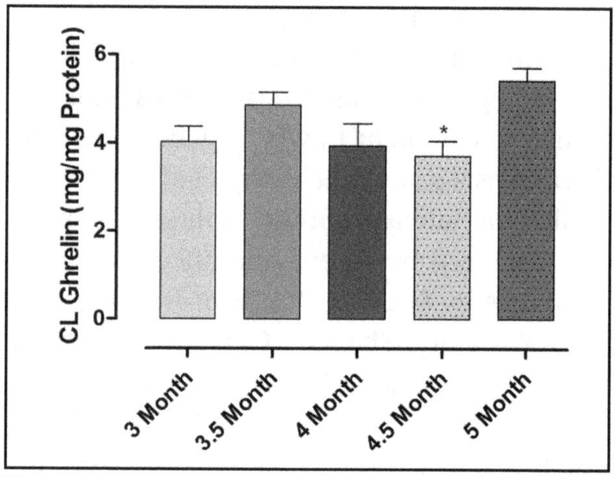

Figure 2. Ghrelin concentration in follicles during second half of ovine pregnancy. Values represent mean± SEM of ghrelin (mg/mg protein of follicle). **Asterisk indicates statistically difference versus 4, 4.5 and 5 months of pregnancy ($p<0.001$).

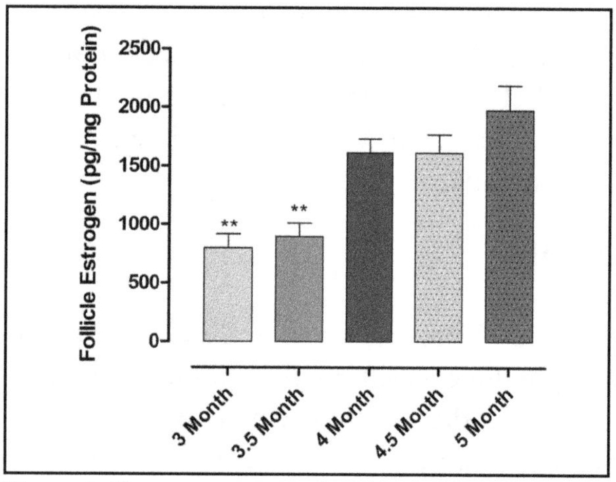

Figure 3. Estrogen concentration in corpus luteum (CL) during second half of ovine pregnancy. Values represent mean± SEM of estrogen (pg/mg protein of CL). **Asterisk indicates statistical difference versus 3, 3.5, 4 and 4.5 months of pregnancy ($p<0.001$).

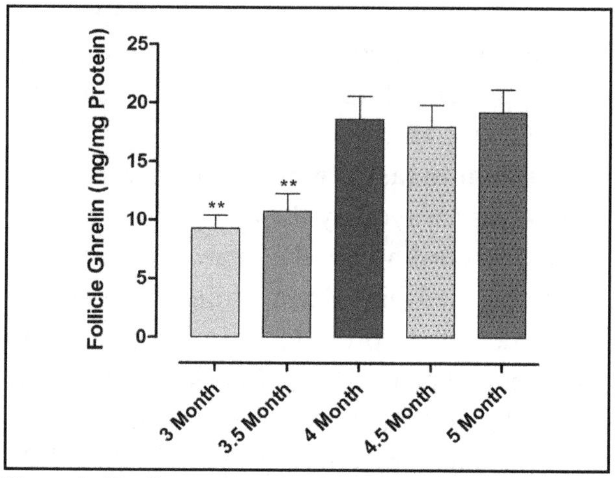

Figure 4. Ghrelin concentration in corpus luteum (CL) during second half of ovine pregnancy. Values represent mean± SEM of ghrelin (mg/mg protein of CL). *Asterisk indicates statistical difference versus 5 month of pregnancy ($p<0.01$).

estrogen concentrations in follicles and corpora lutea, there was a positive linear regression between follicular estrogen and ghrelin during second half of ovine pregnancy ($r=0.97$ and $p=0.004$), while there was no correlation between estrogen and ghrelin in corpus luteum ($p>0.05$).

Discussion

This report is probably the first to show the ghrelin and estrogen relationships during the second half of ovine pregnancy. Our data demonstrate that follicular estrogen concentration increases during second half of ovine pregnancy concomitant with ghrelin concentration. This effect is more noticeable for 4, 4.5 and 5 months in pregnant sheep. Based on the present results, the estrogen concentration in corpus luteum (CL) was only significantly higher in the 5th month of pregnancy as compared to other months. In contrast, the ghrelin concentration in CL significantly decreased in the 4.5 month when compared to the 5th month in pregnant sheep. Therefore, it seems there is a relation between follicular estrogen and ghrelin during second half of pregnancy in the sheep ovary.

As previously mentioned, recent evidence strongly indicates that the ghrelin signal is present in the ovary (Du et al., 2009; Zhang et al., 2008; Miller et al., 2005; Caminos et al., 2003; Gaytan et al., 2003). In the present study, ghrelin concentration within sheep ovarian tissue revealed distribution of ghrelin in both follicles and CL. One of the interesting findings of the current study was the positive correlation between ghrelin and estrogen in ovarian follicles. Based on the results, ghrelin levels are increased when estrogen concentrations are strongly increased from the 4th to 5th month of pregnancy. In this setting, it has been found that estrogen treatment significantly simulated ghrelin mRNA expression and ghrelin production in a dose-dependent manner, indicating that estrogen works on ghrelin gene expression through the α-estrogen receptor (Sakata et al., 2006). Our data showed a significant relation between ghrelin and estrogen in the ovarian follicles. To our knowledge, the source of supply of estrogen precursors is considered to be the gonads or adrenal gland (Lu and Judd 1982; Sakata et al., 2006). Recent studies evidenced that androgens were independent modulators of ghrelin level in the gonads, thus confirming an interaction between ghrelin and sex estrogen synthesis (Rak and Gregoraszczuk 2008; Gambiner et al., 2003; Pagotto et al., 2002). It is well known that aromatase activity, as key enzyme, plays a critical role in estrogen synthesis (Caminos et al., 2003). Moreover, there was a close relation between ghrelin cells and aromatase-expressing cells in the follicular wall, suggesting that ghrelin cells are exposed to estrogen (Du et al., 2010). Therefore, the estrogen concentration increased concomitant with ghrelin level in follicles. In this regard, a previous work demonstrated dependent action of ghrelin on estradiol secretion by follicular cells (Gregoraszczuk et al., 2000). The above and the previous report (Rak and Gregoraszczuk 2008) confirm that ghrelin stimulates estradiol secretion by ovarian follicles and acts on aromatase activity. Therefore, we described a notably dynamic pattern of follicular ghrelin and estrogen with the lowest concentration in 3 and 3.5 months and maximum values in 4, 4.5 and 5 months in pregnant sheep.

To evaluate the relation between ghrelin and estrogen in the CL, measurement of ghrelin and estrogen levels was conducted throughout the 3-5 months of pregnancy in an active CL. Interestingly, despite a persistent decrease of the estrogen concentration in 3-4.5 months of pregnancy, estrogen level significantly increased in the 5th month of pregnancy in potent CL. Indeed, estrogen level reached its highest value when CL entered into its regression phase. Our previous report indicated a decrease of aromatase activity in CL during second half of ovine pregnancy and there was a negative correlation between aromatase activity and stage of pregnancy ($r=-0.69$ and $p<0.05$) (Sokhtehzari et al., 2011). Al-Gubory et al., 1994 also reported that a non-steroidal factor in the ovine CL of late pregnancy directly inhibits aromatase activity in ovarian follicles. Therefore, it seems that the increasing of estrogen concentration is related to the blood estrogen level that was originated from the placenta or elsewhere. In this regard, there was no correlation between ghrelin and estrogen in CL which indicates ghrelin elevation in the 5th month also is related to elevation of blood estrogen since estrogen directly induces ghrelin gene expression and production (Sakata et al., 2006). The previous reports on the biochemistry and structure of the CL, suggest that during late pregnancy the CL is at the very early stage of structural regression, with no changes at the morphological level, but with changes in the molecular and biochemical functions (Du et al., 2009; Caminos et al., 2003). Hence, ghrelin levels decreased in CL at 4.5 month of pregnancy, along with the regression of CL. In the Figure 4, we demonstrated slightly higher ghrelin content for 3.5 months in comparison with 4, and 4.5 months in pregnant sheep, although it was not significant. This result is in agreement with Du et al's., 2009 study in which middle CL (mature CL) indicated higher relative mRNA expression of ghrelin when compared to late CL (Du et al., 2009). It seems elevations of ghrelin and estrogen in late pregnancy are partially related to blood estrogen when estrogen concentration increases at the late stage of pregnancy to induce parturition. Nevertheless, it remains to be established whether ghrelin is actually involved in estrogen synthesis of the CL during 3-5 months of pregnancy.

In conclusion, ghrelin peptide is indicated as quantitative in ovarian follicles and functional CL during pregnancy of sheep. Dynamic changes in the profile of ovarian ghrelin and estrogen were more noticeable during second half of ovine pregnancy. These results further emphasize the potential regulatory role of ghrelin in the reproductive system and open a new window to future studies.

Acknowledgments

This study was financially supported by Lorestan University, Khorram Abad, Iran.

References

1. Al-Gubory, K.H., Driancourt, M.A., Antoine, M., Martal, J., Neimer, N. (1994) Evidence that a non-steroidal factor from corpus luteum of pregnant sheep inhibits aromatase activity of ovarian follicles in vitro. J Reprod Fertil 100: 51-56.
2. Alirezaei, M., Dezfoulian, O., Kheradmand, A. (2015) Novel Antioxidant properties of ghrelin and oleuropein versus lipopolysaccharide-mediated renal failure in rats. Int J Pept Res Ther 21: 411-421.
3. Caminos, J.E., Tena-Sempere, M., Gaytán, F., Sanchez-Criado, J.E., Barreiro, M.L., Nogueiras, R., Casanueva, F.F., Aguilar, E., Diéguez, C. (2003) Expression of ghrelin in the cyclic and pregnant rat ovary. Endocrinology. 144: 1594-602.
4. Du, C., Li, H., Cao, G., Xilingaowa, Wang, C., Li, C. (2010) Expression of the orexigenic peptide ghrelin and the type 1a growth hormone secretagogue receptor in sheep oocytes and pre-implantation embryos produced in vitro. Reprod Domest Anim. 45: 92-8.
5. Du, C., Xilingaowa, Cao. G., Wang, C., Li, H., Zhao. Y., Cao, S., Cao, J. (2009) Expression of the orexigenic peptide ghrelin in the sheep ovary. Domest Anim Endocrinol. 36: 89-98.
6. Dupont, J., Maillard, V., Coyral-Castel, S., Rame, C., Froment, P. (2010) Ghrelin in Female and Male Reproduction. Int J Pept, A rticle ID 158102, 8 pages.
7. Gambineri, A., Pagotto, U., Tschop, M., Vicennati, V., Manicardi, E., Carcello, A., Cacciari, M., De Iasio, R., Pasquali, R. (2003) Anti-androgen treatment increases circulating ghrelin levels in obese women with polycystic ovary syndrome. J Endocrinol Invest. 26: 629-634.
8. Garcia, M.C., Lopez, M., Alvarez, C.V., Casanueva, F.F., Tena-Sempere, M., Diéguez, C. (2007) Role of ghrelin in reproduction. Reproduction. 133: 531-540.
9. Gaytan, F., Barreiro, M.L., Chopin, L.K., Herington, A.C., Morales, C., Pinilla, L., Casanueva, F.F., Aguilar, E., Diéguez, C., Tena-Sempere, M. (2003) Immunolocalization of ghrelin and its functional receptor, the type 1a growth hormone secretagogue receptor, in the cyclic human ovary, J Clin Endocrinol Metab. 88: 879-887.
10. Gnanapavan S., Kola, B., Bustin, S.A., Morris, D.G., McGee, P., Fairclough, P., Bhattacharya, S., Carpenter, R., Grossman, A.B., Korbonits, M. (2002) The tissue distribution of the mRNA of ghrelin and subtypes of its receptor, GHS-R, in humans. J Clin Endocrinol Metab. 87: 2988-2990.
11. Gregoraszczuk, E.L., Bylica, A., Gertler, A.

(2000) Response of porcine theca and granulosa cells to GH during short-term in vitro culture. Anim Reprod Sci. 58: 113-125.
12. Gualillo, O., Lago, F., Gomez-Reino, J., Casanueva, F.F., Dieguez, C. (2003) Ghrelin a widespread hormone: insights into molecular and cellular regulation of its expression and mechanism of action, FEBS Lett. 552: 105-109.
13. Harrison, J.L., Adam, C.L., Brown, Y.A., Wallace., J.M., Aitken, R.P., Lea RG., Miller, DW. (2007) an immunohistochemical of the localization developmental expression of ghrelin and its functional receptor in the ovine placenta. Reprod Biol Endocrinol. 5: 25-32.
14. Kheradmand, A., Alirezaei, M., Birjandi, M. (2010) Ghrelin promotes antioxidant enzyme activity and reduces lipid peroxidation in the rat ovary. Regul Pept. 162: 84-89.
15. Kheradmand, A., Dezfoulian, O., Tarrahi, M.J. (2011) Ghrelin attenuates heat-induced degenerative effects in the rat testis. Regul Pept. 167: 97-104.
16. Kojima, M., Kangawa, K. (2005) Ghrelin: structure and function. Physiol Rev. 85: 495-522.
17. Lowry, O.H., Rosebrough, N.J., Farr, A.L., Randal, R.J. (1951) Protein measurement with the Folin phenol reagent. J Biol Chem. 193: 265-275.
18. Lu, J.K., Judd, H.L. (1982) Silastic implants of progesterone produce high circulating levels of both progesterone and 20 alpha-hydroxyprogesterone in ovariectomized, adrenalectomized rats. Biol Reprod. 26: 385-390.
19. Miller, D.W., Harrison, J.L., Brown, Y.A., Doyle, U., Lindsay, A., Adam, C.L., Lea, RG. (2005) Immunohistochemical evidence for an endocrine/paracrine role for ghrelin in the reproductive tissues of sheep. Reprod Biol Endocrinol. 3: 60-65.
20. Neamati, S., Alirezaei, M., Kheradmand, A. (2011) Ghrelin acts as an antioxidant agent in the rat kidney. Int J Pept Res Ther. 17: 239-245.
21. Obay, B.D., Tasdemir, E., Tumer, Cl., Bilgin, HM., Atmaca, M. (2008) Dose dependent effects of ghrelin on pentylenetetrazole-induced oxidative stress in a rat seizure model. Peptides. 29: 448-455.
22. Pagotto, U., Gambineri, A., Vicennati, V., Heiman, M.L., Tschop, M., Pasquali, R. (2002) Plasma ghrelin, obesity, and the polycystic ovary syndrome: correlation with insulin resistance and androgen levels. J Clin Endocrinol Metab. 87: 5625-5629.
23. Rak, A., Gregoraszczuk, EŁ. (2008) Local feedback loop of ghrelin-GH in the pig ovary: Action on estradiol secretion, aromatase activity and cell apoptosis. Growth Hormone IGF Res. 18: 221-227.
24. Sakata, I., Tanaka, T., Yamazaki, M., Tanizaki, T., Zheng, Z., Sakai, T. (2006) Gastric estrogen directly induces ghrelin expression and production in the rat stomach. J Endocrinol. 190: 749-757.
25. Sirotkin, A.V., Grossmann, R., Mar´ıa-Peon, M.T., Roa, J., Tena-Sempere, M., Klein, S. (2006) Novel expression and functional role of ghrelin in chicken ovary. Mol Cell Endocrinol. 257-258: 15-25.
26. Sivachelvan, M.N., Ali, M.G., Chibuzo, G.A. (1996) Fetal age estimation in sheep and goats. Small Rumin Res. 19: 69-76.
27. Sokhtehzari, A., Alirezaei M., Mirzaei, A., Neamati, Sh. (2011) Ovarian and placental P450-aromatase activity during second half of ovine pregnancy. Online J Vet Res. 15: 381-389.
28. Zhang, W., Lei, Z., Su, J., Chen, S. (2008) Expression of ghrelin in the porcine hypothalamo-pituitary-ovary axis during the estrous cycle. Anim Reprod Sci. 109: 356-367.

Changes in electrocardiographic, hematologic and biochemical indices of Markhoz goat breed in experimental hypocalcemia

Fakour, Sh.[1*]**, Hajizadeh, P.**[2]

[1]*Department of Clinical Sciences, Faculty of Veterinary Medicine, Sanandaj Branch of Islamic Azad University, Sanandaj, Iran*

[2]*Graduated from the Faculty of Veterinary Medicine, Sanandaj Branch of Islamic Azad University, Sanandaj, Iran*

Key words:
experimental hypocalcemia, electrocardiography, hematology, biochemical, Markhoz goat

Correspondence
Fakour, Sh.
Department of Clinical Sciences, Faculty of Veterinary Medicine, Sanandaj Branch of Islamic Azad University, Sanandaj, Iran

Email: fakours@yahoo.com

Abstract:

BACKGROUND: Milk fever in cattle, sheep and goats occurs around the time of parturition and is caused by hypocalcemia. **OBJECTIVES:** The aim of this study was to investigate the physiological effects of experimental hypocalcemia on electrocardiography, hematology and serum biochemical changes in Markhoz goat breed. **METHODS:** Ethylene diamine tetra- acetate solution 4.6% was intravenously infused to 5 healthy goats (experimental group) and 5 healthy goats received 0.9% saline solution (IV) as control group. In both groups, electrocardiogram was recorded in base apex lead and serum was collected before and after infusion. Electrocardiography, biochemical and hematologic parameters were measured. Clinical signs of hypocalcaemia were caused by EDTA infusion. **RESULTS:** The results in experimental group showed a significant decrease in calcium, lactate dehydrogenase, potassium, and increase in glucose concentration, ($p<0.05$).The white blood cells, lymphocytes, eosinophils decreased significantly ($p<0.05$). Magnesium concentration, creatine phosphokinase, alanine transaminase, aspartate transaminase, phosphorus, red blood cells, hemoglobin, hematocrit, Mean cell volume, Mean cell hemoglobin did not show significant change ($p>0.05$), heart rate change, presence of arrhythmias and its type were significant ($p<0.05$). But, QRS pattern, T shape, P, QRS and T amplitude, S-T and Q-T interval waves had no significant change ($p>0.05$). No significant change was seen in control group. **CONCLUSIONS:** The results indicate that evaluating some biochemical, enzymatic, hematological and electrocardiography changes can be helpful in the diagnosis of hypocalcemia.

Introduction

In goats, a depression in serum levels of calcium and phosphorus occurs similar to that in cows but in ewes no such depression occurs at lambing and the intervention of a precipitating factor appears to be necessary to further reduce the serum calcium level below a critical point. Milking goats become affected mostly in the 4-6 years age group (Kenneth et al., 2011). Milk fever may occur in does and goats either prepartum or postpartum because they have both the potential for high milk production and relatively large fetoplacental requirement associated with multiple births (Andreson et al., 2009). Normal parturition in goats is accompanied by mild hypocalcemia (Smith and Sherman 2011). The economic losses of milk fever include milk fever relapses, dystocia and reproductive diseases (Radostits et al., 2014). Mostaghni et al studied experimental hypocalcemia by EDTA on sheep in 2012, while Desmecht et al studied on calf in 1995, and Mellau et al induced the disease in cow and studied it in 2001. Since no research has been done about experimental hypocalcemia for goat by" EDTA infusion", the results of this study can reveal new information related to goat hypocalcemia as species of ruminant and beyond that in one of the Iranian original breeds. The origin of Markhoz goat is Kurdistan province in Iran. They are used as multipurpose animals for the production of milk, meat, hair and hide (Farshad et al., 2008). The aim of this study was to investigate the physiological effects of experimentally induced hypocalcemia on electrocardiography, hematology and serum biochemical changes in Markhoz breed goat.

Materials and Methods

10 female goats of Markhoz breed, weighing 25-30 kg, aged 1.5 to 2 years-old were selected.

Using history and ultrasonography their non-pregnancy was confirmed. Transabdominal ultrasonography was conducted using a real-time B-mode scanner (Emp-820 plus vet, Shenzhen Empror Electronic Technology Co. Ltd., China) equipped with 5 MHz convex transducer (Hesselink and Taveme 1994, Raja et al., 2011, Karaddaev 2015). 10 goats were divided in two groups, the experimental group (n=5) and control group (n=5).

A 4.6% Na 2EDTA (Merck nr. 8418 Pro-analysi, E. Merck) solution was prepared by dissolving 46 gr of salt in 1 liter of sterile distilled water and bringing its PH to 7.4 using sodium hydroxide. In order to induce hypocalcemia, a standardized flow rate of 1.2 ml/kg per hour of a 4.6% solution Na2EDTA was infused for 5 goats (experimental group) intravenously. Simultaneously with any EDTA solution infusion, the heart sounds, heart rate, rectal temperature, rumen activity and respiratory rate were controlled. Intravenous EDTA solution was stopped when the goats showed clinical signs of circulatory collapse manifested by cold extremities, increased heart rate, tachypnea, accumulation of mucus exudation in the nostrils, salivation, ruminal stasis, tympany, ataxia and sternal recumbency. Thereafter, goats were allowed to recover spontaneously from EDTA induced hypocalcemia. 5 healthy goats received 0.9% saline solution (IV) as control group in similar conditions. 10 ml blood sample of jugular vein was collected from two experimental and control groups before and after infusion, 8 ml of which was maintained in tube without anticoagulant for biochemical tests and the remaining 2 ml was maintained in evacuated heparine tubes for hematologic tests.

Electrocardiogram was recorded in standing position from two control and experimental groups before and after infusion, using electrocardiography device (model ECG2000 Bionet made in Korea) on base-apex lead. The paper speed was adjusted to 25 mm/ sec and calibration was 10 mm/ mV. For blood enzyme and biochemical tests, first the blood samples were centrifuged to separate their serum, then serum parameters including calcium, phosphorus, magnesium, potassium, glucose, and ALT, AST, CPK and LDH enzymes were measured by Auto-chemistry Analyzer, (Model DIRUI, CS-T240 made in China) and potassium was measured with (Fater Electronic device, model 620 made in Iran) by flame Photometric method. Blood parameters including the white blood cells, the red blood cells, hemoglobin, hematocrit, MCV, MCH, MCHC and differential count of white blood cells were measured. To study electrocardiography changes, heart rate, the presence of arrhythmias and its type, QRS wave pattern, T wave shape, P amplitude, S-T interval, QRS waves amplitude, T wave amplitude and Q-T interval, were measured.

Initially data were entered in Microsoft Excel and then imported to GraphPad prism (GraphPad Software Inc., USA) version 3.0 where descriptive statistics (Mean, standard deviation of the mean) of the biochemical, hematologic and electrocardiographic analytical variables were determined. The difference between the mean of the variables before and after infusion was analyzed statistically by t- test and arrhythmia by using a nonparametric test of Wilcoxon, and $p \leq 0.05$ was considered significant.

Results

Results obtained from the study for two experimental and control groups has been shown separately in Tables 1 to 6 before and after infusion (after hypocalcemia induction) as the average standard deviation for any of the biochemical, hematologic, electrocardiographic parameters.

As shown in Table 1, decrease in calcium concentration, LDH, potassium, and increase in glucose concentration before and after infusion was significant but magnesium concentration, CPK, phosphorus, ALT, AST has not shown significant change.

As shown in Table 3, the white blood cells, lymphocytes, eosinophils decreased significantly, but the red blood cells, hemoglobin, hematocrit, MCV, MCH, MCHC did not show significant change; as shown in Table 5, heart rate, presence of arrhythmias and its type also had significant change. But, QRS wave pattern, T wave shape, P, QRS, T wave amplitude, S-T and Q-T interval had no significance statistically.

In experimental group before infusion, arrhythmias were seen only in a case which was atrial fibrillation. But after induction of the hypocalcemia, the arrhythmias were diagnosed in all 5 goats and the diagnosed arrhythmias were atrial fibrillation in 3 cases, sinus arrhythmia as well as atrial fibrillation in 1 case and atrial premature beat with atrial fibrillation was seen in 1 case.

In control group before and after infusion no arrhythmias were diagnosed in 3 cases, but in 1 case before infusion, sinus arrhythmia and in another case, the second-degree atrioventricular block were diagnosed though no difference was observed compared to before infusion in 2 cases.

Regarding P value obtained from Wilcoxon test for arrhythmia in experimental group, it can be concluded that among arrhythmias, only the arrhythmia of atrial fibrillation with $P=0.046$ was less than 0.05 and is significant, it means that before and after infusion, it is different.

Discussion

EDTA solution with its chelating proper-

Table 1. The mean ± SD of biochemical parameters in test group. [a,b] Mean with different superscript on the same row are significantly different (p≤0.5).

Time	Ca (mg/dl)	Mg (mg/dl)	K (mg/dl)	P (mg/dl)	GLu (mg/dl)	AST (IU/L)	ALT (IU/L)	CPK (IU/L)	LDH (IU/L
Before	9.52±0.42a	2.54±0.56	4.92±0.38a	4.26±1	54±10	80 ±15	15 ±4.2	147±29	629±685a
After	6.16±1.5b	2.82±1.4	3.82±0.1b	4.7±1.4	61±12	77.8±14	15.2±3.7	192.6±63	608.8±65b

Table 2. The mean ± SD of biochemical parameters in control group.

Time	Ca (mg/dl)	Mg (mg/dl)	K (mg/dl)	P (mg/dl)	GLu (mg/dl)	AST (IU/L)	ALT (IU/L)	CPK (IU/L)	LDH (IU/L
Before	9.58±0.17	2.52±0.37	4.16±015	452±1.2	65±14	86±12	18.6±4	141.8±1	778.2±14
After	9.5±0.1	2.6±0.4	4.18±0.08	4.36±1.1	69±14	86±11	18.2±4.0	144.2±12	767±158

Table 3. The mean ± SD of hematologic parameters in test group. [a,b] Mean with different superscript on the same row are significantly different (p≤0.5).

Time	WBC (103/mm3)	RBC (106/mm3)	Hb (g/dl)	PCV (%)	MCV (Fl)	MCH (pg)	Lym. (103/mm3)	Neut. (103/mm3)	Eos. (103/mm3)
Before	19±1.53a	16.2±1.0	8.46±	25.3±4	15.5±1.9	5.17±o.6	11.2±1.9a	5 ±1.4	2.8±0.2a
After	16±2.5b	16±.82	8.3±1.5	24.9±4.	15.3±2.5	5.1±0.8	9.0±2.1b	5.3±1.0	2.2±0.2b

ties causes calcium in the blood to be away from the body's reactions, as a result hypocalcemia occurs. This property of EDTA was used in the study, and by injecting it, hypocalcemia conditions were induced.

In this survey, also calcium concentration was decreased from 9.52 mg/dl to 6.16 mg/dl ($p<0.05$) which confirmed the results obtained from a study in experimental hypocalcemia on sheep (Mostaghni et al., 2012), a study on calf (Desmecht et al., 1995), and one study's results on cow (Mellau et al., 2001).

Glucose concentration was changed from 54.6 mg/dl to 61 mg/dl after infusion ($p<0.05$) which was similar to results obtained from the other studies (Martinez et al., 2014 and Mostaghni et al., 2012).

Clinical signs observed by infusion EDTA and appearance of hypocalcemia in the study, including weakness, tremor and tetany causes the stress in experimental group, whereas this clinical signs were not observed in control group. The stress leads to increase in the secretion of adrenal corticotrophin hormone (ACTH) from the pituitary followed by increase in the secretion of cortisol from the cortex of adrenal gland.

Following the cortisol secretion increase, provocation for action of gluconeogenesis takes place in amount of 6 to 10 times, and thus promotes the formation of glucose. Cortisol also causes average decreases in the use of glucose by cells throughout the body (John et al., 2016). CPK enzyme was not significant after hypocalcemia induction ($p>0.05$), though the present result confirms Desmecht's et al., 2012 study on calf. Remarkable changes in the enzymes concentration are mostly related to skeletal muscles and cardiac muscle, and the damages to them. In the present study all goats of experimental group were not recumbent but tetany was observed in 5 goats in which CPK increase can be related to tetany caused by hypocalcemia. ALT and AST enzymes did not show significant change after inducing hypocalcemia ($p>0.05$), the results of which are similar to the those obtained in the study done by Mostaghni et al.,2012 and Desmecht et al., 1995 and the similarity was also observed about AST enzyme in

Table 4. The mean ± SD of hematologic parameters in control group.

Time	WBC (103/mm3)	RBC (106/mm3)	Hb (g/dl)	PCV (%)	MCV (Fl)	MCH (pg)	Lym. (103/mm3)	Neut. (103/mm3)	Eos. (103/mm3)
Before	18.9±4.4	16.3±0.5	8.9±0.3	26.8±0.9	16.4±1.0	5.4±0.3	11.2±1.9	5.4 ±3.4	2.3±0.9
After	18±4.0	15±0.4	8.9±0.5	26.9±1.5	16.8±1.1	5.6±0.3	11.0±1.7	4.7±2.9	2.5±0.7

Table 5. The mean ± SD of electrocardiographic parameters in test group. [a,b] Mean with different superscript on the same row are significantly different ($p \leq 0.5$).

Time	Heart rate/min.	ST duration (Sec)	QT duration (Sec)	QRS amplitude (mv)	T amplitude (mv)
Before	96.8±15.14a	0.176±0.036	0.22±0.02	0.36±0.11	0.24±0.21
After	111.8±12.49b	0.200±0.04	0.22±0.02	0.34±0.9	0.16±0.13

Table 6. The mean ± SD of electrocardiographic parameters in control group.

Time	Heart rate/min.	ST duration (Sec)	QT duration (Sec)	QRS amplitude (mv)	T amplitude (mv)
Before	100.4±23.86	0.176±0.022	0.19±0.033	0.34±0.11	0.34±0.11
After	100.2±25.44	0.168±0.018	0.19±0.033	0.40±0.10	0.36±0.13

Daniel's study (1979). Muscular enzymes including AST, CPK and LDH are entered in the blood stream with delay after muscular injuries incidence and for some time their amount remains high, for example, CPK amount reaches its maximum after 2 to 12 hours following muscular injury or AST amount remains high for more than a week after muscular injuries incidence. By continuing sampling in the coming hours, there was the possibility of obtaining conclusions other than the recent results that was not possible in the present study procedure to be examined. No significant change was seen for phosphorus concentration statistically ($p>0.05$) which confirms the results obtained by the other study (Daniel and Moodie, 1979). Change in the concentration of phosphorus plasma is subject to Parathoromone changes, so it can be concluded that the cause of various reports about being significant or not for phosphorus decrease simultaneously with calcium decrease, is due to the difference in reaction of parathyroid glands in animals tested. Also, the amount of hypocalcemic and phosphorus absorption and excretion by animals is regarded as important factors in blood phosphor changes, so that phosphorus decrease was observed in some samples of the study, but the mean had no significance statistically.

LDH enzyme was decreased after infusion and the change was significant statistically ($p<0.05$) which does not confirm the results obtained by the studies done by Desmecht et al., 1995 indicating non-significance of the enzyme changes.

This enzyme exists in all tissues in large quantities, some anticoagulant substances such as EDTA and Oxalates inhibit the enzyme activity indirectly and decrease its amount.

In this study LDH amount had significant decrease unexpectedly, this decrease was not observed in control group, and the reason for this is probably experimental hypocalcemia by injecting EDTA solution that causes the LDH to be decreased indirectly. Therefore, using EDTA solution to measure LDH enzyme changes in experimental hypocalcemia is not appropriate and other methods can be applied.

Potassium was decreased after hypocalcemia induction ($p<0.05$) that is similar to another study (Martinez et al., 2014). Calcium decrease was followed by parathyroid hormone which reduces reabsorption of potassium in proximal tubular and its quick excreting in the urine.

No significant statistical change was observed in Magnesium after hypocalcemia induction ($p>0.05$), which confirms the results obtained in a similar study (Mellau et al., 2001), but does not confirm the result of Martinez et al., (2014) and Yamagishi et al., (1999) in hypocalcemia induced with hemodialysis regarding increase in Magnesium.

Magnesium slightly increased in the study which can be related to parathyroid hormone that increases reabsorption of Magnesium ions and hydrogen ions.

White blood cells, the number of lymphocytes and eosinophils of the blood decreased after hypocalcemia induction and the decrease was significant statistically ($p<0.05$). Cortisol decreases the number of lymphocytes, and subsequent eosinophils in the blood. The reason for this is that T lymphocytes produce eosinopoietine and eosinophil chemotactic anaphylactic factor (ECAF).The first protein to increase production of eosinophil in bone marrow and second protein is chemotaxic for eosinophil. This effect is mediated through the anterior pituitary and adrenocorticol hormones which are increased during stressful situation (Karpoor et al., 2011). Antihistamine and lyses' property of T lymphocyte, margination lymphocytes and eosinophils in blood vessels and establishing them in the tissues is caused by cortisol secretion, these effects start within a few minutes after cortisol secretion and are revealed within a few hours. Decrease in the number of lymphocytes, eosinophils causes the decrease in the number of white blood cells.

Other hematological parameters including the red blood cells, hemoglobin, hematocrit, MCV, MCH and neutrophil have not shown significant changes statistically ($p>0.05$); regarding the number of neutrophils and the red blood cells, it confirms the other study (Matinez et al., 2014).

Although the increase in the number of neutrophils was not significant statistically ($p>0.05$), decreasing neutrophil adhesion to the arteries inner walls and decreasing their migration from the reservoir circulating to the tissue caused by cortisol secretion resulted from stress can be the reasons for this increase (Kenneth et al., 2011).

Regarding the role of calcium on cardiac mechanical activity, it is of particular importance in electrocardiogram changes in which electrocardiogram parameter was evaluated before and after hypocalcemia induction in this study.

In the study, QRS wave pattern, T wave shape and P amplitude, in two groups did not show significant change before and after hypocalcemia induction. Heart rate changes after hypocalcemia induction had significant increase ($p>0.05$). Contractive strength of the heart muscle depends on Calcium ions concentration in extracellular fluids and decrease of extracellular calcium induces disorders for heart natural performances including decrease in contractive strength of the heart, tonicity decrease of the arteries wall leads to peripheral vascular dilation, decreases in blood pressure, increases in heart rate to compensate blood pressure decrease and decrease in intensity of heart sounds.

Moreover, in clinical examination during testing on animals, the heart sound intensity was decreased remarkably that confirms the studies in induced hypocalcemia with hemodialysis (Yamagishi et al., 1999).

T waves amplitude was decreased after

hypocalcemia induction but this decrease had no significant difference statistically (p>0.05). This decrease may be due to individual differences among animals. Changes in QRS waves amplitude had no significant difference before and after hypocalcemia induction (p>0.05). QRS complex indicates ventricles activity in which amplitude and shape depend on the animal heart status. It can be concluded that experimental hypocalcemia has no effect on QRS wave amplitude.

Q-T interval wave did not show significant change statistically before and after hypocalcemia induction (p>0.05), that has no similarity with the results obtained in the study which indicate significant increase in Q-T interval in hypocalcemia (Daniel and Moodie 1979).

Q-T interval wave was increased after hypocalcemia induction, but this increase was not significant statistically (p>0.05).

S-T segment is the distance between ventricular depolarization and ventricular repolarization,this distance is extended in electrolyte abnormalities. Distance extension of S-T segment in experimental hypocalcemia can be a helpful diagnostic tool (Radostits et al., 2014).

Although no significant change was observed in this study, surveying electrocardiography with delay after hypocalcemia may show this change.

Q-T interval has considerable importance in condition of electrolyte changes, so that it increases in hypocalcemia and hypokalemia (Radostits et al., 2014). In this study, Q-T interval increase in one of the goats in experimental group was significant so that the goat's calcium concentration was less than all goats, therefore, it can be concluded that in small amounts of calcium, Q-T interval can be increased.

In this study, there was arrhythmia in one goat in experimental group before hypocalcemia (Atrial Fibrillation). But after inducing hypocalcemia, arrhythmia appeared in all goats. Atrial fibrillation arrhythmia was diagnosed in 3 cases, and atrial fibrillation with sinus arrhythmia in one case, as well as atrial fibrillation with premature atrial beat in another case that confirms the results obtained by Dehkordi et al., (2014) in studying arrhythmia on high and low-yielding dairy cows, in which blood calcium decrease was introduced as an agent causing arrhythmia. Atrial fibrillation was the main arrhythmia type observed after hypocalcemia induction which was significant statistically. Appearance of this arrhythmia type is mostly related to disorder in heart performances and anatomical damage plays no role in its incidence and it mostly associates with metabolic disease and electrolyte abnormalities.

As calcium has a significant role both in the conduction heart system and in heart muscle performance, it can be deduced that calcium amount decrease may lead to appearance of this type of arrhythmia (Bardley and Cunningham 2012). Findings obtained from biochemical, hematologic, electrocardiographic changes caused by experimental hypocalcemia of goat can provide a more complete understanding for pathophysiologic and metabolic process for this disease.

Acknowledgements

The authors gratefully acknowledge the financial support by Sanandaj Islamic Azad University.

References

1. Anderson, D., Rings, E., Michael, D. (2009) Current Veterinary Therapy Food Animal

Practice, Saunders, Missouri, USA.

2. Klein, B.G. (2012) Cunningham's Textbook of Veterinary Physiology. (5th ed.) Elsevier. Philadelphia, USA.
3. Daniel, R.C.W. (1979) The effect of reducing plasma calcium levels on some plasma enzyme levels in cows and sheep. Br Vet J. 135: 30-39.
4. Daniel, R.C.W., Moodie, E.W. (1979) Induced hypocalcemia in cows and sheep. I. Changes in plasma inorganic phosphorus levels. Br Vet J. 135: 440-451.
5. Daniel, R.C.W., Moodie, E.W. (1979) Relationship between plasma calcium and QT interval of electrocardiogram in dairy cows. J Dairy Sci. 62: 1014-1018.
6. Desmecht, D.J.M., Linden, A.S., Godeaut, J.M., Lekeux, P.M. (1995) Experimental production of hypocalcemia by EDTA infusion in calves: A critical appraisal assessed from the profile of blood chemicals and enzymes. Comp Biochem Physiol. 110: 115-130.
7. Farshad, A., Akhondzadeh, S., Zamiri, M.J., Sadeghi, GH. (2008) The estrous cycle of the markhoz goat in Iran. Asian-Aust J Anim Sci. 21: 1411-1415.
8. Hesselink, J.W., Taveme, H.A.M. (1994) Ultrasonography of the uterus of the Goat. Vet Quart. 16: 41-45.
9. Jafari Dehkordi, A., Nasser Mohebi, A., HeidariSoreshjani, M. (2014) Frequency of cardiac arrhythmias in high- and low- yielding dairy cows. Vet Res Forum. 5: 1-5.
10. Hall Guyton, J.E.A.C. (2016) Guyton and Hall Textbook of Medical Physiology. (13th ed.) Saunders. Philadelphia, USA.
11. Karadaev, M. (2015) Pregnancy diagnosis techniques in Goats. Bulg J Vet Med. online-first: 1-11.
12. Karpoor, C.H., Deshpande, D.V., Shettar, S., Nagari, P. (2011) Effect of stress on absolute eosinophil count. Indian J Public Health Res Dev. 2: 38.
13. Latimer, K.S. (2011) Duncan and Prasse's Veterinary Laboratory Medicine: Clinical Pathology. (5th ed.) Wiley-Blackwell. Iowa, USA.
14. Martinez, N., Sinedino, L.D.P., Bisinotto, R.S., Ribeiro, E.S, Gomes, G.C, Lima, F.S, Greco, L. F., Risco, C.A., Galvão, K.N., Taylor-Rodriguez, D., Tatcher, W.W., Santos, J.B.P. (2014) Effect of induced subclinical hypocalcemia on physiological responses and neutrophil function in dairy cows. J Dairy Sci. 97: 874-887.
15. Mellau, L.S.B., Jorgensen, R., Jand Enemark, J.M.D. (2001) Plasma calcium, inorganic phosphate and magnesium during hypocalcemia induced by a standardized EDTA infusion in cows. Acta Vet Scand. 42: 251-260.
16. Mostaghni, Kh., farzinpour, M., Smimi, A.S., taghavi-razavizadeh, A. (2012) Changes in biochemical, enzymatic, and electrolyte indices of sheep in experimental hypocalcemia. J Vet Res. 67: 331-335.
17. Radostits, O.M., Gay, C.C., Hinchcliff, K.W., Constable, R.D. (2014) Veterinary Medicine, A Textbook Of The Diseases Of Cattle, Horses, Sheep, Pigs And Goats. (10th ed.) Saunders Elsevier Company, London, UK.
18. Raja Ili Airina, R.K., Mohd, A.R., Abdullah, R.B., Wan Khadijah W.E. (2011) Using fetal heart size measured from ultrasound scanner images to estimate age for gestation in goat. J Anim Vet Adv. 10: 2528-2540.
19. Smith, M.C., Sherman, D.M. (2011) Goat Medicine. (2th ed.) Wiley- Blackwell Company, Iova, USA.
20. Yamagishi, N., Oishi, A., Sato, J., Sato, R., Naito, Y. (1999) Experimental Hypocalcemia Induced by Hemodialysis in Goats, J Vet Med Sci. 61: 1271-1275.

4

Tissue distribution of artemisinin in broiler chickens following single or multiple oral administration

Habibian Dehkordi, S.[1*], Arab, H.A.[2], Esmaeili, M.[1], Kabutari, J.[1], Shahbazfar, A.A.[3]

[1]Department of Pharmacology, School of Veterinary Medicine, Shahrekord University, Shahrekord, Iran
[2]Department of Pharmacology, Faculty of Veterinary Medicine, University of Tehran, Tehran, Iran
[3]Department of Pathobiology, School of Veterinary Medicine, University of Tabriz, Tabriz, Iran

Key words:
artemisinin, biodisposition, broilers, multiple oral intake, single dose

Correspondence
Habibian Dehkordi, S.
Department of Pharmacology, School of Veterinary Medicine, Shahrekord University, Shahrekord, Iran

Email: habibian@vet.sku.ac.ir

Abstract:

BACKGROUND: Artemisinin is commonly used for the treatment of malaria, but recently has been considered as a potential substance to control poultry coccidiosis. **OBJECTIVES:** The aim of the present study was to determine the tissue distribution of artemisinin following single or multiple oral administration of different doses in broiler chickens. **METHODS:** A total number of 390 one day old Ross broiler chicks were divided randomly into two main groups, in the first group 0, 1, 5, 25, 125, 250, 500 or 1000 mg/kg artemisinin as a single oral dose was administered on day 44, but the second group were treated with 0, 17, 34, 68 or 136 ppm artemisinin from day 8 to day 44. The HPLC system was used to determine the level of artemisinin in different tissue samples. Data were assessed using one way analysis of variance (ANOVA) followed by the Tukey's test ($p<0.05$). **RESULTS:** Maximum concentrations of artemisinin were found in the liver of chickens in both groups in a dose dependent manner. While, the minimum level was determined in the brain and the kidney of chickens received multiple artemisinin administration; in the spleen of those chickens a single oral dose was administered. The concentration of artemisinin in the brain reached a plateau at 68 ppm in multiple administration and 125mg/kg at single dose, no shift was found with dose increment. **CONCLUSIONS:** It can be concluded that tissue accumulation of artemisinin is time and dose dependent. Moreover, redistribution, saturation effect and tissue selectivity were also observed.

Introduction

Artemisinin, a natural product from *Artemisia annua*, has been used against malaria for decades in parts of the world where the disease is endemic. Artemisinin and its semisynthetic derivatives have also been shown to be anthelminthic, antidiarrheal, and antipyretic. Moreover, it is a cytotoxic agent against tumor cells (Moore et al; 1995; Efferth et al., 1996, 2001). Recently, in veterinary medicine, artemisinin, has been considered as a safe and effective agent to control poultry coccidiosis. Several studies have been carried out to explore anticoccidial effects of artemisinin in chickens (Allen et al., 1997; Arab et al., 2006; Kaboutari et al., 2014). However, there are few studies to show the toxicity and pharmacokinetic features of artemisinin in different animals including birds. In an attempt to characterize the single dose toxicity of the drug following oral administration, it has been reported that artemisinin is a relatively safe drug that can be used for poultry coccidiosis. There was not any mortality at high doses, but some mild side effects were found in the kidney, the liver and particularly in the nervous system (Arab et al., 2009). Further study showed that multiple administration of high doses of artemisinin in broiler chickens was not effective on different organs including the heart, the lung, and the spleen; but it induced various changes in the liver, the kidney, and the brain. It was found that, while there was not any relationship between the severity of the liver alteration and the drug administration, the severity of lesions in the brain was dose dependent (Shahbazfar et al., 2011).

Toxicological studies conducted on human and a few animal species indicate that artemisinin has high margin of safety, and the pathological effects resulted from high doses of artemisinin in various tissues of different species are ambiguous. It seems that there is a saturation state in the artemisinin concentration in some tissues that cause resistance against toxic effects of artemisinin (Gordi and Lepist, 2004; Efferth and Kaina, 2010).

This study was conducted to determine the tissue distribution of artemisinin in broiler chickens following single or multiple oral administration of the drug in high doses. The study sought to examine the relationship between concentration of artemisinin and toxicological effects induced in different tissues of poultry.

Materials and Methods

Artemisinin administration: Artemisinin, as colorless crystals with the purity of 99%, was obtained from a commercial company in China (Sichuan Arts and Crafts Import and Export Corporation). The drug was dissolved in ethyl alcohol and then diluted by proper volume of water so that the maximum concentration of alcohol would not increase more than 10% of solution. The drug solution prepared for multiple administration was sprayed on feed with complete mixing (each time, 5 kg of feed for each group was prepared). The single doses of artemisinin were administrated to the chickens via gavage.

Animals and experimental groups: A total number of 390 one day old Ross broiler chicks were purchased from a local hatchery and housed in wire cages. The birds had free access to food and water. Light was on 24h a day throughout the study. Chickens were vaccinated against bronchitis, Newcastle disease, and bursal disease. The birds were divided randomly into two main groups on day 8. The first group was treated with a single oral administration of artemisinin. Chickens in the second group received the test compound for a period of 36 days. The birds in group one received a single dose of 0, 1, 5, 25, 125, 250, 500 or 1000 mg/kg artemisinin in 2 ml solution on day 44. The chicks in second group were continuously exposed to 0, 17, 34, 68, or 136 ppm of artemisinin from day 8 to day 44 (a period of 36 days). Each subgroup of doses consists of three replicates (n=10). All experiments were done in accordance with principles of the NIH Guidelines for Care and Use of

Laboratory Animals and approved by the Ethical Committee of the University.

Sample collection: To evaluate the distribution of artemisinin in different organs, animals were euthanized and tissue samples were collected from the liver, the kidney, the brain, the lung and the spleen of birds from both treated groups. Before euthanizing and tissue sampling, each animal was inspected for any gross changes. Animals in the first group were euthanized 1 hour after the administration of artemisinin on day 44, and animals in the second group were euthanized by the end of day 44. Tissue samples were wrapped in an aluminum paper and stored at -20°C until analysis.

Sample preparation and analysis: The method used to extract artemisinin was based on the procedure described by Rawa-Adkonis et al., 2003 with some modification. One gram tissue was dissolved in 5ml of methanol/10%HCl (60/40, v/v), the solution was sonicated for 1.5 min in 3 cycles, and then centrifuged for 10 min. The supernatant was collected and dissolved again in 5 ml petroleum ether and the artemisinin was extracted and dried using a rotary evaporator at 40°C. The residue was then dissolved in ethanol and hydrolyzed by NaOH as explained elsewhere (Liersch et al., 1986). The prepared samples were filtered and stored at -20°C until analysis by HPLC system.

The HPLC analyzing procedure used to determine the amount of artemisinin in tissues was based on the isocratic analytical method described by Liersch et al., 1986 with some modifications. The system consisted of a Knauer 1001 HPLC pump, an h-2600 UV detector, a 10 cm × 4 mm Nucleosil C18 column, and an autosampler. The mobile phase was prepared from 20 mmol/l phosphate buffer (K2HPO4 + KH-2PO4) and methanol (60:40) adjusted at pH 7.9. The volume of each sample automatically injected into the loop of pump was 100 µl at flow rate of 1.5 ml/min.

Method validation of HPLC system: The method validation was conducted according to the guidelines on validation of analytical methods for selectivity, accuracy, precision, linearity, stability, limit of detection and extracted recovery (Shah et al., 1991). A series of standard solutions with concentrations ranging from 0.1 ng/ml to 500 ng/mL were prepared by dilution of artemisinin in methanol. Different blank and spiked blank samples were obtained from various tissues of six broiler chickens to test the selectivity of method. To ensure test accuracy and precision, the homogenate tissues were spiked with 1, 100 or 500 ng/ml artemisinin. The ratio between the results of the analysis of artemisinin in tissue samples and the standard samples dissolved in methanol were considered as acceptable range of accuracy (recycling percentage). To verify the accuracy of the method, each of the above mentioned concentrations was injected five times to the device. Precision of the method was determined by calculation of relative standard deviation (RDS). The RDS of less than 15% and the minimum detectable concentration of less than 20% were used as acceptable limits of accuracy.

The calibration curves were constructed using linear regression analysis based on the area under curve (AUC) of the peak and different known concentrations of the artemisinin. The curves were obtained from a blank sample and eight non - zero spiked samples covering the expected range including lower limit of quantification (LLOQ). The recovery extraction was determined as the ratio of the peak area of the spiked samples to that of the reference samples prepared in methanol with the same concentrations. The homogenate tissues were spiked with artemisinin at concentrations of 1, 100 and 500 ng/ml, and then extracted according to the above-mentioned extraction procedures. The stability of the Artemisinin in biosamples was assessed at different storage conditions including long term stability, freeze and thaw stability and the room temperature stability. All the samples were analyzed and compared with freshly prepared samples.

Statistical analysis: The statistical analysis of data was performed using SPSS software (SPSS version 19.0 for Windows, Inc., Chicago, IL). Data obtained from analytical tests and in vivo experiments were expressed as Mean ± SEM from at least five (samples for each dose) experiments. The comparison of the mean values obtained from different experimental groups was performed by one way analysis of variance, and was followed by the Tukey's test ($p<0.05$).

Results

Method of analysis validation: Artemisinin was separated well with the retention time of approximately 4.6 min; no interferences were detected from endogenous substances. Figure 1 shows a representative chromatogram of standard artemisinin dissolved in methanol at a concentration of 100 ng/ml, liver tissue sample with no artemisinin (Blank) and liver tissue sample with 50 ng/ml of the artemisinin.

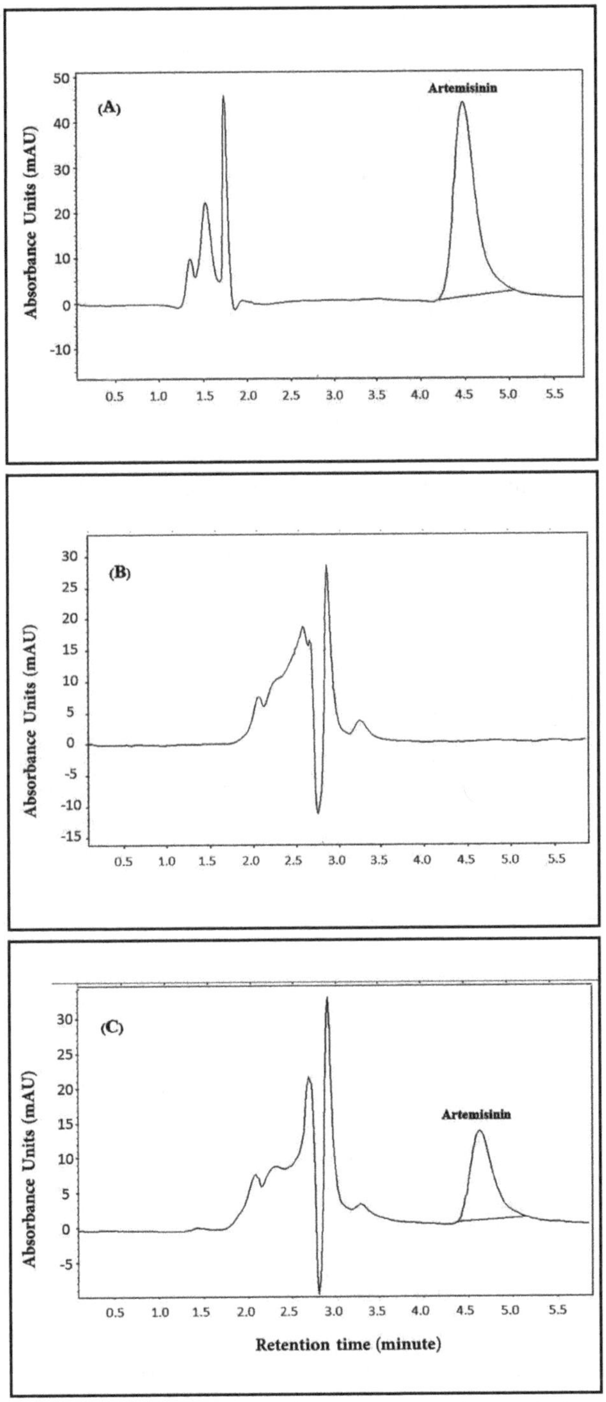

Figure 1. Representative chromatograms obtained from analysis of: A) Standard artemisinin dissolved in methanol at a concentration of 100 ng/mL, B) Liver tissue sample with no artemisinin (Blank), C) Liver tissue sample with 50 ng/mL of the artemisinin.

The range of relative recoveries obtained from different tissue samples was 76.4% to 103.98 %. The RDS of the intra-day precision and the inter-day precision were both less than 17.4%. The standard curves and correlation coefficients of the artemisinin in all tissue samples are listed in Table 1.The calibration plots of artemisinin were linear over the concentration range of 1- to 500 ng/ml. The values obtained in limits of

Table 1. Calibration curves for artemisinin in various tissues.

Biosamples	Liver	Kidney	Lung	Spleen	Brain
Calibration curves	$y = 114.13x + 180.26$	$y = 96.347x + 486.9$	$y = 102.33x + 367.05$	$y = 87.583x + 820.02$	$y = 118.67x + 331.42$
Calibration coefficients (R^2)	$R^2 = 0.9976$	$R^2 = 0.9925$	$R^2 = 0.9946$	$R^2 = 0.9914$	$R^2 = 0.991$

Table 2. Chickens Tissues concentration (ng/g tissue) of artemisinin following a single oral administration. The values presented are Mean ± SD ng/g dry tissue. In each row, different English characters show significant differences ($p<0.05$). In each column, different Greek characters show significant differences ($p<0.05$).

Tissue \ Dose	1 mg/ kg	5 mg/ kg	25 mg/ kg	125mg/ kg	250 mg/ kg	500 mg/ kg	1000 mg/ kg
Liver	$2.85 \pm 0.96^{a\alpha}$	$3.70 \pm 1.34^{a\alpha\beta}$	$15.49 \pm 2.93^{a\alpha}$	$124.02 \pm 13.80^{b\alpha}$	$177.14 \pm 70.46^{b\alpha}$	$326.81 \pm 80.98^{c\alpha}$	$361.88 \pm 116.78^{c\alpha}$
Brain	$2.65 \pm 0.87^{a\alpha\beta}$	$3.28 \pm 1.01^{a\alpha\beta}$	$19.52 \pm 5.23^{a\alpha}$	$41.39 \pm 8.96^{b\beta}$	$47.34 \pm 12.67^{b\beta}$	$51.71 \pm 9.96^{b\beta\gamma}$	$48.77 \pm 13.26^{b\beta}$
Kidney	$3.13 \pm 1.22^{a\alpha}$	$5.168 \pm 1.86^{a\beta}$	$17.22 \pm 3.44^{ab\alpha}$	$46.81 \pm 8.30^{b\beta\gamma}$	$52.92 \pm 12.77^{b\beta}$	$119.38 \pm 22.17^{c\beta}$	$163.66 \pm 48.85^{d\gamma}$
Lung	$3.88 \pm 0.84^{a\alpha}$	$5.284 \pm 1.90^{a\beta}$	$32.50 \pm 6.49^{b\beta}$	$63.10 \pm 13.11^{c\gamma}$	$60.12 \pm 17.68^{c\beta}$	$52.18 \pm 9.69^{bc\beta\gamma}$	$64.83 \pm 19.35^{c\beta\gamma}$
Spleen	$1.13 \pm 0.25^{a\beta}$	$1.04 \pm 0.37^{a\alpha}$	$2.23 \pm 0.46^{a\gamma}$	$3.3 \pm 0.67^{a\gamma}$	$5.74 \pm 2.12^{a\beta}$	$21.65 \pm 7.14^{b\gamma}$	$23.46 \pm 5.60^{b\beta}$

Table 3. Chickens tissues distribution (ng /g tissue) of artemisinin following chronic oral administration. The values presented are Mean ± SD ng /g dry tissue. In each row, different English characters show significant differences ($p<0.05$). In each column, different Greek characters show significant differences ($p<0.05$).

Tissue \ Dose	17 ppm	34 ppm	68 ppm	136 ppm
Liver	$21.24 \pm 4.14^{a\alpha}$	$77.86 \pm 14.54^{b\alpha}$	$71.416 \pm 13.01^{b\alpha}$	$112.23 \pm 23.61^{c\alpha}$
Brain	$12.65 \pm 2.46^{a\beta}$	$21.6 \pm 6.01^{a\beta}$	$44.236 \pm 10.42^{b\beta}$	$44.66 \pm 17.66^{b\beta\gamma}$
Kidney	$6.38 \pm 1.50^{a\beta}$	$34.356 \pm 12.72^{b\beta}$	$38.824 \pm 13.58^{b\beta}$	$29.67 \pm 8.04^{b\gamma}$
Lung	$7.29 \pm 3.19^{a\beta}$	$21.834 \pm 6.87^{a\beta}$	$37.378 \pm 12.28^{b\beta}$	$77.14 \pm 22.30^{c\beta}$
Spleen	$31.77 \pm 7.76^{a\gamma}$	$23.24 \pm 4.88^{a\beta}$	$56.55 \pm 19.31^{b\alpha\beta}$	$71.98 \pm 16.21^{b\beta}$

detection and limits of quantification tests were 0.2 ng/ml and 1 ng/ml, respectively. The level of artemisinin recoveries in liver tissues with three different concentrations (1, 100, 500 ng/ml) was 78.8%, 86.82% and 93.81%, respectively. The artemisinin content of the samples placed in different storage conditions and processed with various procedures was almost identical to those of freshly prepared samples (RSD<12.0%), indicating good stability of this method.

Tissue distribution of artemisinin: The levels of artemisinin determined in different tissue of broiler chickens following single and multiple oral administration are summarized in Table 2 and 3, respectively. The highest concentration of artemisinin following single oral administration was found in the liver. The amount of artemisinin measured in the liver increased significantly following dose increase (doses higher than 125 mg/kg) (Table 2).

The amount of artemisinin detected in the different tissues of chicks that received multiple administration of doses are shown in Table 3. As these show, the accumulation of artemisinin in the liver of chickens exposed to the multiple doses had an increasing pattern, and the groups fed 17 and 136 ppm had a significant difference with each other ($p<0.05$) (Table 3).

Following single oral administration, distribution of artemisinin in brain increased following dose increment at doses lower than 125 mg/kg, however no shift could be found with dose increment at higher doses.

After multiple doses there was a significant difference between the groups fed 17 and 34 ppm with groups fed 68 and 136 ppm ($p<0.05$), and no additional increase was observed after increment of dosage from 68ppm to 136 ppm.

In the kidney following single administration, a significant accumulation was observed at doses higher than 250 mg/kg ($p<0.05$); it appears that at doses higher than 250 mg/kg the excess amount of drug was eliminated via renal routes. On the contrary, the concentration of the drug in kidney samples after multiple doses was even lower at the highest dose (136 ppm) than groups which were fed 34 and 68 ppm.

In the lung samples, following single oral administration, a significant increase was found following dose increment up to 125 mg/kg ($p<0.05$). No dose dependent increment was found at higher doses. However, a significant increase was observed following multiple dose study ($p<0.05$).

Very little artemisinin was found in the spleen samples following single oral administration at doses lower than 125mg/kg. However, at higher doses (500, 1000 mg/kg), concentration of artemisinin in spleen increases surprisingly. In contrast to single dose results, following multiple dose administration the concentration of the drug in the spleen increased significantly.

In general, single oral doses of artemisinin were seen to have a homogenous distribution between various tissues at doses lower than 25 mg/kg, with a significant decline towards the spleen. After single dose of 25 mg/kg, the tissue concentration was the highest in the lung. After that, the distant second was the brain which was closely followed by the liver, the kidney and the spleen. There was no significant difference between the liver, the brain and the kidney ($p>0.05$). At doses of 125 and 250 mg/kg the liver contained the highest dose followed by the lung, the kidney, the brain and the spleen. No significant differences were found between the kidney, the brain and the lung ($p>0.05$). At doses of 500 and 1000 mg/kg the tissue concentrations in various tissues from high to low were the liver, the kidney, the lung, the brain and the spleen. Significant differences were found between liver versus all other tissues and spleen versus all other tissues ($p<0.05$) (Table 2). After multiple administrations, in the group which was fed 17 ppm, the spleen was found to have the highest concentration. The highest level of artemisinin was found in the liver and followed by the spleen, the lung, the brain and the kidney in other groups (Table 3).

Discussion

The present study was conducted to test the relationship between artemisinin dose and tissue distribution following single or multiple administration of compound in broilers. The highest total amount of artemisinin, following multiple or single doses was found in the liver and the accumulation increased following dose increment. Orally administrated artemisinin is metabolized primarily in the liver over time (Ashton et al., 1998). Observations in the liver are considerably in agreement with different studies on tissue distribution of artemisinin in mice and rats (Genovese et al., 1999; Cheeramakara et al., 2008). Toxicopathologic study indicated that only the presence of drug was important in the frequency of lesions occurrences (Arab et al., 2009).

In the brain no increase was observed in the accumulation of artemisinin at high doses following single or multiple oral doses with dose increment. It suggests that binding sites in cerebral cortex and cerebral nuclei are being saturated, and that at high doses uptake into the brain tissues is limited by blood brain barrier. Neurotoxicity is considered as the main side effect of artemisinin and its derivatives, however, its incidence and severity is dependent on dose, period and route of administration (Fishwick et al., 1995),

Drug levels in the kidney were relatively low at doses lower than 250 mg/kg, but increased more at higher doses. Cheeramakara et al. 2008 reported that following intramuscular administration of arteether, an ethyl ether derivative of artemisinin, it was localized mainly in the kidney. The ratio of labeled arteether distribution in the blood: kidney: liver was 1: 5: 2. Higher kidney radioactivity was noted in the cytoplasmic cortex than the medulla (Cheeramakara et al. 2008).

In the present study, following multiple oral doses, a small amount of artemisinin distributed in the kidney. There is evidence that small amount of artemisinin is excreted through kidney without metabolism (Dien et al., 1997). It seems that artemisinin excreted via renal routes in broilers at high doses. This is in agreement with the previous study whichreported that in the microscopic observation the kidney tissues showed some pathologic lesions following single oral doses (Arab et al., 2009).

The distribution in the lung at doses lower than 250 mg/kg increased following an increase in the dose, however, no shift could be found with dose increment. Following single administration, at 25 mg/kg, the tissue concentration was significantly increased. The highest level was observed in the lung followed by the brain, the liver, the kidney, and the spleen. At doses of 125 and 250 mg/kg the liver contained the highest dose followed by the lung, the kidney, the brain and the spleen. No significant differences were found between the kidney, the brain and the lung. At doses of 500 and 1000 mg/kg the tissue concentrations in various tissues from high to low were the liver, the kidney, the lung, the brain and the spleen. Significant differences were found between the liver versus all other tissues and the spleen versus all other tissues.

The result of lung tissue samples from multiple dose study appeared to be inconsistent with the single dose administration. Results suggested that the lung deposition is time dependent and the long half-life of artemisinin in the lung tissue samples is one of the probable reasons.

In the spleen, the lowest level was found following single oral doses, in agreement with this, previous histopathologic studies showed no lesions in the microscopic sections of the spleen following administration of single or multiple doses of artemisinin (Arab et al., 2009; Shahbazfar et al., 2011). However, in the present study, considerable accumulation of artemisinin was observed following administration of multiple doses of artemisinin. It appeared that artemisinin redistributed into the spleen, as it cleared from other tissues, and distribution was time dependent. Results of tissue concentration in the spleen samples obtained from the chicks administrated multiple oral doses are in agreement with the findings from other investigations in rats. Xie et al. 2009 reported that 1h after IV injection of labeled dihydroartemisinin in rats, drug distributed in tissues and after 24h, rapidly declined in all tissues with the exception of spleen (96h). It showed longest residence time in the spleen. This distribution pattern of artemisinin is understandable. The spleen, despite its small size is an important part of the reticuloendothelial system and receives a large percentage of the total cardiac output to filter aging erythrocytes (Smith et al., 1999), and besides, the affinity of artemisinin for heme group of hemoglobin is high (Woerdenbag et al., 1990). Thus the filtration of aging erythrocytes by the red pulp of spleen (Smith et al., 1999) can lead to the accumulation of artemisinin in the spleen following long exposure time.

In this study the tissue distribution of artemisinin in broilers following single or multiple oral administration at different doses was compared. Data obtained in this study allows a comprehensive tissue distribution of artemisinin in broiler chicken at different doses. In general, the results of this study demonstrated considerable complications in terms of artemisinin distribution in chicken tissues, so that tissue accumulation of artemisinin was time and dose dependent, and redistribution, saturation effect and tissue selectivity were observed. Mainly, the results showed highest accumulation in the liver, but the spleen levels were very low following single doses, in contrast, following multiple doses a considerable level of artemisinin was observed in the spleen. Moreover, data suggests that distribution of artemisinin in the brain is saturable, and the drug is eliminated by renal routs at higher doses.

Acknowledgements

This work was supported financially by Shahrekord University and University of Tehran which is gratefully acknowledged.

References

1. Allen, P.C., Lydon, J., Danforth, H.D. (1997) Effects of components of *Artemisia annua* on coccidia infections in chickens. Poult Sci. 76: 1156-163.
2. Arab, H.A., Rahbari, S., Rassouli, A., Moslemi, M.H., Khosravirad, F. (2006) Determination of artemisinin in *Artemisia sieberi* and anticoccidial effects of the plant extract in broiler chickens. Trop Anim Health Prod. 38: 497-503.
3. Arab, H.A., Mardjanmehr, S.H., Shahbazfar, A.A, Rassouli, A., Abdollahi, M., Nekouie, O. (2009) Toxicopathologic effects of artemisinin in broiler chickens following a single oral dose: An LD50 Study. Int J Poultry Sci. 8: 808-812.
4. Ashton, M., Hai, T.N., Sy, N.D., Huong, D.X., Van Huong, N., Niêu, N.T. (1998) Artemisinin pharmacokinetics is time-dependent during repeated oral administration in healthy male adults. Drug Metab Dispos. 26: 25-27.
5. Cheeramakara, C., Khachonsaksumet, V., Suthisai, N., Nakosiri, W., Songmuaeng, K., Saenghirun, C., Phienpicharn, D., Nontprasert, A. (2008) Distribution of C14-labelled arteether in kidneys and livers of experimental mice after intramuscular injection. Southeast Asian J Trop Med Public Health. 39: 195-199.
6. Dien, T.K., de Vries, P.J., Khanh, N.X., Koopmans, R., Binh, L.N., Duc, D.D., Kager, P.A., van Boxtel, C.J. (1997) Effect of food intake on pharmacokinetics of oral artemisinin in

healthy Vietnamese subjects. Antimicrob Agents Chemother. 41: 1069-1072.

7. Efferth, T., Kaina, B. (2010) Toxicity of the antimalarial artemisinin and its dervatives. Crit Rev Toxicol. 40: 405-421.
8. Efferth, T., Dunstan, H., Sauerbrey, A., Miyachi, H., Chitambar, C.R. (2001) The anti-malarial artesunate is also active against cancer. Int J Oncol. 18: 767-773.
9. Efferth, T., Rucker, G., Falkenberg, M., Manns, D., Olbrich, A., Fabry, U., Osieka, R. (1996) Detection of apoptosis in KG-1a leukemic cells treated with investigational drugs. Arzneimittelforschung. 46: 196-200.
10. Fishwick, J., McLean, W.G., Edwards, G., Ward, S.A. (1995) The toxicity of artemisinin and related compounds on neuronal and glial cells in culture. Chem Biol Interact. 96: 263-271.
11. Genovese, R.F., Newman, D.B., Gordon, K.A., Brewer, T.G. (1999) Acute high dose arteether toxicity in rats. Neurotoxicology. 20: 851-859.
12. Gordi, T., Lepist, E.I. (2004) Artemisinin derivatives: toxic for laboratory animals, safe for humans? Toxicol Lett. 147: 99-107.
13. Kaboutari, J, Arab, HA., Ebrahimi, K, Rahbari, S. (2014) Prophylactic and therapeutic effects of a novel granulated formulation of Artemisia extract on broiler coccidiosis. Trop Anim Health Prod. 46: 43-48.
14. Liersch, R., Soicke, H., Stehr, C., Tüllner, H.U. (1986) Formation of artemisinin in *Artemisia annua* during one vegetation period. Planta Med. 5: 387-390.
15. Moore, J.C., Lai, H., Li, J.R., Ren, R.L., McDougall, J.A., Singh, N.P., Chou, C.K. (1995) Oral administration of dihydroartemisinin and ferrous sulfate retarded implanted fibrosarcoma growth in the rat. Cancer Lett. 98: 83-87.
16. Rawa-Adkonis, M., Wolska, L.,Namieśnik, J. (2003) Modern techniques of extraction of organic analytes from environmental matrices. Crit Rev Anal Chem. 33: 199-248.
17. Shah, V.P., Midha, K.K., Dighe, S., McGilveray, I.J., Skelly, J.P., Yacobi, A., Layloff, T., Viswanathan, C.T., Cook, C.E., McDowall, R.D. (1992) Analytical methods validation: bioavailability, bioequivalence and pharmacokinetic studies. Eur J Drug Metab Pharmacokinet. 16: 249-255.
18. Shahbazfar, A.A., Mardjanmehr, S.H., Arab, H.A., Rassouli, A., Abdollahi, M. (2011) Effects of artemisinin in broiler chickens following multilpe oral intake. Trop Anim Health Prod. 43: 843-849.
19. Smith, F.M., West, N.H., Jones, D.R. (1999) The Cardiovascular System. In: Sturkie's Avian Physiology. Whittow, G.C. (ed.). (5th ed.) Academic Press, London, UK. p. 171-172.
20. Woerdenbag, H.J., Lugt, C.B., Pras, N. (1990) *Artemisia annua* L.: a source of novel antimalarial drugs. Pharm Weekbl Sci. 12: 169-181.
21. Xie, L.H., Li, Q., Zhang, J., Weina, P.J. (2009) Pharmacokinetics, tissue distribution and mass balance of radiolabeled dihydroartemisinin in male rats. Malar J. 8, 112: 1-14.

Interactions between histamine H1 and H3 and dopamine D1 receptors on feeding behavior in chicken

Ghand Foroushan, M., Zendehdel, M.*, Babapour, V.

Department of Basic Sciences, Faculty of Veterinary Medicine, University of Tehran, Tehran, Iran

Key words:
chicken, dopamine, food intake, ICV, histamine

Correspondence
Zendehdel, M.
Section of Physiology, Department of Basic Sciences, Faculty of Veterinary Medicine, University of Tehran, Tehran, Iran

Email: zendedel@ut.ac.ir

Abstract:

BACKGROUND: Brain monoamines (such as histamine and dopamine) play an important role in emotions, cognition, reward and feeding behavior. The interactions between histamine and dopamine were studied in many physiological functions but this correlation is unclear in feeding behavior of chickens. **OBJECTIVES:** The aim of this study was to investigate the interaction of central histaminergic and dopaminergic systems on food intake in broiler chicken. **METHODS:** In this study intracerebroventricular (ICV) injection was used for manipulation of histaminergic and dopaminergic systems. In Experiment 1, 3 h-fasted chicks were given an ICV injection of histamine, SCH23390, a D1 receptors antagonist and co-injection of histamine and SCH23390. Experiments 2-5 were similar to experiment 1 except birds were injected with AMI-193, D2 receptors antagonist; NGB2904, D3 receptors antagonist; L-741,742, D4 receptors antagonist and 6-OHDA, 6-hydroxydopamine instead of SCH 23390, respectively. In experiment 6, ICV injection of dopamine, chlorpheniramine, H1 receptors antagonist and co-administration of dopamine and chlorpheniramine were done. Experiments 7-9 were similar to experiment 6, except birds ICV injected with famotidine, H2 receptors antagonist; thioperamide, H3 receptors antagonist and α-FMH, alpha-fluoromethylhistidine in place of chlorpheniramine, respectively. Then cumulative food intake (g) was measured at 30, 60 and 120 min after the injection. **RESULTS:** Histamine decreased food intake compared to the control chicks indicating an inhibitory effect of histamine on food intake and SCH23390 attenuated the effect of histamine on food intake ($p<0.001$). In addition, hypophagic effect of histamine decreased by 6-OHDA ($p<0.001$). Chlorpheniramine and α-FMH significantly attenuated dopamine induced hypophagia ($p<0.001$). However, thioperamide amplified the inhibitory effect of dopamine on food intake($p<0.001$). **CONCLUSIONS:** These results suggest there is relationship between histaminergic and dopaminergic systems on food intake in chicken and H1, H3 and D1 receptors are involved in this interaction.

Introduction

Birds, like mammals, have complex mechanisms regulating food intake. Given a choice between more than one diet, turkeys, broilers, layers, and other avian species display the ability to self-select a diet adequate for growth or pro¬duction (Denbow, 1999). Although compensation may not be complete, if exposed to severe feed restriction early in life, birds compensate by increasing their intake in order to increase weight gain following the restriction. In contrast, force feeding birds twice their ad libitum food intake causes Leghorns to stop eating for 7-10 days until their fat stores approach pre-force-feeding levels. Therefore, clearly, birds have the ability to regulate food intake (Denbow, 1999). A number of peptides comprise a complex network that regulates feeding behavior in avian (Kaneko et al., 2012).

Histamine is one of the well-known amines which contribute in many physiological functions in the central nervous system (CNS) (Blandina et al., 2012). It is reported that paraventricular nucleus (PVN) and ventromedial hypothalamus (VMH) receive afferent projected axons of histaminergic (HA-ergic) neurons from tuberomammillary nucleus (TMN). They send projections organized in functionally distinct circuits impinging on different brain regions and their firing frequency changes according to the behavioral state (Giannoni et al., 2009). Four subtypes of histamine receptors have been classified (H1, H2, H3 and H4), all of these subtypes distributed in several part of CNS (Schneider et al., 2014).

Brain histamine plays a vital role in eating behavior and has been considered as satiety signal that is released during food intake (Rozov et al., 2014). It is known ICV administration of histamine decreases food intake whereas ICV injection of chlorpheniramine (histamine H1 receptor antagonist), or alpha-fluoromethylhistidine (α-FMH, selective inhibitor of histidine decarboxylase) increases food intake in rats (Morimoto et al., 2001) and chicken (Kawakami et al., 2000; Taati et al., 2009).

Dopamine is the predominant catecholamine neurotransmitter in the mammalian brain which controls a variety of functions including locomotoractivity, cognition, emotion, positive reinforcement and food intake (Ikemoto, 2007). Dopamine is a key anorexigenic neurotransmitter modulating reward which acts mainly through its projections from the ventral tegmental area (VTA) into the nucleus accumbens (NAcc) and arcuate nucleus (ARC) (Volkow et al., 2011). Dopaminergic neurons (DAergic) of the Substantia Nigra (SN), Pars Compacta, VTA and hypothalamus give origin to three main pathways, Nigrostriatal, Mesolimbocortical and Tuberoinfundibular in CNS (Cadet et al., 2010). The inhibitory effect of DA on food intake was decreased by SCH23390 pretreatment in chicken (Bungo et al., 2010; Zendehdel et al., 2014). The same observation was reported in mammals in which ICV injection of SKF 38393 (D1 receptors agonist) and apomorphine (D2 receptors agonists) decreased cumulative food intake in rats (Kuo, 2002).

Based on the reports, there is correlation between DAergic and HAergic systems where L-DOPA activates histaminergic neurons in CNS (Yanovsky et al., 2011). For instance, H3 receptor interacts with D1 and D2 receptors in the striatum of patients suffering Parkinson's disease (Yanovsky et al., 2011). It is shown the dopamine D1 and

D2 receptors in the basolateral amygdaloid (BLA) nucleus may be involved in the anxiogenic-like effects induced by histamine in rat model (Bananej et al., 2012). Histaminergic projections innervate VTA, which consists of the cell bodies of dopamine neurons (Montoro et al. 2013). The modulation of monoamines and other neurotransmitters via H3 heterorecepetors has also been described (Schlicker et al. 1994). It is possible that the H3 receptor functions as a heteroreceptor to release monoamines such as NE, and DA.

To date, much progress has been done to identify mediatory effect of neurotransmitters on feeding behavior in mammals but food intake regulation in domestic poultry is not fully studied (Zendehdel and Hassanpour 2014; Hassanpour et al., 2015). It is well documented that central feeding behavior is not regulated via a single neuropeptide and a wide distributed neural network interacts with diversity of neurotransmitters on feeding status (Zendehdel et al., 2016).

The interactions between histamine and dopamine were studied in many physiological functions but this correlation is unclear in feeding behavior of chickens. So, the aim of this study was to investigate the interaction of central histaminergic and dopaminergic systems on feeding behavior in broiler chicken.

Materials and Methods

Animals: A total of 432 one-day-old broiler chickens (Ross 308) were purchased from a local hatchery (Eshragh Co. Iran). At 2 d of age birds were randomly transferred to individual cages and kept at a temperature of 30 ± 1°C with 50 ± 2 percent humidity (Olanrewaju et al., 2006). Birds were housed according to a completely randomized design. During the study birds had ad libitum access to fresh water and a starter diet containing 21% crude protein and 2850 kcal/kg of metabolizable energy (Animal Science Research Institute Co., Iran). Three hours prior to the injections, birds were food deprived (FD3) but had free access to water. Animal handling and experimental procedures were performed according to the Guide for the Care and Use of Laboratory Animals by the National Institutes of Health (USA) and the current laws of the Iranian government for animal care.

Experimental drugs: The histamine, SCH 23390 (D1 receptors antagonist), AMI-193 (D2 receptors antagonist), NGB2904 (D3 receptors antagonist), L-741,742 (D4 receptors antagonist), 6-OHDA (6-hydroxydopamine), dopamine, chlorpheniramine (H1 receptors antagonist), famotidine (H2 receptors antagonist), thioperamide (H3 receptors antagonist), α-FMH (alpha-fluoromethylhistidine) and Evans blue purchased from Sigma Co. (Sigma, USA). Drugs were first dissolved in absolute dimethyl sulfoxide (DMSO) then diluted with 0.85% saline containing Evans blue at a ratio of 1/250. DMSO with this ratio does not have a cytotoxic effect (Blevins et al., 2002; Qi et al., 2008).

Intracerebroventricular injection procedures: Intracerebroventricular (ICV) injections conducted at 5 days of age. A total of 9 experiments were designed to investigate the interconnection of histaminergic and dopaminergic systems on food intake in neonatal birds. Each experiment included 4 treatment groups with 12 replicates per group (n = 48 chickens per experiment). In each experiment, chicks were weighed and allocated into experimental groups based on their body weight so that the average weight (45±5 g) between treatment groups was as uniform as possible. Each chicken received ICV injected once in each experiment. Injections were done using a microsyringe (Hamilton, Switzerland) without anesthesia based on the method described by Davis et al., (1979) and Furuse et al., (1997). In this technique, the head of the chick was held with an acrylic device in which the bill holder was at 45° and the calvarium was parallel to the surface of table (Van Tienhoven and Juhasz, 1962). An orifice was made in a plate that was located over the skull immediately over the right lateral ventricle. The microsyringe was inserted into the ventricle through the orifice in the plate. The tip of the needle perforated only 4 mm below the skin of the skull (Jonaidi and Noori, 2012). There is no physiological stress using this technique in neonatal chicken (Saito et al., 2005). Injections were done in a volume of 10 μl (Furuse et al., 1999). The control group received control solution as 10 μl of saline containing Evan's blue (Furuse et al., 1999). At the end of the experiments, to recognize the accuracy of injection, chicken were killed by decapitation. Accuracy of placement of the injection in the ventricle was verified by the presence of Evans blue followed by slicing the frozen brain tissue. Only data from individuals in which dye was present in their lateral ventricle were used for analysis. All experimental procedures were done from 8:00 A.M. until 3:30 P.M. Also, the time course of food consumption was selected by previous studies (Bungo et al., 2010; Zendehdel et al., 2008, 2014, 2016).

Food intake measurement procedure: In this study, 9 experiments were designed, each with 4 treatment groups (n=48). In Experiment 1, 3 h-fasted chicks were given an ICV injection of histamine (300 nmol), SCH23390 (5 nmol), a D1 receptors antagonist and co-injection of histamine and SCH23390. Experiments 2-5 were similar to experiment 1 except birds were injected with AMI-193 (5 nmol), D2 receptors antagonist; NGB2904 (6.4 nmol), D3 receptors antagonist; L-741,742(6 nmol), D4 receptors antagonist and 6-OHDA (2.5 nmol), 6-hydroxydopamine instead of SCH 23390, respectively. In experiment 6, ICV injection of dopamine (40 nmol), chlorpheniramine (300 nmol), H1 receptors antagonist and co-administration of dopamine and chlorpheniramine were done. Experiments 7-9 were similar to experiment 6, except birds ICV injected with famotidine (82 nmol), H2 receptors antagonist; thioperamide (300 nmol), H3 receptors antagonist and α-FMH (250 nmol), alpha-fluoromethylhistidine in place of chlorpheniramine, respectively. To find the possible relationship between these two systems, effective and sub-effective doses of pharmacologic agents were administered to confront nullifying effects of the agents. In other words, when an effective dose of a system is administered, the sub-effective dose of the other system is considered. Immediately after injection, chickens were returned to their individual cages and provided with access to pre-weighed food ad libitum and water. Cumulative food intake (g) was measured at 30, 60 and 120 min after the injection. Food consumption was calculated as a percentage of body weight (%BW) to minimize impact of body weight on the amount of food intake. Each bird was just used once in each experimental group.

Statistical analysis: Data is presented as mean ± SEM (standard error of the mean). Cumulative food intake (as percentage

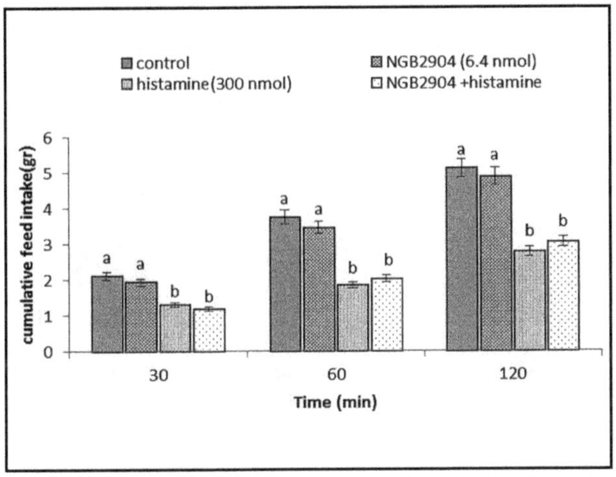

Figure 3. Effect of ICV injection of NGB2904 (6.4 nmol), histamine (300 nmol) and their combination on cumulative food intake in neonatal chicken (n=48). NGB2904: D3 receptor antagonist, Data are expressed as mean ± SEM. Different letters (a and b) indicate significant differences between treatments ($p<0.001$).

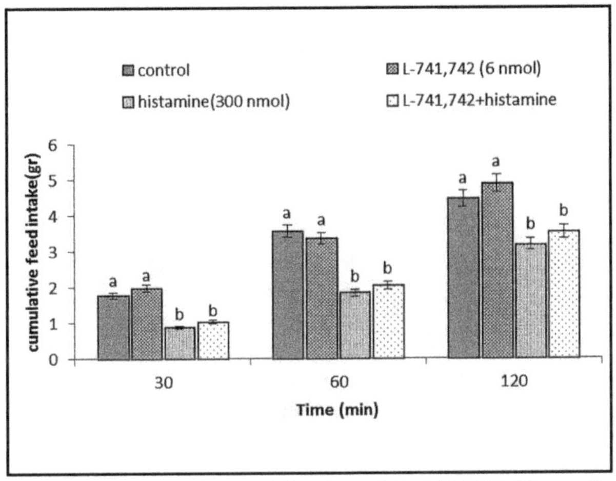

Figure 4. Effect of ICV injection of L-741,742 (6 nmol), histamine (300 nmol) and their combination on cumulative food intake in neonatal chicken (n=48). L-741,742: D4 receptor antagonist, Data are expressed as mean ± SEM. Different letters (a and b) indicate significant differences between treatments ($p<0.001$).

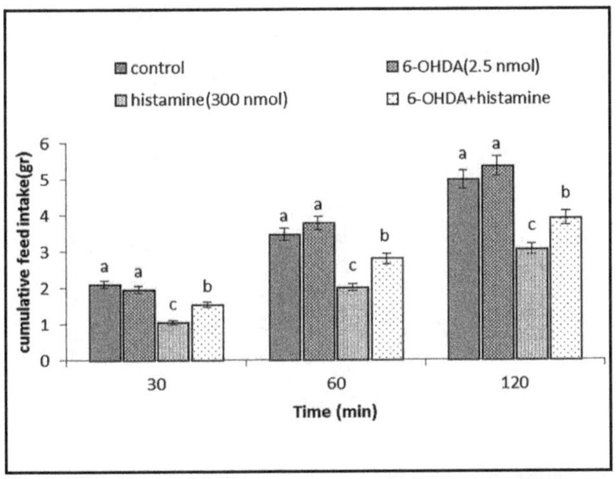

Figure 5. Effect of ICV injection of 6-OHDA (2.5 nmol), histamine (300 nmol) and their combination on cumulative food intake in neonatal chicken (n=48). 6-OHDA: 6-hydroxydopamine, Data are expressed as mean ± SEM. Different letters (a, b and c) indicate significant differences between treatments ($p<0.01$).

Effect of ICV injection of 300 nmol chlorpheniramine, 40 nmol dopamine and their combination on cumulative food intake in neonatal chicken is presented in Fig. 6. According to the results, the ICV injecion of 40 nmol dopamine significantly decreased food intake compared with control group ($p<0.001$) (Fig. 6). Chlorpheniramine administration also significantly decreased the effect of dopamine on food intake in birds ($p<0.001$)(Fig. 6).

As seen in Fig. 7, ICV injection of sub effective dose of famotidine (82 nmol) had no effect on food intake ($p>0.05$). Also, ICV injection of 40 nmol dopamine significantly decreased food intake in neonatal broiler chicken ($p<0.001$). Co-injection of dopamine and famotidine had no effect on food intake compared with dopamine group ($p>0.05$) (Fig. 7).

Based on the results in experiment 8, 300 nmol thioperamide administration significantly amplified dopamine-induced hypophagia in chickens ($p<0.001$) (Fig. 8); but ICV injection of thioperamide alone could not alter food intake in comparison with control group ($p>0.05$) (Fig. 8).

As observed in Fig. 9, ICV injection of sub effective dose of α-FMH (250 nmol) had no effect on feeding behavior in neonatal broiler chicken ($p>0.05$). Also, ICV injecion of dopamine (40 nmol) significantly decreased food intake in neonatal broiler chicken ($p<0.001$). Co-injection of dopamine and α-FMH decreased dopamine-induced hypophagia in neonatal broiler chick-

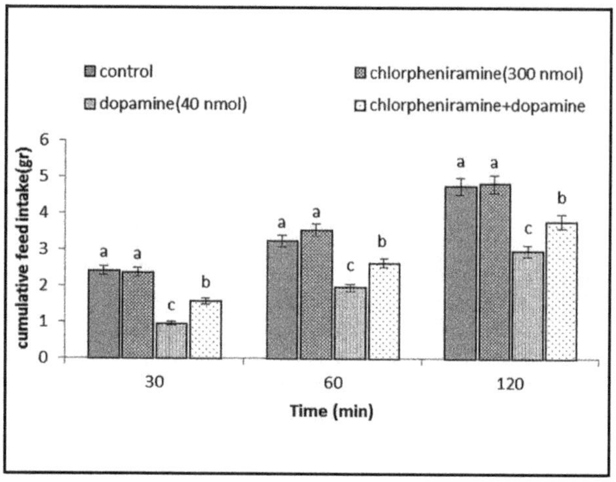

Figure 6. Effect of ICV injection of chlorpheniramine (300 nmol), dopamine (40 nmol) and their combination on cumulative food intake in neonatal chicken (n=48). chlorpheniramine: H1 receptor antagonist, Data are expressed as mean ± SEM. Different letters (a, b and c) indicate significant differences between treatments ($p<0.001$).

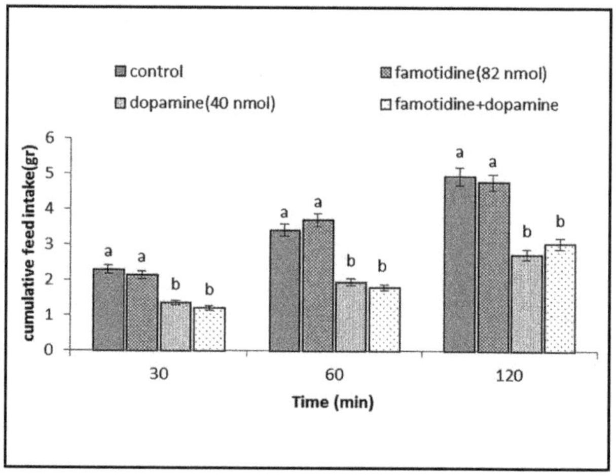

Figure 7. Effect of ICV injection of famotidine (82 nmol), dopamine (40 nmol) and their combination on cumulative food intake in neonatal chicken (n=48). famotidine: H2 receptor antagonist, Data are expressed as mean ± SEM. Different letters (a and b) indicate significant differences between treatments ($p<0.001$).

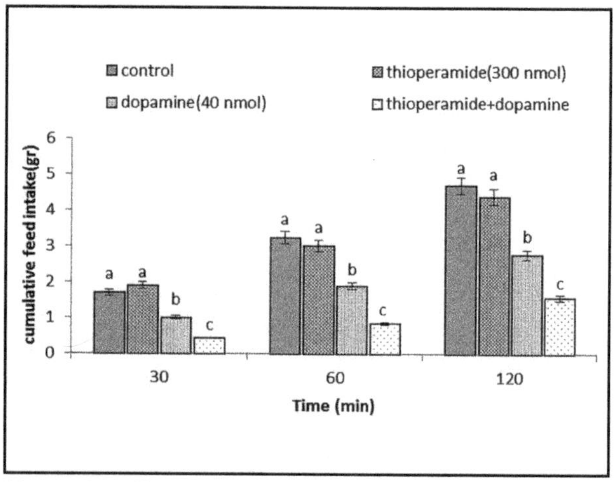

Figure 8. Effect of ICV injection of thioperamide (300 nmol), dopamine (40 nmol) and their combination on cumulative food intake in neonatal chicken (n=48). thioperamide: H3 receptor antagonist, Data are expressed as mean ± SEM. Different letters (a, b and c) indicate significant differences between treatments ($p<0.001$).

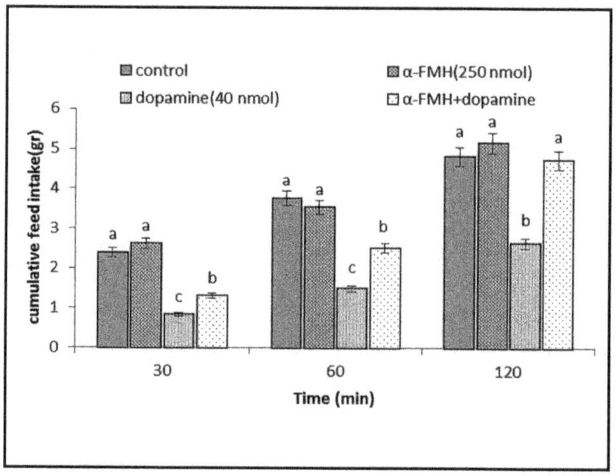

Figure 9. Effect of ICV injection of α-FMH (250 nmol), dopamine (40 nmol) and their combination on cumulative food intake in neonatal chicken (n=48). α-FMH: alpha-fluoromethylhistidine, Data are expressed as mean ± SEM. Different letters (a, b and c) indicate significant differences between treatments ($p<0.001$).

en ($p<0.001$) (Fig. 9). These results showed that dopamine-induced hypophagia is mediated via histaminergic H1 and H3 receptors in neonatal chicks.

Discussion

Based on the literature this paper is the first report on the relationship between DAergic and HAergic systems on food intake in FD3 neonatal broiler chickens. According to the results, there is relationship between two systems via D1, H1 and H3 receptors on central food intake regulation in neonatal broiler chicken. According to the previous studies, the ICV injection of dopamine and L-DOPA (precursor of dopamine) significantly decreased food intake in FD3 broiler cockerels (Zendehdel et al., 2014).

of body weight) was analyzed by repeated measure two-way analysis of variance (ANOVA) using SPSS 16.0 for Windows (SPSS, Inc., Chicago, IL, USA). For treatment, showing a main effect by ANOVA means was compared by Tukey-Kramer test. $p<0.05$ was considered significant difference between treatments.

Results

The results of interaction between central DAergic and HAergic systems on food intake control in neonatal broiler chicks are presented in Figs. 1-9. In experiment 1, ICV injection of an effective dose of histamine (300 nmol) significantly decreased food consumption at 30, 60 and 120 min post-injection ($p<0.001$). ICV injection of sub effective dose of SCH23390 (5 nmol) had no significant effect on food intake compared to control group in FD3 neonatal broiler ($p>0.05$); while co-injection of SCH23390 (5 nmol) and histamine (300 nmol) significantly attenuated histamine-induced hypophagia at 30, 60 and 120 min post-injection ($p<0.001$)(Fig. 1).

As seen in Fig. 2, the ICV injection of sub effective dose of AMI-193 (5 nmol) had no significant effect on food intake compared to control group in FD3 neonatal broiler ($p>0.05$). Also, co-injection of AMI-193 and histamine had no effect on histamine-induced hypophagia in chicken ($p>0.05$) (Fig. 2).

As seen in Figs. 3 and 4 ICV injection of sub effective doses of NGB2904 (6.4 nmol) and L-741,742 (6 nmol) could not alter food intake induced by 300 nmol histamine in neonatal chick ($p>0.05$) (Figs. 3 and 4).

According to the results obtained from experiment 5, post hoc analysis revealed

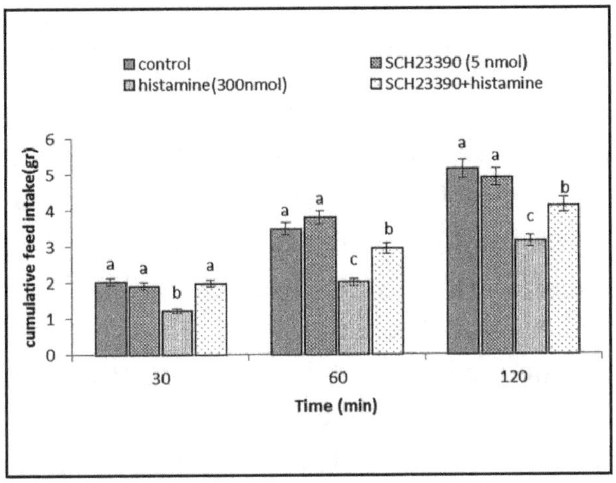

Figure 1. Effect of ICV injection of SCH23390 (5 nmol), histamine (300 nmol) and their combination on cumulative food intake in neonatal chicken (n=48). SCH23390: D1 receptor antagonist, Data are expressed as mean ± SEM. Different letters (a, b and c) indicate significant differences between treatments ($p<0.01$).

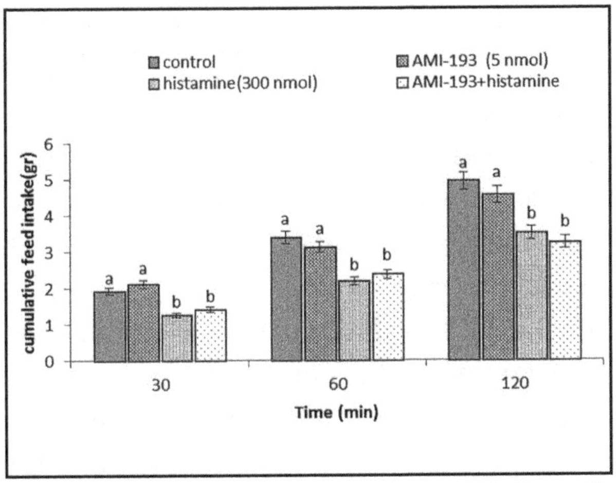

Figure 2. Effect of ICV injection of AMI-193 (5 nmol), histamine (300 nmol) and their combination on cumulative food intake in neonatal chicken (n=48). AMI-193: D2 receptor antagonist, Data are expressed as mean ± SEM. Different letters (a and b) indicate significant differences between treatments ($p<0.01$).

that 6-OHDA (2.5 nmol) administration significantly decreased hypophagic effect of histamine ($p<0.001$) (Fig. 5); however, ICV injection of 6-OHDA (2.5 nmol) alone had no effect on food intake compared with control group($p>0.05$) (Fig. 5). The results obtained from experiments 1-5 revealed that hypophagic effect of histamine is mediated via dopaminergic D1 receptors in neonatal chicks.

A daily decrease on cumulative food intake was reported using D1 (SKF 38393) and D2 (apomorphine) receptors agonists in rats (Kuo 2002). Also, previous studies showed that central injection of histamine H1 receptor antagonist increased cumulative food intake in rat (Morimoto et al., 2001), layer and broiler chickens (2010). Perhaps, histamine mediates food intake in CNS using H1 receptors, but the direct location of this receptor is still unclear in chicken (Taati et al., 2006). Also, in this study, we used sub effective doses of antagonists to determine possible interaction of HAergic and DAergic systems on feeding behavior in neonatal chicken. As observed, sub effective doses of H1-H4 receptors antagonists had no role on food intake in neonatal broiler chicken. Thioperamide is histamine H3 receptor antagonist which increases histaminergic neurons activity. Perhaps thioperamide-induced histaminergic neurons activity occurs via disencumbering negative feedback on histidine decarboxylase enzyme and/or release of histamine (Sakata et al., 1997).

As seen in this study, a relationship was identified between two systems via D1, H1 and H3 receptors on central food intake regulation in neonatal broiler chicken. H3 receptors antagonists are able to stimulate monoamine neurotransmission. Recently it was revealed modulation of DAergic neurons play an important role in functional interactions between histamine and other monoamines (Flik et al., 2015). The ICV injection of histamine into the VTA mimicked the stimulatory effect of thioperamide on DAergic neurons (Flik et al., 2015). So, it seems interaction exists between central DAergic and HAergic systems, our results are in agreement with previous reports.

On the other hand, the stimulatory effect of thiopiramide on DAergic system is mediated by activation of dopamine neurons probably via excitatory histamine H1 receptors (Flik et al., 2011). The ICV injection H1 receptor agonist stimulates mesolimbic and mesocortical dopamine release (Lapa et al., 2005). Thus, activation of the HAergic system by L-DOPA increased histamine and dopamine levels in forebrain areas (Yanovsky et al., 2011). The results of the current study demonstrate that chlorpheniramine attenuated dopamine induced hypophagia while thioperamide increased the effect of dopamine on food intake. This finding is consistent with previous observations. It was reported that thioperamide potentiated L-DOPA and methamphetamine induced DA release in striatum and nucleus accumbens, respectively (Nowak et al., 2008). Other antagonists of H3 receptors, ABT-239 and GSK189254, increased DA levels in PFC and cingulate cortex, respectively (Medhurst et al., 2007).

It was recently shown that H3 receptors form heteromers either with D1 or D2 receptors in the striatum, where histamine is able to decrease sensitivity of the receptor to dopaminergic drugs, while an H3 receptors antagonist increases its sensitivity (Ferrada et al., 2009). Also, there are H3 receptors on dopaminergic neurons terminals as heteroreceptors and modulate dopamine release (Flik et al., 2015). However, scarce information exists on interaction of DAergic and HAergic systems on feeding behavior. So, we are not able to compare our results with them. However, it is reported there are other interactions between DAergic and HAergic systems via GABAergic and/or serotonin where GABA and serotonergic neurons contribute with dopamine neurons in modulation of anxiety behavior (Zarrindast and

Khakpai, 2015). For instance, thioperamide increased serotonin, norepinephrine and dopamine levels in the rat prefrontal cortex (Flik et al., 2015). Also, the H3 receptors are ligands on serotonergic and DAergic neurotransmission (Flik et al., 2015).

In conclusion these results suggest there is a relationship between histaminergic and dopaminergic systems on food intake in chicken and H1, H3 and D1 receptors are involved in this interaction. Based on our knowledge, there was no report on molecular and cellular interaction between DAergic and HAergic systems on feeding behavior in avian. So, further researches are needed to determine molecular pathway(s) for this relationship. Presumably, obtained results can be as base information for further studies on the possible involvement of DAergic and HAergic systems with other neurotransmitters on feeding behavior.

Acknowledgments

This research was supported by a grant from the Research Council of the Faculty of Veterinary Medicine, University of Tehran, Iran.

References

Bananej, M., Karimi-Sori, A., Zarrindast, M.R., Ahmadi, S. (2012) D1 and D2 dopaminergic systems in the rat basolateral amygdala are involved in anxiogenic-like effects induced by histamine. J Psychopharmacol. 26: 564-574.

Blandina, P., Munari, L., Provensi, G., Passani, M.B. (2012) Histamine neurons in the tuberomamillary nucleus: A whole center or distinct subpopulations? Front Syst Neurosci. 6: 33.

Blevins, J.E., Stanley, B.G., Reidelberger, R.D. (2002) DMSO as a vehicle for central injections: tests with feeding elicited by norepinephrine injected into the paraventricular nucleus. Pharmacol Biochem Behav. 71: 277-282.

Bungo, T., Yanagita, K., Shiraishi, J. (2010) Feed intake after infusion of noradrenalin, dopamine or its precursor into the lateral ventricles in neonatal chicks. J Anim Vet Adv. 9: 760-763.

Cadet, J.L., Jayanthi, S., McCoy, M.T., Beauvais, G., Cai, N.S. (2010) Dopamine D1 receptors, regulation of gene expression in the brain, and neurodegeneration. CNS Neurol Disord Drug Targets. 9: 526-538.

Davis, J.L., Masuoka, D.T., Gerbrandt, L.K., Cherkin, A. (1979) Autoradiographic distribution of L-proline in chicks after intracerebral injection. Physiol Behav. 22: 693-695.

Denbow, D.M., Duke, G.E., Chaplin, S.B. (1999) Food intake, gastric secretion, and motility as affected by avian pancreatic polypeptide administered centrally in chickens. Peptides. 9: 449-454.

Ferrada, C., Ferre, S., Casado, V., Cortes, A., Justinova, Z., Barnes, C., Canela, E.I., Goldberg, S.R., Leurs, R., Lluis, C., Franco, R. (2008) Interactions between histamine H3 and dopamine D2 receptors and the implications for striatal function. Neuropharmacol. 55: 190-197.

Flik, G., Dremencov, E., Cremers, T.I., Folgering, J.H., Westerink, B.H. (2011) The role of cortical and hypothalamic histamine-3 receptors in the modulation of centralhistamine neurotransmission: an in vivo electrophysiology and microdialysis study. Eur J Neurosci. 34: 1747-1755.

Flik, G., Joost Folgering, H.A., Thomas Cremers, I.H.F., Westerink, B.H.C., Dremencov, E. (2015) Interaction Between Brain Histamine and Serotonin, Norepinephrine, and Dopamine Systems: In Vivo Microdialysis and Electrophysiology Study. J Mol Neurosci. 56: 320-328.

Furuse, M., Ando, R., Bungo, T., Ao, R., Shimo-JO, M., Masuda, Y. (1999) Intracerebroventricular injection of orexins does not stimulate food intake in neonatal chicks. Br Poult Sci. 40: 698-700.

Furuse, M., Matsumoto, M., Saito, N., Sugahara, K., Hasegawa, S. (1997) The central corticotropin-releasing factor and glucagon-like peptide-1 in food intake of the neonatal chick. Eur J Pharmacol. 339: 211-214.

Giannoni, P., Passani, M.B., Nosi, D., Chazot, P.L., Shenton, F.C., Medhurst, A.D., Munari, L., Blandina, P. (2009) Heterogeneity of histaminergic neurons in the tuberomammillary nucleus of the rat. Eur J Neurosci. 29: 2363-2374.

Hassanpour, S., Zendehdel, M., Babapour, V., Charkhkar, S. (2015) Endocannabinoid and nitric oxide interaction mediates food intake in neonatal chicken. Br Poult Sci. 56: 443-451.

Jonaidi, H., Noori, Z. (2012) Neuropeptide Y-induced feeding is dependent on GABAA receptors in neonatal chicks. J Comp Physiol A. 198: 827-832.

Kaneko, K., Yoshikawa, M., Ohinata, K. (2012) Novel orexigenic pathway prostaglandin D2-NPY system-involvement in orally active orexigenic d opioid peptide. Neuropeptides. 46: 353-357.

Kuo, D. (2002) Co-administration of dopamine D1 and D2 agonists additively decreases daily food intake, body weight and hypothalamic neuropeptide Y level in rats. J Biomed Sci. 9: 126-32.

Lapa, G.B., Mathews, T.A., Harp, J., Budygin, E.A., Jones, S.R. (2005) Diphenylpyraline, a histamine H1 receptor antagonist, has psychostimulant properties. Eur J Pharmacol. 506: 237-240.

Medhurs, A.D., Atkins, A.R., Beresford, I.J., Brackenborough, K., Briggs, M.A., Calver, A.R., Cilia, J., Cluderay, J.E., Crook, B., Davis, J.B., Davis, R.K., Davis, R.P., Dawson, L.A., Foley, A.G., Gartlon, J., Gonzalez, M.I., Heslop, T., Hirst, W.D., Jennings, C., Jones, D.N., Lacroix, L.P., Martyn, A., Ociepka, S., Ray, A., Regan, C.M., Roberts, J.C., Schogger, J., Southam, E., Stean, T.O., Trail, B.K., Upton, N., Wadsworth, G., Wald, J.A., White, T., Witherington, J., Woolley, M.L., Worby, A., Wilson, D.M. (2007) GSK189254, a novel H3 receptor antagonist that binds to histamine H3 receptors in alzheimer's disease brain and improves cognitive performance in preclinical models. J Pharmacol Exp Ther 321: 1032-1045.

Morimoto, T., Yamatodani, Y., Yamatodani, A. (2001) Brain histamine and feeding behavior. Behav Brain Res. 124: 145-150.

Montoro, J., Bartra, J., Sastre, J., Dávila, I., Ferrer, M., Mullol, J., del, Cuvillo, A., Jáuregui, I, Valero, A. (2013) J Investig Allergol Clin Immunol. 23(Suppl. 1): 17-26.

Nowak, P., Bortel, A., Dabrowska, J., Biedka, I., Slomian, G., Roczniak, W., Kostrzewa, R.M., Brus, R. (2008) Histamine H(3) receptor ligands modulate L-dopa-evoked behavioral responses and L-dopa derived extracellular dopamine in dopamine-denervated rat striatum. Neurotox Res. 13: 231-240.

Olanrewaju, H.A., Thaxton, J.P., Dozier, W.A., Purswell, J., Roush, W.B., Branton, S.L. (2006) A review of lighting programs for broiler production. Int J poult Sci. 5: 301-308.

Qi, W., Ding, D., Salvi, R.J. (2008) Cytotoxic effects of dimethyl sulphoxide (DMSO) on cochlear organotypic cultures. Hear Res. 236: 52-60.

Rozov, S.V., Zant, J.C., Karlstedt, K., Porkka-Heiskanen, T., Panula, P. (2014) Periodic properties of the histaminergic system of the mouse brain. Eur J Neurosci. 39: 218-228.

Saito, E.S., Kaiya, H., Tachibana, T., Tomonaga, S., Denbow, D.M., Kangawa, K., Furuse, M. (2005) Inhibitory effect of ghrelin on food intake is mediated by the corticotropin-releasing factor system in neonatal chicks. Regul Pept. 125: 201-208.

Schneider, E.H., Neumann, D., Seifert, R. (2014) Modulation of behavior by the histaminergic system: lessons from HDC-, H3R- and H4R-deficient mice. Neurosci Biobehav Rev. 47: 101-121.

Schlicker, E., Kathmann, M., Detzner, M., Exner, H.J., Gothert, M. (1994) H3 receptor- mediated inhibition of noradrenaline release: an investigation into the involvement of Ca2+ and K+ ions, G protein and adenylate cyclase. Naunyn Schmiedebergs Arch Pharmacol 350: 34-41.

Taati, M., Nayebzadeh, H., Khosravinia, H., Cheraghi, J. (2010) The role of the histaminergic system on the inhibitory effect of ghrelin on feed intake in broiler chickens. Iran J Vet Res. 11: 38-45.

Van Tienhoven, A., Juhasz, L.P. (1962) The chicken telencephalon, diencephalon and mesencephalon in sterotaxic coordinates. J Comp Neurol. 118: 185-197.

Volkow, N.D., Wang, G.J., Baler, R.D. (2011) Reward, dopamine and the control of food intake: implications for obesity. Trends Cogn Sci. 15: 37-46.

Yanovsky, Y., Li, S., Klyuch, B.P., Yao, Q., Blandina, P., Passani, M.B., Lin, J., Haas, H.L., Sergeeva, O.A. (2011) L-Dopa activates histaminergic neurons. J Physiol. 589: 1349-1366.

Zarrindast, M.R., Khakpai, F. (2015) The modulatory role of dopamine on anxiety behavior. Arch Iran Med. 18: 591-603.

Zendehdel, M., Babapour, V., Jonaidi, H. (2008) Effects of central histamine receptor blockade on GABAa agonist-induced food intake in broiler cockerels. Pakistan J Biol Sci. 11: 416-421.

Zendehdel, M., Ghashghayi, E., Hassanpour, S., Baghbanzadeh, A., Jonaidi, H. (2016) Interaction between opioidergic and dopaminergic systems on food intake in neonatal layer type chicken. Int J Pept Res Ther. 22:83-92.

Zendehdel, M., Hasani, K., Babapour ,V., Seyedali Mortezaei, S., Khoshbakht, Y., Hassanpour, S. (2014) Dopamine-induced hypophagia is mediated by D1 and 5HT-2c receptors in chicken. Vet Res Commun. 38: 11-19.

Zendehdel, M., Hassanpour, S. (2014) Ghrelin-induced hypophagia is mediated by the β2 adrenergic receptor in chicken. J Physiol Sci. 64: 383-391.

Circulating metabolic hormones in different metabolic states of high producing Holstein dairy cows

Chalmeh, A.[*]**, Hajimohammadi, A.**

Department of Clinical Sciences, School of Veterinary Medicine, Shiraz University, Shiraz, Iran

Key words:
dairy cows, herd management, metabolic hormones, normal value, physiologic states

Correspondence
Chalmeh, A.
Department of Clinical Sciences, School of Veterinary Medicine, Shiraz University, Shiraz, Iran

Email: achalmeh81@gmail.com

Abstract:

BACKGROUND: Information regarding the metabolic hormones in different metabolic states of high producing dairy cows can aid high producing herds to manage and resolve the metabolic and production problems. Furthermore, it can be considered as a tool to evaluate metabolic status of dairy cows. Herd managers can also evaluate the energy input-output relationships by assessing the metabolic profile to prevent and control negative energy balance, metabolic disorders and nutritional insufficiencies. **OBJECTIVES:** The present study was performed to clarify the metabolic hormone profile in each metabolic state of high producing Holstein dairy cows. The results of this research can reveal the normal metabolic state of these animals. **METHODS:** 25 multiparous Holstein dairy cows were divided to 5 equal groups containing early, mid and late lactations, far-off and close-up dry periods. Blood samples were collected from all cows and sera were analyzed for concentrations of triiodothyronine (T3), thyroxine (T4), free T3 (fT3), free T4 (fT4), cortisol and insulin like growth factor-1 (IGF-1). **RESULTS:** Serum T3 concentration in early lactation group was significantly higher than other ones ($p<0.05$). T4 levels in early and mid lactation dairy cows were lower than other studied groups, significantly. The cows in early lactation and close-up dry periods had the highest and the lowest serum fT3 concentrations, respectively ($p<0.05$). fT4 in far-off dry cows was significantly higher than others. The highest and the lowest circulating levels of cortisol were detected in mid and late lactation periods, respectively ($p<0.05$). The lowest concentrations of IGF1 were detected in early lactation period and its highest levels were seen in mid and late lactation and far-off dry cows ($p<0.05$). **CONCLUSIONS:** Metabolic hormones change in different metabolic states of high producing Holstein dairy cows. The presented metabolic hormone profile can be considered as criteria to monitor the metabolic status of dairy cows at different metabolic states.

Introduction

Dairy cows pass different physiological states during their producing life. Metabolic characteristics in each state are different from others. Transitional period is one of these states which includes 3 weeks before and 3 weeks after calving when metabolic processes are adapted to providing energy for parturition and lactogenesis (Overton and Waldron, 2004). Subsequently, in early lactation, as a state causes negative energy balance, a high mobilization of lipids from body fat reserves as well as hypoglycemia occur (Reist et al., 2002). The negative energy balance is continued to mid lactation period and in this period the cow has the highest amount of milk production. At the end of lactation period, the dry matter intake is parallel to milk synthesis; hence in late lactation the negative energy balance is resolved (Van Knegsel et al., 2007)

Negative energy balance is defined as disproportion between input-output relationships which can cause metabolic diseases. Metabolic diseases may be created due to an imbalance between the rates of input of dietary nutrients and output of production (Quiroz-Rocha et al., 2009). When the imbalance is continued, it may lead to change in the amount of body reserves of certain metabolites (Radostits et al., 2007). Excess negative energy balance, fat mobilization and subsequent elevations in ketone body concentrations play a contributing role in the expression of metabolic diseases such as fatty liver syndrome and clinical ketosis (Goff and Horst, 1997). A severe negative energy balance during some metabolic states of high producing dairy cows may also increase the risk of retained placenta, metritis, and mastitis through impaired immune function (Kim et al., 2005).

The hormonal activities in each metabolic state are different from the other ones. Metabolic hormones such as thyroid hormones, insulin like growth factors and cortisol have important roles in each metabolic period for determining cell metabolism intensity, metabolism of lipids and carbohydrates and the lactation courses (Nikolic et al., 1997). Under the conditions of negative energy balance and high lipid mobilization, the circulatory concentrations of metabolic hormones can change in dairy cows (Pezzi et al., 2003; Reist et al., 2002).

Determining metabolic hormones can be a reliable tool for early diagnosis of nutritional deficiency or metabolic disease that would be a major forward step in attempting to optimize flock production and obtain maximum yields at minimum costs (Radostits et al., 2007). Therefore, information regarding circulating metabolic hormones is considered as a useful diagnostic aid to uncover the problems in difficult herd situations (Găvan et al., 2010). Furthermore, the genetically superior cows may be selected via evaluating their circulating metabolic hormones (Rowlands et al., 1973).

There are several literatures on metabolic hormones in transition and pre parturition periods in dairy cows (Nikolic et al., 1997; Roberts et al., 1997; Djoković et al., 2007) but based on the author's knowledge, comprehensive information about circulating metabolic hormones in different metabolic states of high producing Holstein dairy cows is lacking. Determining the normal base line values of circulating metabolic hormones in early, mid and late lactation and far-off and close-up dry cows and comparing them together in a single comprehensive study were the aims of the present research.

Materials and Methods

Animals: The present study was carried out in winter 2014 on 25 multiparous Holstein dairy cows from a high producing industrial dairy farm around Shiraz, southwestern Iran. These cows were housed in open-shed barns with free access to water and shade. The total mixed rations were formulated and prepared for all animals according to National Research Council (NRC) requirements. At this farm, a dry period of 60 days has been considered for late pregnant cattle. Milk production was about 10,000 kg for one year, an average of 3.6 of milk fat %, and 3.3 of milk protein %. All the animals were clinically healthy, had no history of debilitating disease, and were free from internal and external parasites due to routine antiparasitic programs at this farm. Body condition score (BCS) of these animals was estimated based on 0 to 5 system (Alapati et al., 2010). Cattle were divided to 5 equal groups containing early (30.2±5.7 days after calving, with 3.25±0.25 BCS), mid (108.1±8.4 days after calving, with 3.25±0.25 BCS) and late lactations (184.5±5.7 days after calving, with 3.5±0.25 BCS), far-off (281.9±5.4 days after calving, 228.4±8.6 days of pregnancy, with 3.5±0.25 BCS) and close-up dry periods (312.1±8.3 days after calving, 255.6±6.3 days of pregnancy, with 3.5±0.25 BCS).

Blood sampling and hormonal assays: Blood samples were collected from all cows through jugular venipuncture in plain tubes. Immediately after blood collections, sera were separated by centrifugation for 10 minutes at 3,000 g and stored at -22°C until assayed. Serum triiodothyronine (T3) concentrations were determined using a competitive enzyme immunoassay kit (Padtan Elm Co., Tehran, Iran). The intra- and inter-assay CVs of the assays were 12.6% and 13.2%, respectively. The sensitivity of the test was 0.2 ng/mL. Serum thyroxine (T4) concentrations were measured using a competitive enzyme immunoassay kit (Monobind Inc., CA, USA). The intra- and inter-assay CVs of the assays were 3.0% and 3.7%, respectively. The sensitivity of the test was 0.4 mg/dl. Serum free T3 (fT3) and free T4 (fT4) concentrations were determined by the fT3 and the fT4 ELISA kits (DiaPlus Inc., San Francisco, CA, USA). The intra- and inter-assay CVs of the fT3 assays were 4.1% and 5.2%, respectively. The sensitivity of the test was 0.05 pg/mL. The intra- and inter-assay CVs of the fT4 assays were 4.5% and 3.7%, respectively. The sensitivity of the test was 0.05 ng/dL. Serum cortisol concentrations were determined by Enzyme Immunoassay Colormetric method (AccuBind® ELISA kit; Monobind Inc., CA, USA). The sensitivity of the test was 0.25 µg/dl. Serum levels of insulin like growth factor-1 (IGF-1) were evaluated by ELISA kit (ImmunoDiagnosticSystem®) with the sensitivity equal to 3.1 µg/l.

Statistical analyses: All data are presented as mean ± standard deviation (SD). Differences among the averages of concentrations of serological factors in the different groups were analyzed by one-way ANOVA and the least significant difference (LSD) test was used to find differences using SPSS software (SPSS for Windows, version 20, SPSS Inc, Chicago, IL, USA). The level of significance was set at $p<0.05$.

Results

The levels of circulating metabolic hormones (mean±SD) in different metabolic states of high producing Holstein dairy cows are presented in Table I. Serum T3 concentration in early lactation group was significantly higher than other ones ($p<0.05$). T4 levels in early and mid lactation dairy cows

Table 1. Circulating metabolic hormones (mean±SD) in different metabolic states of high producing Holstein dairy cows (n=5). Different letters indicate significant differences in each row ($p<0.05$).

Hormones	Early lactation	Mid lactation	Late lactation	Far-off dry	Close-up dry
T3 (ng/dl)	143.00±22.15^{a}	122.60±8.14^{b}	141.25±9.50^{b}	128.00±20.79^{b}	126.20±17.75^{b}
T4 (µg/dl)	3.61±0.68^{a}	3.64±0.80^{a}	4.11±0.27^{b}	4.17±0.78^{b}	4.09±1.18^{b}
fT3 (ng/l)	3.29±0.67^{a}	2.82±0.13^{b}	2.90±0.26^{b}	2.83±0.20^{b}	2.52±0.31^{c}
fT4 (ng/l)	4.50±0.79^{a}	4.91±1.29^{a}	5.31±0.90^{a}	6.34±1.61^{b}	4.99±2.64^{a}
IGF1 (µg/l)	53.40±12.21^{a}	84.20±18.00^{b}	84.50±36.78^{b}	86.20±27.73^{b}	67.80±43.60^{c}
Cortisol (ng/ml)	15.02±7.51^{a}	21.58±6.26^{b}	6.32±4.34^{c}	16.76±3.65^{a}	11.68±6.12^{a}

were lower than other studied groups, significantly. The cows in early lactation and close-up dry periods had the highest and the lowest serum fT3 concentrations, respectively ($p<0.05$). fT4 in far-off dry cows was significantly higher than others. The highest and the lowest circulating levels of cortisol were detected in mid and late lactation periods, respectively ($p<0.05$). The lowest concentrations of IGF1 were detected in early lactation period and its highest levels were seen in mid and late lactation and far-off dry cows ($p<0.05$).

Discussion

Physiological systems of dairy cows work together to challenge with energy intake and output in order to maintain adipose tissue. Furthermore, adipose tissue secretes leptin and cytokines, which induces satiety and has been linked to hormones such as thyroid hormones, cortisol and IGF-1. Thus, adipose tissue is acted upon by a number of physiological stimuli, including hormones, and simultaneously, is an active component in the regulation of its own lipid content (Van Knegsel et al., 2007). All of the hormones mentioned above are associated with each other in changing metabolic states. Hencc, the present study was performed to clarify the levels of thyroid hormones, cortisol and IGF-1 as metabolic biomarkers in different metabolic states of high producing Holstein dairy cows.

Thyroid gland produces the thyroid hormones containing T3 and its prohormone T4, which are tyrosine-based hormones. Thyrotropes of the anterior pituitary gland secrete thyroid stimulating hormone and this hormone regulates the production of T3 and T4 by follicular cells of the thyroid gland. T4 is the major circulating thyroid hormone which has a longer half-life than T3. T4 is changed to the active T3 and T3 is more potent than T4. Circulating fT3 and fT4 represent the amount of T3 and T4 that are not bound to proteins. Evaluating the fT3 and fT4 can be used to assess and manage disorders of the thyroid gland (Yen, 2001).

Thyroid hormones are primarily responsible for metabolism regulation. They increase the metabolic rate, change protein synthesis, regulate osteoblasts and nervous system maturation and increase the sensitivity to catecholamines. The proper circulating levels of thyroid hormones are necessary for developing and differentiation of all cells. These hormones also are responsible for regulation of protein, fat, carbohydrate and vitamin metabolism. Numerous physiological, pathological and pharmacological stimuli influence thyroid hormonc metabolism (Tan et al., 1998; Taylor et al., 2004).

The results of the present study showed that circulating levels of thyroid hormones in each metabolic state were different from others (Table 1). The characteristics of each metabolic state of dairy cows, with emphasis on negative energy balance, can interfere with the thyroid hormone levels and activities. The intensity of oxidation in mitochondria of cells is closely linked with the functional state of the thyroid gland, so it is justifiably considered that the conditions of negative energy balance and the increased lipid mobilization from body fat reserves result in lipid infiltration of liver cells (Djoković et al., 2007). The reason is the decreased capacity of mitochondria to oxidize fatty acids in the conditions of low concentrations of thyroid hormones in blood (Johannsen et al., 1993).

Djoković et al. (2007)suggested that a hypothyroidal status was established in ketotic cows and that the blood concentrations of free fatty acids, triacylglycerols, total cholesterol and glucose served as major biochemical indicators in determining liver steatosis in the dairy cows in transitional period. Thyroid hormones are important for maintenance of pregnancy and for a normal ensuing lactation cycle. It is found that thyroid hormone is a necessary hormone in the development of mouse mammary tissue (Vonderhaar and Greco, 1979).

Based on our research, T3 and T4 levels were decreased near to parturition. In the dairy cow, plasmaT4 levels gradually decrease around the time of parturition. There is a gradual rise following calving with prepartum levels ofT4significantly higher compared to postpartum concentrations (Goff and Horst, 1997). Levels of T3 and T4 were measured in Estonian cows during different stages of lactation. During early lactation, plasma thyroid hormone concentrations were lower and progressively increased as lactation continued (Tiirats, 1996).

Cortisol is the major stress hormone produced by the adrenal glands in the ruminant (Hunter et al., 1970). Based on our finding the highest levels of cortisol were seen in mid lactation period when the cows had the high milk yield. It may be suggested that the negative energy balance in this period can be considered as a stress factor to induce the elevation of circulating cortisol. Hunter et al. (1970) mentioned that during the transition period, cortisol is elevated prior to, during and following parturition, signifying an increased release of the adrenocorticotropin (ACTH). A normal response to stressful conditions is activation of the hypothalamic-pituitary-adrenal axis (Christison and Johnson, 1972). Physiological stressors cause the release of the hypothalamic corticotropin releasing factor which increases ACTH (Collins and Weiner, 1968). During the periparturient period, stressors are above what the cow normally experiences, eliciting an increased release of ACTH (Hunter et al., 1970).

Several studies mentioned that at the time of parturition, cortisol peaks, followed by a sharp drop in concentrations in early lactation (Hunter et al., 1970; Goff and Horst, 1997). The current study showed that after parturition, serum cortisol concentrations were elevated in early lactation period. Beerda et al. (2004) have shown that high yielding dairy cows have lower cortisol response to ACTH administration than low yielding cows. One possible reason could be difficulties in synthesizing cortisol when their energy demands increase in peak lactation.

Growth hormone is in control of metabolism in the dairy cow in all stages of lactation (Sjaastad et al., 2010). The effect of growth hormone on lactation is discussed to be only partly direct and instead mediated by IGF-1 (Svennersten-Sjaunja and Olsson, 2005). Receptors for IGF-1 can be found in all mammary cells and release of IGF-1 is stimulated by binding of growth hormone to hepatocytes in the liver (Tucker, 2000), which is the main source of circulating IGF-1 (Akers, 2002).

The concentration of IGF-1 can be seen as an indicator of the metabolic state of the dairy cow (Taylor et al., 2004). The results of the current study showed that the lowest circulating levels of IGF-1 were in early lactation period. Abribat et al. (1993) showed that the levels of IGF-1 are lower at the start of lactation and increase during the whole lactation, inversely related to milk yield.

Based on Roberts et al.'s study (1997), determining the circulating concentrations of growth hormone and IGF-1 may provide a clinical approach for evaluating the nutritional status of individual cows within herd basis. Under adequate dietary availability, circulating concentrations of IGF-1 are under positive regulation by growth hormone (Vicini et al., 1991).

The concentrations of IGF-1 were decreased near to parturition in close up dry cows (Table 1). As previously demonstrated, circulating concentrations of IGF-1 decline at parturition and gradually increase over time, whereas concentrations of growth hormone increase at parturition and then decline over time (Vicini et al., 1991; Roberts et al., 1997). The magnitude in decline and duration of time required for IGF-1 levels to return to prepartum levels are greater in animals subjected to dietary restriction (Hunter et al. 1970) and may interact with genetic potential for milk production (Roberts et al., 1997).

Finally, the present research revealed the circulating baseline levels of some metabolic hormones in dairy cows.

In conclusion, it could be stated that metabolic hormones change in different metabolic states of high producing Holstein dairy cows. These changes are induced commonly by metabolic alterations of cow's body systems such as lactogenesis, pregnancy and parturition.

Acknowledgments

Hormonal analysis was kindly performed with the cooperation of Professor Saeb Specialized Hormone Laboratory, Shiraz, Iran.

References

1. Abribat, T., Brazeau, P., Davignon, I., Garrel, D.R. (1993) Insulin-like growth factor-l blood levels in severely burned patients: effects of time post injury, age of patient and severity of burn. Clin Endocrinol. 39: 583-589.
2. Akers, R.M. (2002) Lactation and the Mammary Gland. (1st ed.) Iowa State Press, Ames, Iowa, USA.
3. Alapati, A., Kapa, S.R., Jeepalyam, S., Rangappa, S.M., Yemireddy, K.R. (2010) Development of the body condition score system in Murrah buffaloes: validation through ultrasonic assessment of body fat reserves. J Vet Sci. 11: 1-8.
4. Beerda, B., Kornalijnslijper, J., Van der Werf, J., Noordhuizen-Stassen, E., Hopster, H. (2004) Effects of milk production capacity and metabolic status on HPA function in early postpartum dairy cows. J Dairy Sci. 87: 2094-2102.
5. Christison, G., Johnson, H. (1972) Cortisol turnover in heat-stressed cows. J Anim Sci. 35: 1005-1010.
6. Collins, K.J., Weiner, J.S. (1968) Endocrino-

logical aspects of exposure to high environmental temperatures. Physiol Rev. 48: 785-839.

7. Djoković, R., Šamanc, H., Jovanović, M., Nikolić, Z. (2007) Blood concentrations of thyroid hormones and lipids and content of lipids in the liver of dairy cows in transitional period. Acta Vet Brno. 76: 525-532.
8. Găvan, C., Retea, C., Motorga, V. (2010) Changes in the hematological profile of Holstein primiparous in periparturient period and in early to mid lactation. SPASB. 43: 244-246.
9. Goff, J., Horst, R. (1997) Physiological changes at parturition and their relationship to metabolic disorders. J Dairy Sci. 80: 1260-1268.
10. Hunter, D., Erb, R., Randel, R., Garverick, H., Callahan, C., Harrington, R. (1970) Reproductive steroids in the bovine. I. Relationships during late gestation. J Anim Sci. 30: 47-59.
11. Johannsen, U., Menger, S., Staufenbiel, R., Klukas, H. (1993) Investigations on morphology and function of the liver of high-yielding cows 2 weeks postpartum. Deut Tierarztl Woch. 100: 177-181.
12. Kim, I.H., Na, K.J., Yang, M.P. (2005) Immune responses during the peripartum period in dairy cows with postpartum endometritis. J Reprod Dev. 51: 757-764.
13. Nikolic, J., Samanc, H., Begovic, J., Damjanovic, Z., Dokovic, R., Kostic, G., Krsmanovic, J., Resanovic, V. (1997) Low peripheral serum thyroid hormone status independently affects the hormone profile of healthy and ketotic cows during the first week post partum. Acta Vet Beograd 47: 3-13.
14. Overton, T., Waldron, M. (2004) Nutritional management of transition dairy cows: strategies to optimize metabolic health. J Dairy Sci. 87: E105-E119.
15. Pezzi, C., Accorsi, P., Vigo, D., Govoni, N., Gaiani, R. (2003) 5′-deiodinase activity and circulating thyronines in lactating cows. J Dairy Sci. 86: 152-158.
16. Quiroz-Rocha, G.F., LeBlanc, S.J., Duffield, T.F., Wood, D., Leslie, K.E., Jacobs, R.M. (2009) Reference limits for biochemical and hematological analytes of dairy cows one week before and one week after parturition. Can Vet J. 50: 383-388.
17. Radostits, O.M., Gay, C., Hinchcliff, K.W., Constable, P.D. (2007) Veterinary Medicine: A Textbook of the Diseases of Cattle, Horses, Sheep, Pigs and Goats. (10th ed.) Saunders. London, UK.
18. Reist, M., Erdin, D., Von Euw, D., Tschuemperlin, K., Leuenberger, H., Chilliard, Y., Hammon, H., Morel, C., Philipona, C., Zbinden, Y. (2002) Estimation of energy balance at the individual and herd level using blood and milk traits in high-yielding dairy cows. J Dairy Sci. 85: 3314-3327.
19. Roberts, A., Nugent, R., Klindt, J., Jenkins, T. (1997) Circulating insulin-like growth factor I, insulin-like growth factor binding proteins, growth hormone, and resumption of estrus in postpartum cows subjected to dietary energy restriction. J Anim Sci. 75: 1909-1917.
20. Rowlands, G., Payne, J., Dew, S.M., Manston, R. (1973) A potential use of metabolic profiles in the selection of superior cattle. Vet Rec. 93: 48-49.
21. Sjaastad, Ø., Hove, K., Sand, O. (2010) The endocrine system. In: Physiology of Domestic Animals. (2nd ed.) Scand Vet Press, Oslo, Norway. p. 248-251.
22. Svennersten-Sjaunja, K., Olsson, K. (2005) Endocrinology of milk production. Domes Anim Endocrinol. 29: 241-258.
23. Tan, K., Shiu, S., Kung, A. (1998) Effect of

thyroid dysfunction on high-density lipoprotein subfraction metabolism: roles of hepatic lipase and cholesteryl ester transfer protein 1. J Clin Endocrinol Metab. 83: 2921-2924.
24. Taylor, V., Cheng, Z., Pushpakumara, P., Wathes, D. Beever, D. (2004) Relationships between the plasma concentrations of insulin-like growth factor-I in dairy cows and their fertility and milk yield. Vet Rec. 155: 583-588.
25. Tiirats, T. (1996) Thyroxine, triiodothyronine and reverse-triiodothyronine concentrations in blood plasma in relation to lactational stage, milk yield, energy and dietary protein intake in Estonian dairy cows. Acta Vet Scand. 38: 339-348.
26. Tucker, H. (2000) Hormones, mammary growth, and lactation: a 41-year perspective. J Dairy Sci. 83: 874-884.
27. Van Knegsel, A., Van den Brand, H., Graat, E., Dijkstra, J., Jorritsma, R., Decuypere, E., Tamminga, S., Kemp, B. (2007) Dietary energy source in dairy cows in early lactation: metabolites and metabolic hormones. J Dairy Sci. 90: 1477-1485.
28. Vicini, J.L., Buonomo, F.C., Veenhuizen, J.J., Miller, M.A., Clemmons, D.R., Collier, R.J. (1991) Nutrient balance and stage of lactation affect responses of insulin, insulin-like growth factors I and II, and insulin-like growth factor-binding protein 2 to somatotropin administration in dairy cows. J Nutr. 121: 1656-1664.
29. Vonderhaar, B.K., Greco, A.E. (1979) Lobulo-alveolar development of mouse mammary glands is regulated by thyroid hormones. Endocrinology 104: 409-418.
30. Yen, P.M. (2001) Physiological and molecular basis of thyroid hormone action. Physiol Rev. 81: 1097-1142.

Peppermint and pennyroyal essential oil effect on performance, rumen microbial population and some blood parameters of sheep

Mohamadi, R.[1], **Rahchamani, R.**[2*], **Ghanbari, F.**[2], **Farivar, F.**[2]

[1]*Graduated Student of Animal Physiology, College of Agriculture and Natural Resources, University of Gonbad Kavous, Gonbad Kavous, Iran*

[2]*Department of Animal Sciences, College of Agriculture and Natural Resources, University of Gonbad Kavous, Gonbad Kavous, Iran*

Key words:
blood metabolites, *Mentha piperita* oil, *Mentha pulegium* oil, microbial population, sheep

Correspondence
Rahchamani, R.
Department of Animal Sciences, College of Agriculture and Natural Resources, University of Gonbad Kavous, Gonbad Kavous, Iran

Email: r_rahchamani@yahoo.com

Abstract:

BACKGROUND: The use of antibiotics as feed additive in animal feeds due to the appearance of residues in milk and meat and their effects on human health is restricted. Two essential oils with high potential for use in ruminant diet are *Mentha piperita* (peppermint) and *Mentha pulegium* (pennyroyal) essential oil. **OBJECTIVES:** This study was conducted to investigate the effects of essential oils of peppermint and pennyroyal on performance, ruminal microbial population and some blood parameters of sheep. **METHODS:** For this purpose, 9 Dallagh sheep were used in a change-over design experiment in three 21-d periods (14 days as adaptation and 7 days for sample collection). Experimental treatments were 1) basal diet without additive (control), 2) basal diet + 110 mg/d *Mentha piperita* essential oil and 3) basal diet +110 mg/d *Mentha pulegium* essential oil. Sheep were kept in individual cages and had free access to food and water. Rumen fluid was collected before, 4 h and 8 h after morning feeding and a blood sample was obtained 3 h after morning feeding at the last day of each period. **RESULTS:** Essential oils had no effect on performance, blood parameters, pH, ammonia, protozoa, and total viable bacterial count of rumen. Coliforms of rumen fluid significantly decreased at 4 h and increased 8 h after morning feeding following peppermint and pennyroyal supplementation, respectively ($p<0.05$). Acid lactic bacteria count was significantly higher at before and 4 h after morning feeding in pennyroyal treatment compared with other treatments. **CONCLUSIONS:** Although essential oils of *Mentha piperita* and *Mentha pulegium* had some effects on rumen microbial population they had no significant effects on performance and blood metabolites of Dallagh sheep.

Introduction

The use of antibiotics as feed additive in animal feeds due to the appearance of residues in milk and meat and their effects on human health is restricted (Ouwehand, 2010; Vakili, 2013; Anantasook, 2013). In the last few years there has been increasing attention to the potential of phytogenic and herbal products as alternative for feed antibiotics and growth promoters in ruminant nutrition (Wallace, 2004; Steiner, 2009; Giannenas, 2011).

Essential oils (EO) are a blend of secondary metabolites that have antimicrobial effect on bacteria, fungi and protozoa. EO are aromatic compounds present in many plants that are generally extracted by steam and/or water distillation and common chemically composed terpenoids including monoterpenes, sesquiterpenes and diterpenes. EO may also include a variety of low-molecular aliphatic hydrocarbons, acids, alcohols, aldehydes, lactones, nitrogen and sulfur containing compounds, coumarins and phenylpropanoides (Dorman and Deans, 2000; Wanapat, 2013). Most of these EOs are safe and can be used as feed additive according to antibacterial, antifungal and antioxidant properties (Cawan, 1999). These compounds have been shown to favorably manipulate ruminal fermentation and improve nutrient utilization in ruminants (Greathead, 2003).

Two EOs with high potential for use in ruminant diet are *Mentha piperita* (peppermint) and *Mentha pulegium* (pennyroyal). Peppermint is a perennial plant in lamiaceae family and the principal components of the peppermint oil are menthol (31.53%), 1, 8 cineole (10.67%), menthon (8.2%), menthyl acetate (3.54%), β-caryophyldene (2.8%) and piperitone (0.77%) (Rafii and Shahverdi, 2007). The flowering aerial parts of Pennyroyal have been traditionally used for its antimicrobial properties in the treatment of common cold, sinusitis, bronchitis, cholera, food poisoning and tuberculosis. Most of the plant parts contain compounds with antilatulent, carminative, expectorant, diuretic, antitussive and menstruation agent. *Mentha piperita* and *Mentha pulegium* possess antimicrobial, antioxidant, cytotoxic and abortifacient properties (Ghalamkari et al., 2012; Nobakht, 2011).

However, most researches conducted on EO have been laboratory based (i.e., in vitro). There are very limited in vivo studies that have evaluated effectiveness of these plants EO in sheep. Therefore the aim of present study was to determine the effects of supplementation to the diet of sheep with these herbs on performance, blood metabolites and ruminal fermentation.

Material and Methods

Animals and dietary treatments: Nine Adult male Dallagh sheep with an average initial BW of 32±3 kg were used in a change-over design. The experiment consisted of three 21-day periods (14 days as adaptation and 7 days as sampling) and there were 3 treatments, each consisting of 9 replicates. At the start of the experiment sheep were weighted and randomly assigned to 1 of 3 treatments: 1) basal diet with no additive (control), 2) basal diet supplemented with 100mg/day peppermint EO and 3) basal diet supplemented with 110mg/day pennyroyal EO.

Essential oils: Essential oils were purchased from Barij Essence Pharmaceutical Company (Kashan- Iran). Major compounds of peppermint EO were carvone (55.87%), limonene (23.88%), menthol (3.38%), pinene (2.34%) and pennyroyal EOs were piperiton (33.60%), pippeirtenone (28.71%), α-terpineol (5.52%), eucalyptol (5.01%), piperitenone oxide (3.94%), menthone (3.39%) and α-pinene (3.03%).

Diets and Animal Management: The

basal diet was composed of 30% roughage and 70% concentrate, and the ingredients and nutrient composition of the basal diet (DM basis) is given in Table 1.

Diets were fed as total mixed rations (TMR) and formulated according to NRC (1996) recommendations. The experimental diets were offered twice (08:00 and 18:00 h) daily for ad libitum intake (10% refusals) with one-half of the daily feed allotment offered at each feeding. The essential oils were mixed with a small amount of concentrate and once daily top dressed onto the TMR before feeding to ensure that sheep would consume the full amount offered. Amounts of feed offered and refused were recorded daily for each animal throughout the trial. Body weight was measured at the beginning and the end of each period. The sheep were housed in individual stalls on mattresses bedded with straw in pens (2m× 1.5m) equipped with a water bowl. The pens were located in a covered barn. Each animal had free access to water at all times.

Measurements, sample collection and analysis: Average daily weight gain was calculated throughout the trail. Feed conversion ratio was calculated as the ratio between feed intake and weight gain.

Ruminal fluid was collected from animals at the last day of each period before morning feeding, and 4 h and 8 h after morning feeding via the esophagus using a 60 ml gavage syringe and a lubricated rubber tube. The first 20 ml of ruminal fluid content was discarded to ensure they were not polluted with saliva and then squeezed through four layers of cheesecloth. Rumen pH was measured immediately with a portable pH meter (Metrohm 691, Switzerland).

A 5-ml portion of the strained ruminal fluid was mixed with 5 ml of 0.2 N HCL. All samples were stored at -20oC for subsequent analyses. The ruminal fluid concentration of NH3-N was determined using spectrophotometry by the phenol hypochlorite method of Broderick and Kang (1980). Serial 10-fold dilutions of strained ruminal fluid were prepared and used as inoculum on plate count agar (PCA), Modified Rogosa and Sharp Agar (MRSA) and Violent Red Bile Agar (VRBA) medium for total viable bacteria, acid lactic bacteria and coliforms count respectively (Ghoorchi et al., 2009).

Blood samples were collected at non-heparinized tube from the jugular vein at the end of each period (3 h after the morning feeding), samples were centrifuged (Denley BS400, England) at 10,000 rpm for 10 min and collected serum was frozen at -20°C until analysis. Serum concentration of glucose, total protein and triglyceride were determined using the commercial kits of Darmanfaraz Company (Isfahan, Iran) by spectrophotometry.

A 1-ml portion of the strained ruminal fluid was preserved using 9 ml of MFS (methyl green- formaldehyde- saline) solution for enumeration of protozoa. Protozoa samples were stored at room temperature in the dark until counting. Protozoa were enumerated microscopically in a Neubauer cytometer at ×40 magnification. Each sample was counted twice and if the average of the duplicates differed by more than 10%, the counts were repeated (Cedrola et al., 2015).

Statistical analysis: All data were statistically analyzed according to a randomized complete block design using the general linear model (GLM) procedure of SPSS software (version18). Significant differences between means of treatments were assessed by the tukey test, and the differences among treatments were declared significant at $p<0.05$. Initial weight of sheep was used as covariate for weight gain data analysis.

Results

Dry matter intake and performance data are presented in Table 2. Initial and final BW did not differ among the experimental treatments and consequently, daily weight gain was not affected by treatments. The mean DM intakes ranged from 0.29 to 0.35 kg/d and were similar for sheep fed basal diet and those consuming diets supplemented with additives. Similarly, feed conversion ratio, expressed as feed: gain ratio (DMI to average daily gain ratio), was similar among treatments.

Mean of the blood metabolites are shown in Table 3. Concentrations of serum glucose, total protein and triglyceride were not affected by additive treatments.

Table 4 represents the effect of experimental treatments on rumen fluid pH, NH3-N and protozoa. Rumen fluid pH was not affected by treatments at before morning feeding, 4 h and 8 h after morning feeding. There was no significant difference in ruminal NH3-N concentration among treatments. No significant influence of experimental diet on rumen protozoa at before morning feeding, 4h and 8 h after morning feeding was observed.

Table 5 summarizes data obtained on the effects of experimental diets on rumen microbial population. Total viable bacterial count had no significant difference before feeding, 4 h and 8 h after feeding. Acid lactic bacteria were influenced by treatments. Before morning feeding and 4 h after morning feeding acid lactic bacteria count significantly increased in pennyroyal treatment compared with control and peppermint treatment. But at 8 h after feeding

Table 1. Ingredient and nutrient composition of basal diet (DM basis). [1] Contained: 21 g/kg Mg, 0.3 g/kg Zn, 2.2 g/kg Mn, 3 g/kg Fe, 0.3 g/kg Cu, 0.001 g/kg Se, 0.1 g/kg Co, 0.12 g/kg I, 195 g/Kg Ca, 80 g/Kg P, 600 IU/g of vitamin A, 200 IU/g of vitamin D, and 2.5 IU/g of vitamin E.

Ingredient	%	Nutrient composition	%
Barley grain, ground	38.34	Dry matter	64.5
Corn silage	25	Crud protein	14
Wheat straw	5	NDF	28.8
Wheat bran	15	Metabolizable energy (Mcal/Kg)	2.76
Soybean meal	15		
salt	0.36		
Mineral-vitamin premix[1]	1		
Pearl powder	0.3		

Table 2. Effect of experimental treatments on performance. * Treatments include: CON: basal diet; PEP: basal diet supplemented with peppermint oil (110 mg/sheep daily); PEN: basal diet supplemented with pennyroyal oil (110 mg/sheep daily).* Standard error of means.

Item	Treatments*			SEM*	p- value
	CON	PEP	PEN		
Initial weight (kg)	33.60	30.37	32.90	2.69	0.94
Final weight (kg)	46.90	54.70	45.67	2.57	0.33
Average daily gain (kg)	0.29	0.32	0.35	0.01	0.34
Dry matter intake (g)	1594	1623	1564	23.94	0.23
Feed conversion ratio	5.38	4.94	4.36	0.03	0.68

Table 3. Effect of experimental treatments on blood metabolites. * Treatments include: CON: basal diet; PEP: basal diet supplemented with peppermint oil (110 mg/sheep daily); PEN: basal diet supplemented with pennyroyal oil (110 mg/sheep daily).* Standard error of means.

Item	Treatments*			SEM*	p-value
	CON	PEP	PEN		
Glucose (mg dl^{-1})	85.47	89.84	76.62	6.43	0.35
Total protein (g dl^{-1})	6.87	6.04	7.52	1.12	0.65
Triglyceride (mg dl^{-1})	86.34	114.16	73.60	15.86	0.20

Table 4. Effect of experimental treatments on pH, NH3-N and protozoa of rumen fluid. * Treatments include: CON: basal diet; PEP: basal diet supplemented with peppermint oil (110 mg/sheep daily); PEN: basal diet supplemented with pennyroyal oil (110 mg/sheep daily). * Standard error of means.

Item	Time	Treatment*			SEM*	p-value
		CON	PEP	PEN		
pH	Before feeding	6.76	6.96	6.93	0.09	0.25
	4 h after feeding	6.35	6.57	6.33	0.09	0.15
	8 h after feeding	6.44	6.29	6.45	0.10	0.48
NH3-N	Before feeding	5.67	5.74	5.74	0.065	0.626
(mg dl^{-1})	4 h after feeding	5.70	5.74	5.69	0.064	0.822
	8 h after feeding	5.67	5.79	5.80	0.060	0.227
Protozoa	Before feeding	6.55	5.55	6.43	0.81	0.64
($\times 10^5$ ml^{-1})	4 h after feeding	6.88	7.68	5.60	0.75	0.16
	8 h after feeding	6.35	7.98	7.83	0.95	0.42

Table 5. Effect of experimental treatments on rumen bacterial population (log cfu/ml). * Treatments include: CON: basal diet; PEP: basal diet supplemented with peppermint oil (110 mg/sheep daily); PEN: basal diet supplemented with pennyroyal oil (110 mg/sheep daily). $^{a-b}$ Means within the same row without common letters differ significantly ($p<0.05$). * Standard error of means.

Item	Time	Treatments*			SEM*	p-value
		CON	PEP	PEN		
Total viable bacteria	Before feeding	6.72	6.79	6.84	0.03	0.06
	4 h after feeding	6.78	6.83	6.76	0.06	0.06
	8 h after feeding	6.67	6.76	6.79	0.03	0.09
Acid lactic bacteria	Before feeding	5.19^a	5.11^a	5.39^b	0.04	0.00
	4 h after feeding	5.19^a	5.02^a	5.29^b	0.03	0.00
	8 h after feeding	5.18	5.21	5.30	0.04	0.18
coliforms	Before feeding	3.59	3.44	3.67	0.06	0.04
	4 h after feeding	3.62^a	3.45^b	3.72^a	0.04	0.02
	8 h after feeding	3.51^a	3.42^a	3.73^b	0.05	0.00

there was no significant difference among treatments. Coliforms count was not influenced by treatments before morning feeding but at 4 h after morning feeding in peppermint treatment was significantly lower than control group. Pennyroyal supplementation significantly increased coliforms at 8 h after morning meal.

Discussion

Feed intake and performance: There is little information on the effects of peppermint and pennyroyal EO on DMI and performance in sheep. The findings of present study for DMI was in line with previous researches in growing lambs (Chaves et al., 2008a), sheep (Distel et al., 2007; Nolte and Provenza, 1992) and cattle (Benchaar et al., 2007; Beauchemin and Mcginn, 2006) who found no effect of EO on DMI. In contrast with our results, Demir et al. (2003) reported that pennyroyal EO increased nutrient absorption, growing and weight gain. Also, Lewis et al. (2003) found that pennyroyal EO and canola oil improved daily weight gain in male broiler chicken because of antimicrobial and positive effect on intestinal micro flora. In some researches low levels of EO improved ruminal fermentation and growing performance (Borek, 2001). Our result confirmed the report which showed that *Leucaena leucocephalaon* and *Salix babylonica* had no effect on weight gain in growing lamb (Salem et al., 2011). The effects of EO on DMI might vary with EO source, type of diet, diet interaction or adaptation of rumen microbial population to EO (Yang et al., 2010a; b; Geraci et al., 2012). Furthermore, it has been reported that it can be affected by a number of dietary or management factors such as body weight, animal growth stage, specific physical and chemical characteristics of diet or rumen fermentation metabolites (Allen, 2000; Yang et al., 2010b).

Blood metabolites: These results are in agreement with some studies that declared peppermint EO feeding did not affect blood metabolites significantly (Hosoda et al., 2006; Ahmadi Naghadehi et al., 2014). Plasma triglyceride concentration is lipid transfer index and triglycerides are lipids that conserve energy in animal tissues (Hatfield et al., 1998). In our study serum triglyceride was not affected by treatments, which was similar to some researches (Hosoda et al., 2006; Ahmadi Naghadehi et al., 2014). The result of total serum protein in this study was in agreement with Ahmadi Naghadehi et al. (2014) who reported that 100 and 200 mg peppermint EO did not significantly changed total serum protein of sheep. It has been reported that concentration of some blood metabolites such as triglycerides can be influenced by EO supplementation via changing of feed intake (Yang et al., 2010b) and no change in blood metabolites in present study may be contributed to lack of DMI alteration by EO.

Rumen pH, NH3-N and protozoa: Rumen pH is a resultant of produced volatile fatty acids (acetate, propionate and lactate), ammonia, rumen buffers and saliva (Vansoet, 1994) and an index for fermentation. In some previous studies it was shown that VFA production decreased and rumen pH increased following EO feeding because of inhibitory effect of phenolic compounds on rumen flora (Benchaar et al., 2007). 100 and 200 mg peppermint EO feeding did not affect rumen pH in sheep (Ahmadi Naghdahi et al., 2014). In agreement with our result peppermint feeding at 5% DM (Hodoso et al., 2006) had no effect on rumen pH in steers. In contrast with our study, peppermint feeding (200 g/day) decreased rumen pH and protozoa count in steers (Ando et al., 2003). Variable effects of EO on rumen pH can result from different diets and levels of EO in studies as when EO was added to diets with higher roughage/concentrate ratio, rumen pH increased (Meyer et al., 2009).

Similarly, supplementation with 0.2g/kg (DM basis) of carvacrol and cinnamaldehyde did not alter ruminal ammonia in growing lamb (Chaves et al., 2008b). In contrast, Hosoda et al. (2006) reported that peppermint feeding at 5% of the diet (DM basis) significantly increased rumen ammonia in Holstein steers. Ruminal ammonia concentration has been reflected in the balance of nitrogen and energy supplies into the rumen, which is associated with microbial activity (McDonald et al., 2002). Also, this is in disagreement with the in vitro results of Newbold et al. (2004), who observed a decrease in ruminal ammonia when rumen contents of cows or sheep supplemented with EO and acid hydrolyzed protein were incubated for 24-48 h in strained ruminal fluid (1 or 110 mg/d, respectively).

EO dose is an important factor for rumen effects (Fraser et al., 2007). Busquet et al.

(2005) showed in vivo that 200 g peppermint powder decreased rumen protozoa. In a study it was reported that peppermint decreased rumen protozoa and ammonia nitrogen (Bach et al., 2005). Our result was in agreement with some researchers (Newbold et al., 2004; Benchaar et al., 2007) who reported that EO feeding had no effect on rumen protozoa in sheep. Similarly, Djouvino et al. (1997) reported that 450 g/d peppermint did not influence protozoa count in sheep.

Rumen bacteria: Rumen bacteria are influenced by diet changes, feed additives, feeding program and physical status. These factors can alter or destroy appearance of new rumen bacteria. The antimicrobial activity of plant extracts is attributed to a number of secondary metabolites, such as saponines, terpenoides (such as carvacrol, carvone, thymol, and terpinen-4-ol) and phenylpropanoides (such as cinnamaldehyde, eugenol, or anethol) compounds, present in the essential oil fraction of many plants (Busquete et al., 2005). Considering the large number of different groups of chemical compounds present in essential oils, it is most likely that their antibacterial activity is not attributable to one specific mechanism but that there are several targets in the cell (Brenes and Roura, 2010). In a study a mixed EO did not change rumen microbial population (Benchaar et al., 2007). Also, Wallas et al. (2002) observed that 100 mg mixed EO had no effect on rumen bacteria in sheep. Also, it was reported that EO inhibited rumen bacteria (Mcintosh et al., 2003). Factors such as EO type, diet property, species, and geographical situation affect variability and bacterial count including lactic acid bacteria of rumen (Dehority et al., 2003). Our result was in disagreement with a study that showed clove and garlic EO did not affected rumen coliforms (Ghoorchi et al., 2009).

Conclusions: The results of this study showed that although pennyroyal EO increased coliform and acid lactic bacteria of rumen, pennyroyal and peppermint EO had no effect on performance, blood metabolites, rumen pH, NH3-N and protozoa count. More in vivo studies are required to investigate the effects of different supplementations levels on rumen microbial fermentation and blood metabolites to improve nutrient utilization and growth performance in sheep.

Acknowledgments

This work was financially supported by University of Gonbad Kavous, Iran which is gratefully acknowledged.

References

Ahmadi Naghadehi, A.A., Pirmohammadi, R., Sahrae Belverdi, M., Parsaemehr, K. (2014) Effect of peppermint (*Mentha piperita*) on digestibility and rumen fermentation of Makuei sheep. Iranian J Animal Sci. 106: 65-70. (In Persian).

Allen, M.S. (1997) Relationship between fermentation acid production in the rumen and the requirement for physically effective fiber. J Dairy sci. 80: 1447-1462.

Ando, S., Nishida, T., Ishida, M., Hosoda, K., Bayaru, E. (2003) Effect of peppermint feeding on the digestibility, ruminal fermentation and protozoa. Livest Prod Sci. 82: 245–248.

Anantasook, N., Wanapat, M., Cherdthong, A., Gunun, P. (2013) Effect of plants containing secondary compounds with Ppalm oil on feed Iintake, digestibility, microbial protein synthesis and microbial population in dairy cows. Asian Australas. J Anim Sci. 26: 820–826.

Bach, A., Calsamiglia, S., Stern, M.D. (2005) Nitrogen metabolism in rumen. J Dairy Sci. 88: 9-21.

Beauchemin, K.A., McGinn, S.M. (2006) Methane emissions from beef cattle: Effects of fumaric acid, essential oil, and canola oil. J Anim Sci. 84: 1489–1496.

Benchaar, C., Calsamiglia, S., Chaves, A.V., Fraser, G.R., Colombatto, D., McAllister, T.A., Beauchemin, K.A. (2007) A review of plant-derived essential oils in ruminant nutrition and production. Anim Feed Sci Technol. 145: 209–228.

Borek, C. (2001) Antioxidant health effects of aged garlic extract. Trop Anim Health Prod. 42: 961-968.

Brenes, A., Roura, E. (2010) Essential oils in poultry nutrition: main effects and mod of actions. Anim Feed Sci Technol. 158: 1-14.

Broderick, G.A., Kang, G.H. (1980) Automated simultaneous determination of ammonia and total amino acids in ruminal fluid and in vitro media. J Dairy Sci. 63: 64-75.

Busquet, M.S., Calsamiglia, A., Kamel, C. (2005) Screening for the effects of natural plant extracts and secondary plant metabolites on rumen microbial fermentation in continuous culture. Anim Feed Sci Technol. 123: 597–613.

Cawan, M.M. (1999) Plant Products as Antimicrobial Agents. Clin Microbiol Rev. 12: 564-580.

Cedrola, F., Rossi, F., Dias, R.J.P., Martinele, M. and Agosto, M. (2015) Methods for taxonomic study of rumen ciliates (Aleolata: Ciliofora): a brief review. Zool Sci. 32: 8-15.

Chaves, A.V., Stanford, K., Dugan, M.E.R., Gibson, L.L., McAllister, T.A., Van Herk, F., Benchaar, C. (2008a) Effects of cinnamaldehyde, garlic and juniper berry essential oils on rumen fermentation, blood metabolites, growth performance, and carcass characteristics of growing lambs. Livest Sci. 117: 215–224.

Chaves, A.V., Stanford, K., Gibson, A.A., Mcallister T.A., Benchaar, C. (2008b) Effects of caracole and cinnamldehyde on intake, rumen fermentation, growth performance, and carcass characteristic of growing lambs. Anim Feed Sci Technol. 145: 396-408.

Dehority, B.A. (2003) Rumen Microbiology. (1st ed.) Nottingham University Press. Nottingham, UK.

Demir, E., Sarica, S., Ozcan, M.A., Suimez, M. (2003) The use of natural feed additives as alternative for an antibiotic growth promoter in broiler diets. Br Poult Sci. 44: S44-45.

Distel, R.A., Iglesias, R.M.R., Arroquy, J., Merino, J. (2007) A note on increased intake in lambs through diversity in food flavor. Appl Anim Behav Sci. 130: 232–237.

Djouvinov, D., Palvov, D., Ilchev, A., Envev E. (1997) Peppermint (*Mentha piperita* Huds.) and basil (*Ocimum basilicum* L.) etheric oil by-products as roughage for sheep feeding. Anim Feed Sci Technol. 68: 287-294.

Dorman, H.J.D., Deans, S.G. (2000) Antimicrobial agents from plants: antibacterial activity of plant volatile oils. J Appl Microbiol. 88: 308-316.

Fraser, G.R., Chaves, A.V., Wang, Y., McAllister, T.A., Beauchemin, K.A., Benchaar, C. (2007) Assessment of the effects cinnamon leaf oil on rumen microbial fermentation using two continuous culture systems. J Dairy Sci. 90: 2315-2328.

Geraci, G.I., Garciarene, A.C., Gagliostro, G.A., Beauchemin, K.A., Colombato, D. (2012) Plant extract containing cinnamaldehyde, eugenol and capsicum oleoresin added to feedlot cattle diet: ruminal environment, short term intake pattern and animal performance. Anim Feed Sci Technol. 176: 123-130.

Ghalamkari, G.R., Toghyani, M., Landy, N., Tavalaeian, E. (2012) Investigation the effects using different levels of *Mentha pulegium* L. (pennyroyal) in comparison with an antibiotic growth promoter on performance, carcass traits and immune responses in broiler chickens. Asian Pac J Trop Biomed. 2: S1396-S1399.

Ghoorchi, T., Ghanbari, F., Khamiri M., Ebrahimi, T. (2009) Survey on effects of clove and garlic essential oils on degradability of dry matter and rumen microbial population in sheep. Gorgan University of Agricultural Sciences and Natural Resources. Research report. 62 p. (In Persian).

Giannenas, I., Skoufos, J., Giannakopoulos, C., Wiemann, M., Gortzi, O., Lalas, S., Kyriazakis, I. (2011) Effects of essential oils on milk production, milk composition, and rumen microbiota in Chios dairy ewes. J Dairy Sci. 94: 5569–5577.

Greathead, H. (2003) Plants and plant extracts for improving animal productivity. Proc Nutr Soc. 62: 279-290.

Hosoda, K., Kuramoto, K., Eruden, B., Nishida, T., Shona, S. (2006) The effects of three herbs as feed supplements on blood metabolites, hormones, antioxidant activity, IgG concentration and ruminal fermentation in Holstein steers. J Anim Sci. 19: 35-41.

Hatfield, P.G., Hopkins, J.A., Shawn R., Wand, G.A. (1998) Effects of level of protein and type of molasses on digesta kinetics and blood metabolites in sheep. Small Rumin Res. 28: 161-170.

Lewis, M.R., Rose, S.P., Mackenzie, A.M., Tucker, L.A. (2003) Effects of dietary inclusion of plant extracts on growth performance of male broiler chickens. Br Poult Sci. 44: S43-44.

McDonald, P., Edwards, R.A., Greenhalgh, G.F.D., Morgan, C.A. (2002) Animal Nutrition. (6th ed.) Pearson education limited, Exsex, England.

Mcintosh, F.M., Williams, P., Losa, R., Wallace, R.J., Beever, D.A., Newbold, C.J. (2003) Effect of essential oils on ruminal microorganisms and their protein metabolism. J Appl Environ Microbiol. 69: 5011-5014.

Meyer, N.F., Erickson, G.E., Klopfenstein, T.J., Greenquist, M.A., Luebbe, M.K., Williams, P., Engstrom, M.A. (2009) Effect of essential oils, tylosin, and monensin on finishing steer performance, carcass characteristics, liver abscesses, ruminal fermentation, and digestibility. J Anim Sci. 87: 2346-2354.

Newbold, C.J., McIntosh, F.M., Williams, P., Losa, R., Wallace, R.J. (2004) Effects of a specific blend of essential oil compounds on rumen fermentation. Anim Feed Sci Technol. 114: 105–112.

Nobakht, A., Solimanzadeh, E., Pishjangh, J. (2011) Effects of varying levels of nettle (*Urtica dioica* L.), pennyroyal (*Mentha pulegium* L.) medicinal plants and enzyme on performance and egg traits of laying hens. Glob Vet. 7: 491–496.

Nolte, D.L., Provenza, F.D. (1992) Food preferences in lambs after exposure to flavors in solid foods. Appl Anim Behav Sci. 32: 337-347.

Ouwehand, A.C., Tiihonen, K., Kettunen, H., Peuranen, S., Schulze, H., Rautonen, N. (2010) In vitro effects of essential oils on potential pathogens and beneficial members of the normal microbiota. Vet Med. 55: 71–78.

Rafii, F., Shahverdi, A. (2007) Comparison of essential oils from three plants for enhancement of antimicrobial activity of nitrofurantoin against enterobacteria. Chemotherapy. 53: 21-25.

Salem, A., Olivares, M., Lopez, S., Gonzalez-Ronquillo, M., Rojo, R., Camacho, L., Cerrillo, S., Mejia, H. (2011) Effect of natural extracts of *Salix babylonica* and *Leucaena leucocephalaon* on nutrient digestibility and growth performance of lambs. Anim Feed Sci Technol. 170: 27-34.

Steiner, T. (2009) Phytogenics in Animal Nutrition: Natural Concepts to Optimize Gut Health and Performance. Nottingham University Press. Nottingham, UK. 8: 2-19.

Van Soest, P.J. (1994) Nutritional Ecology of the Ruminant. Cornel University Press. Ithaca, New York, USA.

Vakili, A.R., Khorrami, B., Mesgaran, M.D., Parand, E. (2013) The effects of thyme and cinnamon essential oils on performance, rumen fermentation and blood metabolites in holstein calves consuming high concentrate diet. Asian Australas J Anim Sci. 26: 935–944.

Wallace, R.J. (2004) Antimicrobial properties of plant secondary metabolites. Proc Nutr Soc. 63: 621–629.

Wallace, R.J., McEvan, N.R., McIntosh, F.M., Teferedegne, B., Newbold, C.J. (2002) Natural products as manipulators of rumen fermentation. Asian Australas. J Anim Sci. 15: 1458-1468.

Wanapat, M., Kang, S., Khejornsart, P., Wanapat, S. (2013) Effects of plant herb combination supplementation on rumen fermentation and nutrient digestibility in beef cattle. Asian Australas J Anim Sci. 26: 1127–1136.

Yang, W.Z., Ametaj, B.N., He, M.L., Benchaar, C., Beauchemin, K.A. (2010a) Cinnamaldehyde in feedlot cattle diet: intake, growth performance, carcass characteristics, and blood metabolites. J Anim Sci. 88: 1082-1092.

Yang, W.Z., Benchaar, C., Ametaj, B.N., Beauchemin, K.A. (2010b) Dose response to eugenol supplementation in growing beef cattle ruminal fermentation intestinal digestion. Anim Feed Sci Technol. 158: 57-64.

Dopamine-induced hypophagia is mediated via NMDA and mGlu1 receptors in chicken

Taheriyan, M.R., Baghbanzadeh, A.*, Zendehdel, M.

Department of Basic Sciences, Faculty of Veterinary Medicine, University of Tehran, Tehran, Iran

Key words:
chicken, dopamine, food intake, glutamate

Correspondence
Baghbanzadeh, A.
Department of Basic Sciences, Faculty of Veterinary Medicine, University of Tehran, Tehran, Iran

Email: abaghban@ut.ac.ir

Abstract:

BACKGROUND: Feeding behavior is regulated by a complex network which interacts via diverse signals from central and peripheral tissues. It is known dopaminergic and glutamatergic systems have crucial role on food intake regulation but scarce reports exist on their interaction in appetite regulation in broilers. **OBJECTIVES:** The present study was designed to examine the role of glutamatergic system on dopamine-induced hypophagia in neonatal meat-type chicken. **METHODS:** In experiment 1, chicks received ICV injection of control solution, dopamine (40 nmol), MK-801 (NMDA glutamate receptors antagonist, 15 nmol) and co-injection of dopamine + MK-801. In experiment 2, birds were ICV injected with saline, dopamine (40 nmol), CNQX (AMPA glutamate receptors antagonist, 390 nmol) and co-injection of dopamine + CNQX. In experiment 3, chicks received ICV injection of control solution, dopamine (40 nmol), AIDA (mGLUR1 glutamate receptors antagonist, 2 nmol), dopamine + AIDA. Experiments 4 and 5 were similar to experiment 3, except birds were injected with LY341495 (mGLUR2 glutamate receptors antagonist, 150 nmol) and UBP1112 (mGLUR3 glutamate receptors antagonist, 2 nmol) instead of AIDA. Then the cumulative food intake was measured until 120 min post injection. **RESULTS:** According to the results, ICV injection of dopamine significantly decreased food intake ($p<0.001$). Co-injection of dopamine and MK-801 decreased dopamine induced hypophagia ($p<0.001$). Moreover, the food intake of chicks was significantly increased by co-injection of AIDA and dopamine ($p<0.001$). **CONCLUSIONS:** These results suggest dopamine-induced hypophagia is mediated via NMDA and mGlu1 receptors in chicken.

Introduction

Appetite is modulated by complex neurochemical pathways in different parts of the brain, such as the striatum, hypothalamus and amygdala. To date frequent neuropeptides and neurotransmitters in the brain have been discovered that regulate food intake (Boswell, 2005). Dopamine (DA) is one of the main neurotransmitters in the brain and regulates several physiological functions such as motion, motivation, novelty, memory and reward (Ladepeche et al., 2013).

Dopaminergic (DAergic) system plays a crucial role on appetite regulation in both mammalian and avian. For instance, D1 and

D2 agonist diminish food intake in rats (Volkow et al., 2011). DA-induced hypophagia mediates by D1 receptors in chicken while other receptors (D2, D3 and D4) may have no role in appetite regulation (Zendehdel et al., 2014b). It is well documented that central feeding behavior is not regulated via a single neuropeptide and a wide distributed neural network interacts with a diversity of neurotransmitters on feeding status (Irwin et al., 2008).

Glutamate is the main excitatory neurotransmitter in the central nervous system (CNS) and plays a role in reward in the different reward and hypothalamic centers (McFadden et al., 2014). Glutamate receptors are classified into two groups, based on their pharmacology and mechanism. The ionotropic receptors including inotropic include N-methyl-D-aspartate (NMDA), Kainate, AMPA receptors and the metabotropic receptors (mGluRs) with different subtypes (Charles et al., 2014). It is reported that of the lateral hypothalamic AMPA receptors, glutamate ionotropic receptors induced feeding in rats (Hettes et al., 2010). In addition, injection of NMDA and AMPA-kainite receptor antagonists into ventral striatal and ventral pallidal areas of the pigeon induced food intake (Da Silva et al., 2003). Also, the ICV injection of DL-AP5 (NMDA receptor antagonist) increased food consumption in FD3 broiler dose dependently (Taati et al., 2011).

A relation between central DA and Glutaminergic systems has been reported. It is reported that dopamine D1 receptor interacts with NMDA mediated signaling in NMDAR-mediated signaling and working memory in the CNS (Ladepeche et al., 2013). For instance, D1 and NMDA receptors interact on the Volitional consumption of ethanol in rats (McMillen et al., 2013) while, blockade of D1 receptors had no changes in the dynamics of glutamate release, blockade of D2 receptors increased glutamate levels during food consumption in rat (Mikhailova et al., 2003).

Despite numerous investigations about the role of neurotransmitters on ingestion, different aspects of appetite regulation in poultry are unclear (Denbow, 1994).There is evidence that central mechanisms for food intake regulation are different between mammalian and birds (Zendehdel and Hassanpour 2014a). So, it will be useful to study the regulatory mechanisms of neurotransmitters in feeding behavior in birds (Furuse, 2002, Zendehdel and Hassanpour 2014b). To the best of our knowledge, no report exists on the role of glutamatergic system on DA-induced hypophagia in domestic fowls. Hence, this study was to determine the possible involvement of the glutamatergic system on DA-induced hypophagia in neonatal meat-type chicken.

Materials and Methods

Animals: In this study, a total of 240 one-day-old broiler chickens (Ross 308) were purchased from local hatchery (Mahan Co. Iran). Birds were kept as flocks for 2 and then randomly transferred into individual cages at a temperature of 30 ± 1°C with 50 ± 2 percent humidity (Olanrewaju et al., 2006). A commercial diet was provided during the study containing 21 % crude protein and 2850 kcal/kg of metabolizable energy (Chineh Co. Iran). All birds received food and fresh water ad libitum during the study. Just 3 h prior to ICV injections, chicken were food deprived (FD3) though they had free access to water. The injections were applied to all birds at 5 days of age. Animal handling and experimental procedures were performed according to the Guide for the Care and Use of Laboratory animals by the National Institutes of Health (USA) and Institutional Ethical Committee of the Iranian government for animal care.

Experimental drugs: Drugs including dopamine, MK-801 (NMDA glutamate receptors antagonist), CNQX (AMPA glutamate receptors antagonist), AIDA (mGLUR1 glutamate receptors antagonist), LY341495 (mGLUR2 glutamate receptors antagonist), UBP1112 (mGLUR3 glutamate receptors antagonist) and Evans blue were purchased from Sigma Co. (Sigma, USA) and Tocris Co. (UK). Drugs were first dissolved in absolute dimethyl sulfoxide (0.08% DMSO) then diluted with 0.85% saline containing Evans blue at a ratio of 1/250. DMSO with this ratio does not have cytotoxic effect (Blevins et al., 2002; Qi et al., 2008).

ICV injection procedures: In this study, 5 experiments were designed to investigate interconnection of DAergic and glutamatergic systems on cumulative food intake in neonatal broiler birds (each experiment includes 4 groups with 3 replicates (n=12). Prior to each experiment, the chicks were weighed and based on their body weight divided into experimental groups so the average weight between treatment groups was as uniform as possible. ICV injection was applied using a microsyringe (Hamilton, Switzerland) without anesthesia according to the technique previously described by Davis et al., (1979) and Furuse et al., (1997). Briefly, the head of the birds was held by acrylic device, the bill holder was 45° and calvarium parallel to the surface of table (Van Tienhoven and Juhasz, 1962). A hole was drilled in acrylic device over the right lateral ventricle of the skull. A microsyringe was inserted into the right ventricle via the hole and tip of the needle penetrated 4 mm beneath the skin of the skull. It is shown that, there is no injection-induced physiological stress using this method in neonatal chicks (Saito et al., 2005). Each chick received a 10 µl ICV injection of vehicle or drug (Furuse et al., 1999). There was no increased intracranial pressure using ICV injections of 2, 5 and 10 µl of saline or solution (Furuse et al., 1999). The control group received control solution (saline containing Evan's blue 10 µl) (Furuse et al., 1999). Right away after injection, FD3 birds returned to their individual cages and supplied fresh water and food (pre-weighed). Cumulative food intake (gr) was measured at 30, 60 and 120 min after the injection. Food consumption was calculated as a percentage of body weight to minimize impact of body weight on the amount of food intake. Each bird was used just once in each experimental group. At the end of the experiments, accuracy of placement of the injection in the ventricle was verified by presence of Evans blue followed by slicing the frozen brain tissue. In each group, 12 birds received injection, but just data of those individuals where dye was present in their lateral ventricle (9-12 chickens per group) were used for analysis. All experimental procedures were done from 8:00 A.M. until 3:30 P.M (Jonaidi and Noori, 2012; Zendehdel and Hassanpour 2014; Hassanpour et al., 2015).

Feeding experiments: In experiment 1, four groups of FD3 chicks received a dose of either the ICV injection of A: control solution (saline containing Evan's blue), B: dopamine (40 nmol), C: MK-801 (NMDA glutamate receptors antagonist, 15 nmol), D: combination of dopamine + MK-801. In experiment 2, group A: ICV injected with saline, B: dopamine (40 nmol), C: CNQX (AMPA glutamate receptors antagonist, 390 nmol), D: combination of dopamine + CNQX. In experiment 3, FD3 chicks received ICV injection of control solution (A), dopamine (40 nmol), AIDA (mGLUR1 glutamate receptors antagonist, 2 nmol), D: dopamine + AIDA. In experiment 4, group A: ICV injected with saline, B: dopamine (40 nmol), C: LY341495 (mGLUR2 glutamate receptors antagonist, 150 nmol), D: dopamine + LY341495. In experiment 5, group A: ICV injected with saline, B: dopamine (40 nmol), C: UBP1112 (mGLUR3 glutamate receptors antagonist, 2 nmol), D: dopamine + UBP1112. Each bird was injected once only. The injection procedure is described in Table 1. These doses of drugs were determined according to the previous (Zeni et al., 2000; Antunes et al., 2005; Baghbanzadeh and Babapour, 2007 Zendehdel et al., 2009, 2012, 2014a).

Statistical analysis: Data were presented

as mean ± SEM (standard error of the mean). Cumulative food intake (as percent of body weight) was analyzed by repeated measure two-way analysis of variance (ANOVA) using SPSS 16.0 for Windows (SPSS, Inc., Chicago, IL, USA). For treatment showing a main effect by ANOVA, means were compared by Tukey-Kramer test. P<0.001 was considered as significant difference between treatments.

Results

Effects and interactions of central DAergic and glutamatergic systems on cumulative food intake in FD3 neonatal meat-type chicks are shown in Figs. 1-5.

In this study to examine the possible interaction between these two systems, effective and sub-effective doses of their antagonists were administered to confront nullifying effects of the agents. In other words, for interactions the effective dose antagonists were injected with the sub-effective dose of the antagonist of the other system. According to the results, ICV injection of an effective dose of DA (40 nmol) significantly decreased cumulative food intake in FD3 compared to control group (p<0.001) (Figs 1-5).

In experiment 1, ICV injection of sub effective dose of the NMDA glutamate antagonist (MK-801, 15 nmol) had no significant effect on food intake in FD3 birds (p>0.05) while co-injection of dopamine and MK-801 attenuated DA-induced hypophagia (p<0.001).

In experiment 2, ICV injection 390 nmol of CNQX (AMPA glutamate antagonist) had no effect on feeding behavior in FD3 neonatal meat-type chicken (p>0.05). Also, co-administration of CNQX + DA had no effect on DA-induced hypophagia in FD3 neonatal meat-type chicken (p>0.05).

In experiment 3, no significant effect was observed on food intake after ICV administration of AIDA (mGLUR1 glutamate antagonist, 2 nmol) in FD3 neonatal meat-type chicken

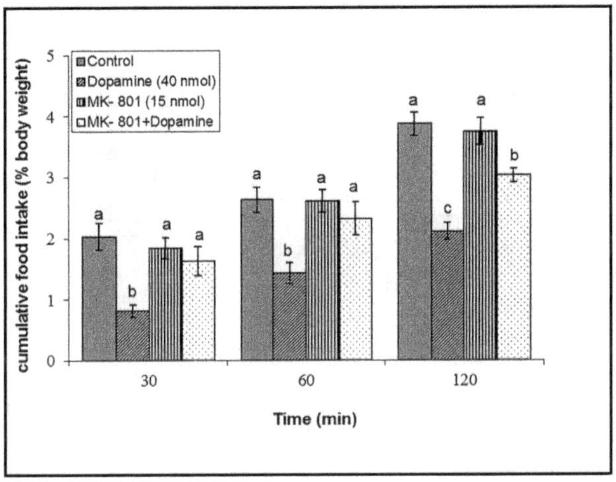

Figure 1. Effects of intracerebroventricular injection of control solution, dopamine, MK-801 and a combination of dopamine plus MK-801 on cumulative food intake (% BW) in neonatal chicks. MK-801: NMDA glutamate receptors antagonist. Data are expressed as mean ± SEM. Different letters (a and b) indicate significant differences between treatments at each time(p<0.001).

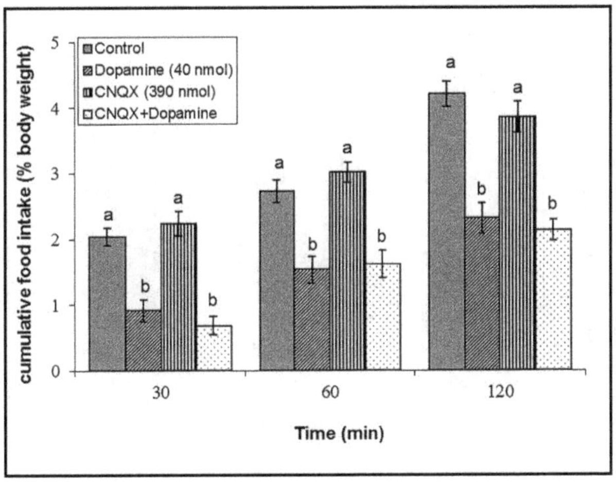

Figure 2. Effects of intracerebroventricular injection of control solution, dopamine, CNQX and a combination of dopamine plus CNQX on cumulative food intake (% BW) in neonatal chicks. CNQX: AMPA glutamate receptors antagonist. Data are expressed as mean ± SEM. Different letters (a and b) indicate significant differences between treatments at each time (p<0.001).

(p>0.05) but, DA-induced hypophagia significantly attenuated by co-injection of DA and AIDA (p<0.001).

In experiment 4, ICV injection of (mGLUR2 glutamate antagonist, 150 nmol) was not able to impress significant change on appetite regulation in birds (p>0.05). Also, combination of DA and LY341495 was not able to decrease

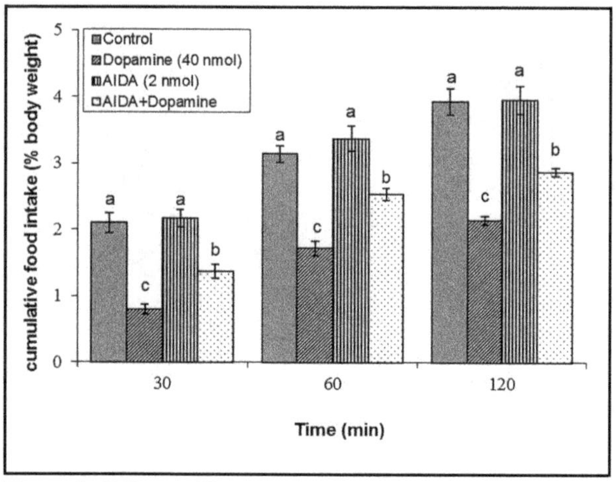

Figure 3. Effects of intracerebroventricular injection of control solution, dopamine, AIDA and a combination of dopamine plus AIDA on cumulative food intake (% BW) in neonatal chicks. AIDA: mGLUR1 glutamate receptors antagonist. Data are expressed as mean ± SEM. Different letters (a, b and c) indicate significant differences between treatments at each time (p<0.001).

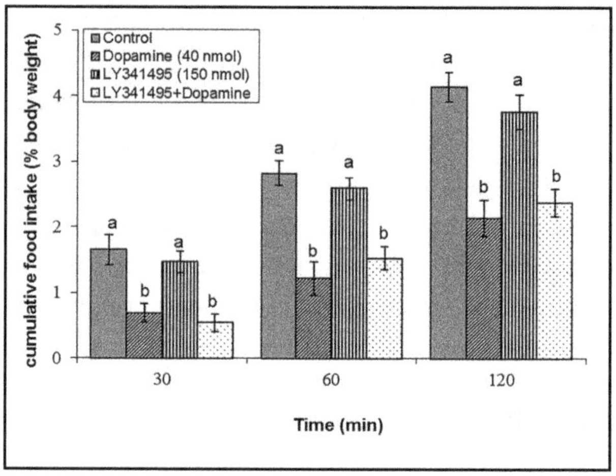

Figure 4. Effects of intracerebroventricular injection of control solution, dopamine, LY341495 and a combination of dopamine plus LY341495 on cumulative food intake (% BW) in neonatal chicks. LY341495: mGLUR2 glutamate receptors antagonist. Data are expressed as mean ± SEM. Different letters (a and b) indicate significant differences between treatments at each time (p<0.001).

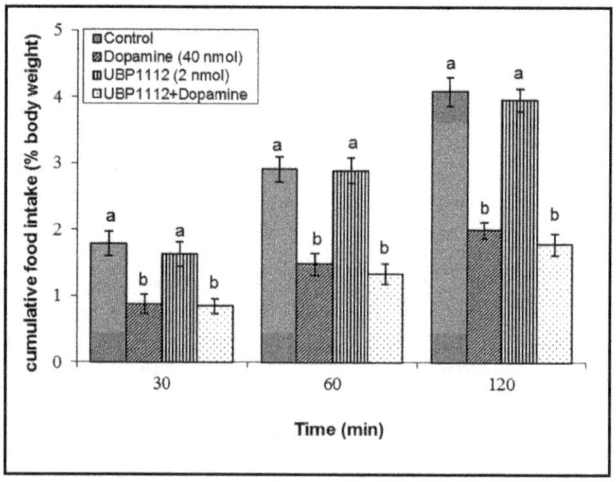

Figure 5. Effects of intracerebroventricular injection of control solution, dopamine, UBP1112 and a combination of dopamine plus UBP1112 on cumulative food intake (% BW) in neonatal chicks. UBP1112: mGLUR3 glutamate receptors antagonist. Data are expressed as mean ± SEM. Different letters (a and b) indicate significant differences between treatments at each time (p<0.001).

the hypophagic effect of DA in FD3 neonatal meat-type chicks in comparison to control group (p>0.05).

In experiment 5, ICV of DA significantly decreased feeding behavior (p<0.001) and injection of UBP1112 (mGLUR3 glutamate antagonist, 2 nmol) had no effect on cummulative food intake in meat-type chicks (p>0.05). Co-injection of DA + UBP1112 was not able to diminish DA-induced hypophagia in FD3 neonatal meat-type chicks compared to control group (p>0.05).

Discussion

To the best of our knowledge, this is the first report on interactions between DAergic and glutamatergic systems on neonatal broiler feed intake. According to the results (Figs. 1, 2, 3, 4 and 5), ICV injection of the DA significantly decreased food intake in FD3 neonatal meat-type chicken. A daily decrease on cumulative food intake was reported using D1 (SKF 38393) and D2 (apomorphine) agonists in rats (Kuo Dy et al., 2002). A dose dependent decrease in food intake was detected using D1 agonist (SKF 38393) in both food deprived and non-deprived rats (Terry et al., 1992). The result of current study was similar to our previous study which reported the ICV injection of the DA decreased food intake in broiler chickens (Zendehdel et al., 2014a).

As observed from the results, co-injection of dopamine and MK-801 (NMDA glutamate antagonist) decreased dopamine induced hypophagia in FD3 neonatal meat-type chicken (Fig. 1). The glutamatergic and the DAergic system plays key role in several brain functions, such as motion and reward. Over the past decades several researches have been done to discover the direct mechanism responsible for the central DA and glutaminergic systems interaction. Release of the DA activates postsynaptic membrane DA1/5 receptors which can affect NMDA receptors signaling in striatal and hippocampal neurons in the rat (Ladepeche et al., 2013). High concentrations of glutamate receptors in the food regulation regions of the brain have a significant effect on DA release (McFadden et al., 2014). Lateral hypothalamic injection of ionotropic glutamate receptors amplifies feeding while NMDA receptor antagonist suppresses natural feeding (Stanley et al., 1996).

There is little information about interaction of DA and glutamatergic systems in the brain. DAergic neurons can be protected against neurotoxic levels of amphetamines via NMDA receptor antagonist, MK-801(McMillen et al., 2013). It is suggested that D1 receptor agonist activate DARPP-32 through the cAMP/PKA pathway while NMDA agonist blockade this effect via increasing the intracellular Ca2+ and activation of calcineurin (McMillen et al., 2013). Based on the literature they were not able to investigate interaction of other neurotransmitters with DA-glutamatergic on food intake regulation. We think merit researches needed to determine a direct cellular and molecular mechanism for interaction of DA-glutamatergic systems on feeding behavior.

Herein, food intake increased by co-injection of AIDA (mGLUR1 glutamate antagonist) and dopamine in FD3 neonatal meat-type chicken (Fig. 3). In this regard, it was reported that food consumption elicits via lateral hypothalamic mGluR1 and/or mGluR5 in rat (Charles et al., 2014). Stimulation of food consumption followed by reduction of elicited feeding using mGluR1 and mGluR5 antagonists, suggests feeding behavior is mediated by mGluRs, specifically the R1 and R5 subtypes (Charles et al., 2014). There are interesting reports on indirect involvement and mediatory role of the ionotropic receptors on mGluRs-induced feeding. For example, activation of mGluR5 can modify NMDA synaptic currents within lateral hypothalamus melanin-concentrating hormone (MCH) neurons (Charles et al., 2014). As seen from the Fig.1 vs. Fig.3, NMDA antagonists strongly minimized DA-induced hypophagia (Fig.1) while mGluR1 antagonist had partial effect (Fig.3). In this study, there was no interaction between DA and other mGluRs (mGLUR2 and mGLUR3).

There is limited information about involvement of mGluRs with DAergic system on feeding behavior. Although there was a difference in central regulation in feeding behavior between broilers and layer chicken, no report was found on interaction of these systems in layer-type chicken. In our previous study, we found that mGLUR2 and mGLUR3 receptors had no effect on the 5-HT induced hypophagia in FD3 chickens (Seyedali Mortezaei et al., 2013). It seems that metabotropic receptors have partial interaction with other neurotransmitters in food intake regulation in broilers. The mGluR1 mechanically acts via phospholipase C activation which leads to the formation of IP3 and diacylglycerol, intracellular release of Ca2+ and stimulation of protein kinase C, while mGLUR2 and mGLUR3 receptors coupled to adenylyl cyclase and cyclase respectively. Different subtypes in each mGluR group have different functional roles. We think the observed differences might relate to the different cellular mechanism of actions of the mGLURs. However, merit studies need to determine direct cellular and molecular interaction of mGLURs with other neurotransmitters.

However, the role of DA in feeding behaviors is complex and varies by brain region. Perhaps DA-glutamatergic system interaction on food intake mediates via other neurotransmitters such as GABA (Richard and Berridge, 2011), orexin and neuropeptide Y (NPY) (Charles et al., 2014) and opioids (Madhavan et al., 2013). For example, pre-treatment with nicotine decreased the NMDA-induced dopamine release from nucleus accumbens nerve terminals (Salamone et al., 2014). Because of the limitation of this study, we were not able to investigate interaction of other neurotransmitters with DA-glutamatergic on food intake regulation. To our knowledge, there has been no previous study on the role of central DAergic and glutamatergic systems on food intake in avian. So, we were not able to compare our results with it. Most research on central food intake regulation has been done with rat models, whereas few investigations have been done on birds. These observations can be used as base information on central food intake regulation in birds. Finally, the authors recommend further merit investigations be done to clarify direct cellular and molecular signaling pathways of the DAergic and glutamatergic systems with other receptors in physiology of food intake regulation in poultry.

Acknowledgments

This research was supported by a grant from the Research Council of the Faculty of Veterinary Medicine, University of Tehran, Iran.

References

1. Antunes, F., Nunes, C., Laranjinha, J., Cadenas, E. (2005) Redox interactions of nitric oxide with dopamine and its derivatives. Toxicol. 208: 207-212.
2. Baghbanzadeh, A., Babapour, V. (2007) Glutamate ionotropic and metabotropic receptors affect feed intake in broiler cockerels. J Vet Res. 62: 125-129.
3. Blevins, J.E., Stanley, B.G., Reidelberger, R.D. (2002) DMSO as a vehicle for central injections: tests with feeding elicited by norepinephrine injected into the paraventricular nucleus. Pharmacol Biochem Behav. 71: 277-282.
4. Boswell, T. (2005) Regulation of energy balance in birds by the neuroendocrine hypothalamus. J Poult Sci. 42: 161-181.
5. Charles, J.R., Duva, M.A., Ramirez, G.J., Lara, R.L., Yang, C.R., Stanley, B.G. (2014) Activation of lateral hypothalamic mGlu1 and mGlu5 receptors elicits feeding in rats. Neuropharmacol. 79: 59-65.
6. Da Silva, A.A., Marino-Neto, J., Paschoalini, M.A. (2003) Feeding induced by microinjections of NMDA and AMPA-kainite receptor antagonists into ventral striatal and ventral pallidal areas of the pigeon. Brain Res. 966: 76-83.
7. Davis, J.L., Masuoka, D.T., Gerbrandt, L.K., Cherkin, A. (1979) Autoradiographic distribution of L-proline in chicks after intracerebral injection. Physiol Behav. 22: 693-695.
8. Denbow, D.M. (1994) Peripheral regulation of food intake in poultry. J Nutr. 124: 1349S-1354S.
9. Furuse, M. (2002) Central regulation of food intake in the neonatal chick. Anim Sci J. 73: 83-94.
10. Furuse, M., Ando, R., Bungo, T., Ao, R., ShimoJO, M., Masuda, Y. (1999) Intracerebroventricular injection of orexins does not stimulate food intake in neonatal chicks. Br Poult Sci. 40: 698-700.
11. Furuse, M., Matsumoto, M., Saito, N., Sugahara, K., Hasegawa, S. (1997) The central corticotropin-releasing factor and glucagon-like peptide-1 in food intake of the neonatal chick. Eur J Pharmacol. 339: 211-214.
12. Hassanpour, S., Zendehdel, M., Babapour, V., Charkhkar, S. (2015) Endocannabinoid and nitric oxide interaction mediates food intake in neonatal chicken. Br Poult Sci. 56: 443-451.
13. Hettes, S.R., Gonzaga, W.J., Heyming, T.W., Nguyen, J.K., Perez, S., Stanley, B.G. (2010) Stimulation of lateral hypothalamic AMPA receptors may induce feeding in rats. Brain Res. 1346: 112-120.
14. Irwin, N., Hunter, K., Frizzell, N., Flatt, P.R.

(2008) Antidiabetic effects of sub-chronic administration of the cannabinoid receptor (CB1) antagonist, AM251, in obese diabetic (ob/ob) mice. Eur J Pharmacol. 581: 226-233.

15. Jonaidi, H., Noori, Z. (2012) Neuropeptide Y-induced feeding is dependent on GABAA receptors in neonatal chicks. J Comp Physiol A. 198: 827-832.
16. Kuo, Dy. (2002) Co-administration of dopamine D1 and D2 agonists additively decreases daily food intake, body weight and hypothalamic neuropeptide Y level in rats. J Biomed Sci. 9: 126-32.
17. Ladepeche, L., Yang, L., Bouchet, D., Groc, L. (2013) Regulation of dopamine D1 receptor dynamics within the postsynaptic density of hippocampal glutamate synapses. PLoS ONE. 8: e74512.
18. Madhavan, A., Argilli, E., Bonci, A., Whistler, J.L. (2013) Loss of D2 dopamine receptor function modulates cocaine-induced glutamatergic synaptic potentiation in the ventral tegmental area. J Neurosci. 33: 12329-12336.
19. McFadden, K.L., Cornier, M.A., Tregellas, J.R. (2014) The role of alpha-7 nicotinic receptors in food intake behaviors. Frontiers In Psychol. 5: 1-7.
20. McMillen, B.A., Lommatzsch, C.L., Sayonh, M.J., Williams, H.L. (2013) Interactions of a dopamine D1 receptor agonist with glutamate NMDA receptor antagonists on the volitional consumption of ethanol by the mHEP rat. Pharmaceuticals. 6: 469-479.
21. Mikhailova, M.O. (2003) Comparison of changes in glutamate levels in the nucleus accumbens of the rat brain during food consumption in conditions of blockade of dopamine D1 and D2 receptors. Neurosci Behav Physiol. 33: 431-434.
22. Olanrewaju, H.A., Thaxton, J.P., Dozier, W.A., Purswell, J., Roush, W.B., Branton, S.L. (2006) A review of lighting programs for broiler production. Int J poult Sci. 5: 301-308.
23. Qi, W., Ding, D., Salvi, R.J. (2008) Cytotoxic effects of dimethyl sulphoxide (DMSO) on cochlear organotypic cultures. Hear Res. 236: 52-60.
24. Ricahrd, J.M., Berridge, K.C. (2011) Nucleus Accumbens dopamine/glutamate interaction switches modes to generate desire versus dread: D1 alone for appetitive eating but D1 and D2 together for fear. J Neurosci. 31: 12866-12879.
25. Saito, E.S., Kaiya, H., Tachibana, T., Tomonaga, S., Denbow, D.M., Kangawa, K., Furuse, M. (2005) Inhibitory effect of ghrelin on food intake is mediated by the corticotropin-releasing factor system in neonatal chicks. Regul Pept. 125: 201-208.
26. Salamone, A., Zappettini, S., Grilli, M., Olivero, G., Agostinho, P., Tomé, A.R., Chen, J., Pittaluga, A., Cunha, R.A., Marchi, M. (2014) Prolonged nicotine exposure down-regulates presynaptic NMDA receptors in dopaminergic terminals of the rat nucleus accumbens. Neuropharmacology. 79: 488-497.
27. Seyedali Mortezaei, S., Zendehdel, M., Babapour, V., Hasani, K. (2013) The role of glutamatergic and GABAergic systems on serotonin- induced feeding behavior in chicken. Vet Res Commun. 37: 303-310.
28. Stanley, B.G., Willett, V.L., Doniasm H.W., Dee, M.G., Duva, M.A. (1996) Lateral hypothalamic NMDA receptors and glutamate as physiological mediators of eating and weight control. Am J Physiol. 270: 443-449.
29. Taati, M., Nayebzadeh, H., Zendehdel, M. (2011) The effects of DLAP5 and glutamate on ghrelin-induced feeding behavior in 3- h food-deprived broiler cockerels. J Physiol Biochem. 67: 217-223.
30. Terry, P., Katz, J.L. (1992) Differential antagonism of the effects of dopamine D1-receptor agonists on feeding behavior in the rat. Physiopharmacology. 109: 403-409.
31. Van Tienhoven, A., Juhasz, L.P. (1962) The chicken telencephalon, diencephalon and mesencephalon in sterotaxic coordinates. J Comp Neurol. 118: 185-197.
32. Volkow, N.D., Wang, G.J., Baler, R.D. (2011)

Reward, dopamine and the control of food intake: implications for obesity. Trends Cogn Sci. 15: 37-46.

33. Zendehdel, M., Baghbanzadeh, A., Babapour, V., Cheraghi, J. (2009) The effects of bicuculline and muscimol on glutamate-induced feeding behaviour in broiler cockerels. J Comp Physiol A. 195: 715-720.
34. Zendehdel, M., Hasani, K., Babapour, V., Seyedali Mortezaei, S., Khoshbakht, Y., Hassanpour, S. (2014a) Dopamine-induced hypophagia is mediated by D1 and 5HT-2c receptors in chicken. Vet Res Commun. 38: 11-19.
35. Zendehdel, M., Hassanpour, S. (2014) Ghrelin-induced hypophagia is mediated by the β2 adrenergic receptor in chicken. J Physiol Sci. 64: 383-391.
36. Zendehdel, M., Hassanpour, S. (2014b) Central regulation of food intake in mammals and birds: a review. Neurotransmitter. 1: 1-7.
37. Zendehdel, M., Taati, M., Jonaidi, H., Amini, E. (2012) The role of central 5-HT (2C) and NMDA receptors on LPS-induced feeding behavior in chickens. J Physiol Sci. 62: 413-419.
38. Zeni, L.A., Seidler, H.B., De Carvalho, N.A., Freitas, C.G., Marino-Neto, J., Paschoalini, M.A. (2000) Glutamatergic control of food intake in pigeons: effects of central injections of glutamate, NMDA, and AMPA receptor agonists and antagonists. Pharmacol Biochem Behav. 65: 67-74.

A study of the employment of melatonin supplementation and darkness regime on reducing the negative effects of acute heat stress and mortality in broiler chickens

Hassanzadeh, M.[1*], Moghimi Niaki, A.A.[1], Babapour, V.[2], Mohit, A.[3], Mirzaie, S.[4]

[1]*Department of Avian Diseases, Faculty of Veterinary Medicine, University of Tehran, Tehran, Iran*
[2]*Department of Basic Sciences, Faculty of Veterinary Medicine, University of Tehran, Tehran, Iran*
[3]*Department of Animal Sciences, Faculty of Agriculture, University of Guillan, Rasht, Iran*
[4]*Institute for Agricultural Research of Iranian Organization for Sciences and Technology, Tehran, Iran*

Key words:
broiler chickens, corticosterone, heat stress, melatonin, T3/T4

Correspondence
Hassanzadeh, M.
Department of Avian Diseases, Faculty of Veterinary Medicine, University of Tehran, Iran

Email: mhzadeh@ut.ac.ir

Abstract:

BACKGROUND: Heat stress is one of the most important environmental stressors challenging poultry production worldwide. Understanding and controlling environmental stressors is crucial for successful poultry production. **OBJECTIVES:** The aim of the present study was to investigate the effects of melatonin supplementation and darkness regime on reducing the negative effects of heat stress in broiler chickens. **METHODS:** A total of 400 broiler chickens (Arian) were obtained and subjected to four different groups. The control chickens were grown in normal conditions without receiving any treatment. The positive control birds were grown similar to the control but exposed to an acute heat stress for 6 h/d from days 35 to 40. The dark group chickens were reared under a dark schedule and exposed to heat stress. The birds of the fourth group were reared similar to the positive control but received 40 ppm melatonin in the diet from days 30 to 40 of age. Dead birds were autopsied. The weekly growth performance of chickens was determined and blood samples were taken for hormonal analysis. **RESULTS:** The number of dead birds due to heat stress was significantly decreased in chickens subjected to the dark program and/or those which received melatonin in the diet compared with those of positive control chickens. Such differences were accompanied with the significantly lower levels of plasma T3, T3/T4 and corticosterone in these groups of chickens. Additionally, plasma thiobarbituric acid reacting substances level was significantly higher in positive control broilers compared to their counterparts. **CONCLUSIONS:** Our findings indicate a reduction of metabolic rate and heat production in dark regime and melatonin supplementation that can reduce the side effects of heat stress and, therefore, reduce the mortality rate.

Introduction

Genetic selection for a faster growth rate in broiler chickens has predisposed them to physiological and metabolic disorders resulting in more sensitivity to harsh environmental conditions including heat stress. Within the thermoneutral zone, the body temperature of birds is maintained by thermal equation. Heat stress occurs when ambient temperature goes above the thermoneutral zone which is between 18 to 22°C for grown broilers (Charles, 2002).

As a consequence of environmental temperature increment, the extra heat could be lost by evaporating the moisture of the respiratory tract through increased respiration rate or panting. In contrast, carbon dioxide would be lost during panting and the bicarbonate buffer system would lower the concentration of hydrogen ions, developing a condition known as respiratory alkalosis (Calder and Schmidt-Neilsen, 1967). During the respiratory alkalosis, the shift in blood pH increasingly depresses the feed intake and adversely affects the overall performance and also health of the birds (Ahmad and Sarwar, 2006). The excessive levels of reactive oxygen forms can be stimulated by stressful situations, e.g., heat stress and clinical conditions (Lara and Rostagno, 2013; Dröge, 2002). These result in the disturbance of balance between the oxidation and antioxidant defense systems, causing lipid peroxidation and oxidative damages to cell membranes, proteins, and DNA (Halliwell and Gutteridg, 1989). This could lead to higher mortality in chickens (Naughton et al., 2002; Gharib et al., 2008).

Hormonal changes occur in broilers under heat stress conditions and the stress responses in poultry are excited mainly by the activation of hypothalamic-pituitary-adrenal axis and of the nervous system (Ben Nathan et al., 1976). Previous studies have indicated that plasma triiodothyronine (T3) concentration of heat-stressed chickens may decrease or remain unchanged (Yahav and McMurtry, 2001; May et al., 1986). One of the mechanisms involved in the improved thermotolerance is modulation of heat production through changes in circulating T3 (Bowen et al., 1984; Yahav and Hurwitz, 1996). Lin et al. (2004) pointed a clear positive relationship between circulating corticosterone levels and plasma lipid peroxidation, which is a direct indication of oxidative cellular damage in broiler chickens (Iqbal et al., 1990).

Melatonin is a neural hormone which is secreted mainly by the pineal gland during the darkness in chickens as in other animals. This hormone is involved in many biological functions including thermoregulation mechanism, reproductive and cardiopulmonary systems, and behaviors of birds (Apeldoorn et al., 1999; Ambriz-Tututi et al., 2009).

Several studies have shown that discontinuous lighting or darkness regime would improve the feed conversion rate and decrease the mortality rate of metabolic disorders such as leg problems, ascites, and sudden death syndrome (Blair et al., 1993; Özkan et al., 2000; Stub and Vestegaard, 2001; Sanotra et al., 2002; Hassanzadeh et al., 2012, 2014).

While most researchers have studied the physiological and/or metabolic changes in heat-stressed birds, only a few of them have implemented management activities to control heat-stressed mortality by taking the darkness regime. Based on these, the aim of the present study was to investigate the effects of melatonin supplementation and darkness regime on reducing the negative consequences of heat stress and its related mortality rate in broiler chickens.

Materials and Methods

A total of 400-day-old fast growing broiler chickens (GGP stock of Pure Sir Broiler Line, Arian Co., Babolkenar, Iran) were reared under a nearly continuous lighting schedule (23 L: 1D) until day 9 of age. Thereafter, they were randomly divided over four equal-sized rooms (6×3 m2), each containing four floor pens (25 chicks per pen) and housed in a low altitude farm 50m above the sea level in the north of Iran. The chickens were reared for six weeks on wood shavings under standard conditions and provided ad libitum access to water and a standard ration (Starter: 2850 kcal/kg metabolizable energy and 210 g/kg crude protein, Grower: 2950 kcal/kg metabolizable energy and 200 g/kg crude protein, Finisher: 3050 kcal/kg metabolizable energy and 190 g/kg crude protein formulated) to meet the requirements for broilers (National Research Council, 1994). In the first room, chickens of the negative control (ConN) group received 23L:1D lighting regime up to the end of the study. The positive control (ConP) chickens were grown similar to the ConN birds up to 35 days of age, but from days 35 to 40, these chickens were exposed to an acute heat stress for 6 h/d. Each day, the temperature was gradually raised up to 38±1°C during the first hour and the degree was kept for the next 5 hours. In the third room (Dark), lighting schedules were provided as presented in Fig 1. Briefly, the dark-length schedules in this group consisted of: 1 to 9 days, 23L:1D; 10 to 11 days, 20L:4D; 12 to 13 days, 19L:5D; 14 to 31 days, 18L:6D; 32 to 33 days, 19L:5D; 34 to 35 days, 20L:4D; 36 to 41 days, 21L:3D and 41 to 42 days, 23L:1D. The birds of the fourth group (Melat) were reared similar to the ConN up to the 30th day, but they received 40 ppm melatonin (Vitane pharmaceutical) in the diet (Apeldoorn et al., 1999) from days 30 to 40 of age. In this study, chickens of the Dark and Melat groups were also exposed to an acute heat stress simultaneously in similar conditions, as already explained for ConP birds. The body weight, feed intake, and feed conversion ratios (FCR) were measured weekly and the mortality rate was recorded daily for each group separately. Blood samples of 10 birds from each group of chickens were randomly taken on days 10, 20, 30, 35, 38 and 42 of age in heparinized tubes. The plasma was separated and stored in aliquots at -20°C for further analysis.

The plasma samples were sent to the Department of Biosystems, Catholic University Leuven, Belgium, for determining the levels of thyroid hormones (T3, T4), corticosterone, and thiobarbituric acid reacting substances (TBARS). Thyroid hormones and corticosterone levels were measured by radioimmunoassay according to the method described earlier (Decuypere et al., 1983, 1994; Hassanzadeh et al. 2004).

Plasma lipid peroxidation was estimated by the spectrophotometric determination of TBARS as reported by Lin et al. (2006). TBARS were expressed as nanomoles of malondialdehyde (MDA) per milliliter of plasma.

Statistical analysis was performed using the "General linear model procedure" (SAS Institute Inc., 2008). If a significant overall effect ($p<0.05$) was found, treatment means were compared using the Scheffe test.

Results

The total number of dead birds due to acute heat stress, mean body weight, the feed intake, and FCR of the different groups of treated birds are summarized in Table 1.

During the 6 weeks of the experiment, 28 (7%) of 400 chickens died (Table 1). Of these, 19 (4.8%) died due to acute heat stress from days 35 to 41 of age . While the other 9 (2.3%) dead birds observed over the first 5 weeks of the growing period were due to neonatal infections (3 birds), arthritis (2 birds), sudden death syndrome (1 bird) and ascites (3 birds). Between days 35 to 41 of the study, 10 of 100 birds (10%) which have been reared under ConP program died due to heat stress, while the rate of heat-stressed mortality declined under the dark condition (5/100 birds) and also when 40 mg melatonin was supplied in the diet (4,100 birds).

Imposing birds to the dark conditions reduced the absolute body weight of chickens compared to the other three groups of birds at days 14 onwards but the difference was only

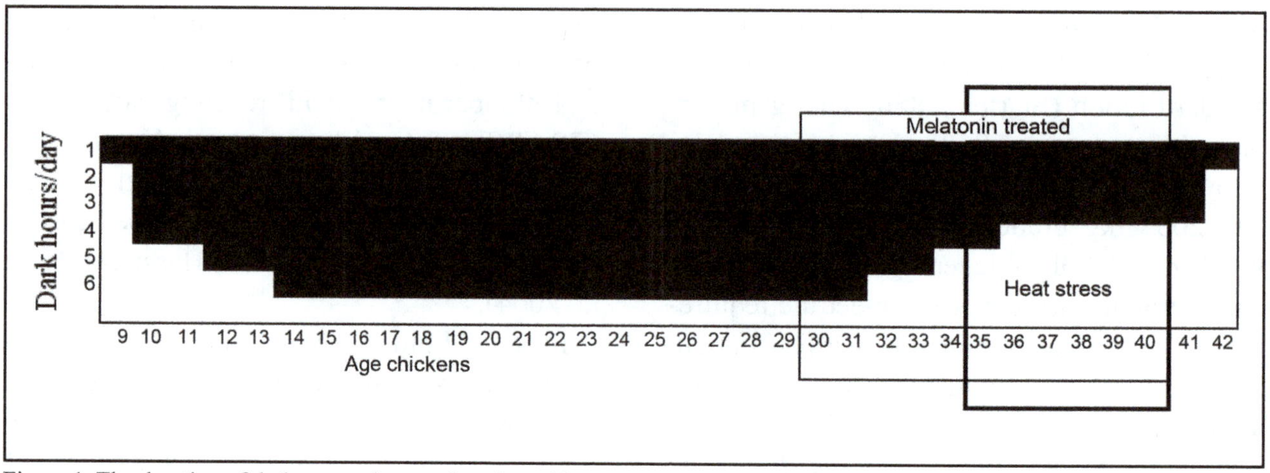

Figure 1. The duration of darkness regime, melatonin and heart stress treatments in experiment.

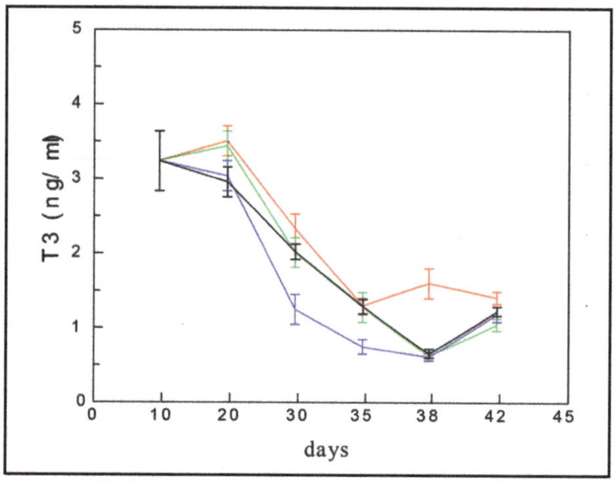

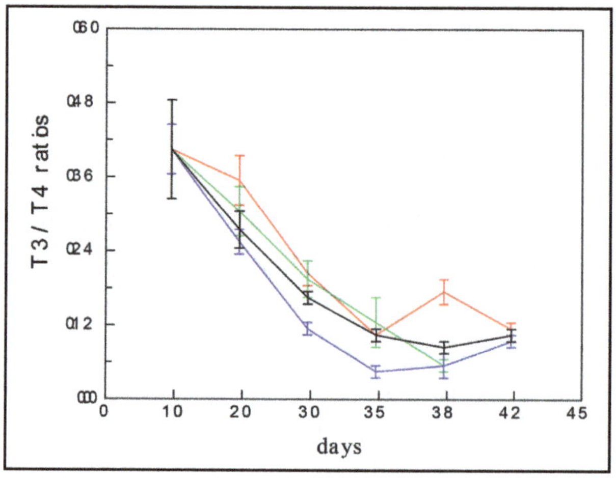

Figure 2. Effects of melatonin supplementation, darkness regime and acute heat stress on plasma T_3. (ng/ml) concentrations and T_3/T_4 ratios. ConN —— ConP —— Dark —— Melat ——

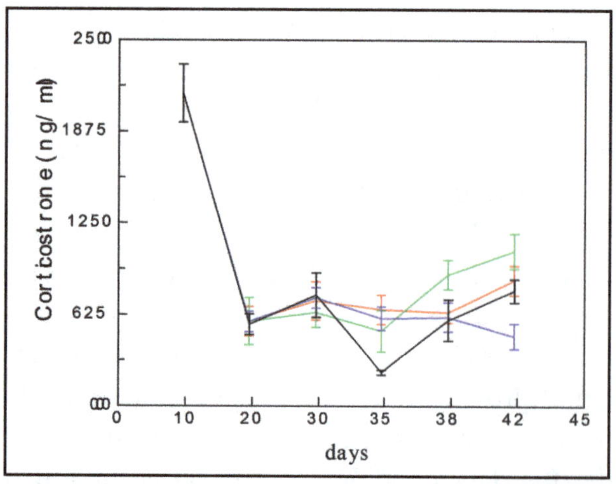

Figure 1. Effects of melatonin supplementation, darkness regime and acute heat stress on plasma corticosterone (ng/ml) concentration. ConN —— ConP —— Dark —— Melat ——

significant at day 35 ($p<0.001$) of age. Meanwhile, melatonin and short period exposure to heating stress had no significant effects on the body weight of chickens (Table 1). Restricting lighting programs and melatonin had also no significant effects on feed intake or feed conversion ratios in all ages. However, feed consumption of dark-reared group chickens tended to be lower from day 14 on, but no significant influence was seen.

At days 30 and 35 of age, mean plasma T3 levels of Dark-reared birds were significantly ($p<0.0001$) lower than the ConN, ConP, and Melat groups. From day 35 onward, plasma T3 concentrations of ConP and Melat groups declined. Therefore, the T3 levels of these two groups of chickens were the same as the darkness regime birds and were significantly ($p<0.0001$) lower compared with the ConN at day 38 of age. Also on day 42, no significant difference was observed between the T3 levels

Table 1. Effects of melatonin supplementation and darkness regime on body weight (BW), feed intake (FI) and FCR of broiler chickens and the number of dead birds due to acute heat stress. (*) number of dead birds to 100 birds. Within rows in each age, means with no common superscripts are significantly different (p<0.05).

Parameters/ age	ConN	ConP	Dark	Melat	p- Values
Dead /total birds*	0/100	10/100	5/100	4/100	-
BW (g) Day 14	388 ± 4	368 ± 8	362 ± 9	383 ± 6	NS
Day 28	1184 ± 13	1210 ± 34	1167 ± 28	1226 ± 23	NS
Day 35	1853 ± 16^a	1842 ± 15^a	1765 ± 17^b	1859 ± 17^a	0.001
Day 42	2275 ± 43	2269 ± 35	2208 ± 37	2264 ± 39	NS
FI (g) Day 1-14	495 ± 3	494 ± 4	497 ± 3	493 ± 2	NS
Day 14-28	1527 ± 44	1505 ± 29	1478 ± 80	1549 ± 31	NS
Day 28-35	1372 ± 20	1381 ± 88	1291 ± 16	1372 ± 32	NS
Day 35-42	1194 ± 56	1217 ± 69	1177 ± 41	1182 ± 55	NS
Day 1-42	4588 ± 66	4597 ± 46	4443 ± 49	4593 ± 67	NS
FCR Day 1-14	1.48 ± 0.05	1.61 ± 0.09	1.60 ± 0.08	1.49 ± 0.12	NS
Day 14-28	1.91 ± 0.11	1.77 ± 0.07	1.83 ± 0.05	1.84 ± 0.06	NS
Day 28-35	2.04 ± 0.05	2.18 ± 0.04	2.16 ± 0.03	2.14 ± 0.07	NS
Day 35-42	2.64 ± 0.21	2.74 ± 0.18	2.65 ± 0.15	2.97 ± 0.18	NS
Day 1-42	2.06 ± 0.11	2.07 ± 0.13	2.05 ± 0.08	2.07 ± 0.14	NS

Table 2. Effects of melatonin supplementation, darkness regime and acute heat stress on plasma TBARS levels. Within rows in each age, means with no common superscripts are significantly different (p<0.05).

Age	ConN	ConP	Dark	Melat	p-Values
TBARS (nm/L)					
Day 10	2.14 ± 0.26	2.17 ± 0.20	2.10 ± 0.19	2.11 ± 0.25	NS
Day 20	2.19 ± 0.38	1.99 ± 0.29	1.85 ± 0.12	1.95 ± 0.26	NS
Day 30	1.53 ± 0.16	1.39 ± 0.11	1.26 ± 0.12	1.46 ± 0.11	NS
Day 35	1.26 ± 0.11	1.43 ± 0.17	1.52 ± 0.21	1.44 ± 0.13	NS
Day 38	1.22 ± 0.05^b	1.51 ± 0.09^a	1.02 ± 0.06^b	1.03 ± 0.08^b	0.05
Day 42	1.25 ± 0.09	1.20 ± 0.10	1.36 ± 0.15	1.27 ± 0.14	NS

of the four groups (Fig. 2).

The results of T3/T4 ratios were almost similar to the T3 levels. Dark-reared birds showed significantly lower T3/T4 ratios than the other three groups on days 30 (p<0.01) and 35 (p<0.001) of age. On day 38, acute heat stress, dark exposure, and melatonin supplementation significantly (p<0.0001) decreased T3/T4 ratios compared to the control birds. No significant difference was pronounced among the T3/T4 ratios of the different groups at the end of the study (Fig. 2).

As shown in Fig. 3, no significant differences were found between the corticosterone values of chickens between the four groups in the first 30 days of the growing period, but melatonin-treated birds had significantly (p<0.0001) lower plasma corticosterone levels at day 35 of age. At day 42 of age, Dark-reared chickens showed significantly (p<0.005) lower plasma corticosterone levels compared to the other three group chickens,

Darkness and melatonin had no significant effects on plasma TBARS in the current study. However, exposure to heat stress had a significant (p<0.05) influence on plasma TBARS levels, only at day 38 of age. At this age, the plasma TBARS level was significantly (p<0.05) higher in ConP broilers compared to their counterparts (Table 2).

Discussion

Heat stress causes a series of physiological and metabolic changes in broiler chickens such as elevated body temperature, panting, and respiratory alkalosis (Deyhim and Teeter, 1991). This results in significant direct economic losses to the broiler industry due to the ruined feed efficiency of the flock and higher mortality rate at farm, especially at marketing ages (Cooper and Washburn, 1998; Naughton et al., 2002; Gharib et al., 2008; Kusandi and Djulardi, 2011). Data in the current study demonstrated that rearing fast growing broiler chickens under darkness regime or feeding with melatonin-supplemented diets leads to a reduction of the mortality rate of broiler chickens when being exposed to acute heat stress. It could be explained by different mechanisms.

Imposing dark schedules reduced the absolute body weight of chickens which coincided with a temporary lower tendency in feed intake (Table 1). This difference in growth rate results in a more concave growth pattern which decreased the heat production of the birds (Buyse et al., 1994; Buys et al., 1998; Julian, 2005) and, consequently, heat-induced mortality (Al-Masri, 2010). Such a claim has already been made in our previous works on ascites syndrome (Buys et al., 1998; Hassanzadeh et al., 2000, 2003, 2005, 2012, 2014), namely that limiting the number of hours of daily light would slightly slow the growth rate, especially at an earlier age. It also reduces the activity of birds that requires additional oxygen. Hence, it would diminish metabolic demands and extra heat production which predisposes chickens to develop metabolic disorders (Julian, 2005; Hassanzadeh et al., 2012, 2014).

It is well known that thyroid hormones play crucial roles in thermoregulation in avian species, and plasma T3 levels are positively correlated with heat production (Buyse et al., 1992; Decuypere and Kühn, 1984, 1988). It is an indicator for the metabolic demand acceleration of the basal metabolic rate by causing an increase in the mitochondria mass, mitochondria cytochrome content, and respiratory rate (Decuypere and Kühn, 1984; Hassanzadeh et al., 2014). In the current study, the decrease of acute heat-induced mortality was accompanied with the diminished T3 and T3/T4 levels at days 30, 35, and 38 of age, in chickens reared under the dark regime (Fig. 1). These are again strengthening the view that a lower metabolic rate had a positive correlation on the side effects of heat-stressed birds. Such an idea is supported by the earlier hypothesis (Apeldoorn et al., 1999; Abbas et al., 2007; Gharib et al., 2008) which stated that restricting light schedules is triggered for heat tolerance, thermoregulation, and hence, health of chickens.

Many biochemical reactions increase with high temperature; it is, thus, very likely that elevated body temperature, in heat stress conditions, would enhance the generation of free radicals via accelerated metabolic reactions in cells and tissues. Lin et al. (2000) suggested that the increased generation of oxygen-free radicals and cytotoxicity of oxidants may mediate in part, heat-induced cellular damage through the lipid peroxidation. In contrast, melatonin, a pineal gland-derived hormone, plays an important role in the antioxidant defense system (Pieri et al., 1994; Barlow-Walden et al., 1995) and has an effective free-radical-scavenging activity (Ozturk et al., 2002). An additional mechanism that could be claimed to be effective in controlling the disadvantages of heat stress is the melatonin treatment of chickens.

Siegel (1995) reported that elevation of plasma corticosterone levels is recognized as an indicator of stress in avian species. Ben Nathan et al. (1976) have argued that exposure to high environmental temperatures will activate the hypothalamo-pituitary-adrenal-axis in chickens that culminates in increased plasma corticosterone levels. Our data showed that the broiler chickens exposed to acute heat stress but fed with a melatonin-supplemented diet (35 d) or reared under the dark program (42 d) had significantly lower plasma corticosterone levels than the ConP group chickens (Fig. 3).

Based on this phenomenon, it is reasonable to hypothesize that these two groups of birds had less difficulty to cope with high environmental temperature and had better tolerance, resulting in numerically reduced dead birds. There is also evidence that melatonin is able to modulate stress at both central and peripheral levels by exerting its inhibitory role in the hypothalamo-pituitaryadrenal axis of chickens and by suppressing hypothalamic gene expression of proopiomelanocortin that encodes ACTH (Decuypere et al., 1989; Rasmussen et al., 2003). The mechanisms might be involved in the current study, since in both Dark and Melat groups heat-induced mortality decrement was accompanied with a significant decrease of plasma corticosterone levels.

A significant elevation of plasma TBARS concentrations observed in ConP but not in the other chicken groups on day 38 of age (Table 2), is included in the studies of Lin et al. (2000) and Mahmoud and Edens (2003), since plasma lipid peroxidation is estimated by determining plasma TBARS (Lin et al., 2004ab). These results proved a disturbance of the equilibrium between the generation and reduction of oxidants that was led to increase lipid peroxidation in ConP birds compared to their counterparts. In contrast, it also means that a positive correlation might exist between dark and melatonin treatments with lipid peroxidation in heat-stressed chickens.

Plasma T3 levels of ConP chickens was significantly lower than the ConN chickens on day 38 of age (Fig. 2), and this is supported by previous studies which have reported that T3 concentrations consistently decrease in high temperature conditions (Geraert et al., 1996; Star et al., 2008). It appears that high temperature conditions improve thermotolerance by enhancing the ability to reduce T3 concentration followed by reducing the heat production of birds (Bowen et al., 1984; Yahav and Hurwitz, 1996).

Overall, no significant effect of melatonin on absolute body weight, feed intake, or feed consumption ratios of chickens was observed throughout the study which is confirmed by Apeldoorn et al. (1999) and Brennan et al. (2002). However, it is inconsistent with the previous reports (Osei et al., 1989; Clark and Classen, 1995) and such differences could be due to the age of birds and/or the duration of melatonin use.

Significant negative effects of high ambient temperature on the growth performance of poultry have been widely reported (Cooper and Washburn, 1998; Sahin et al., 2003; Abbas et al., 2007). However, such results were not observed in our study. Thus, differences were most probably due to the method and the duration of heat exposure to the chickens. In the current study, acute heat stress has been applied for a few hours in the last days of the growing period. Therefore, we observed more acute stress responses, e.g., mortality and hormonal changes when compared with the chronic heat stress response, e.g., the ruined feed efficiency of birds.

Many authors have reported that the change of continuous to restricted lighting schedule is followed by initial growth depression. This depression is, however, followed by a period of compensatory growth in a way that the birds reared in alternative light reached almost the same final body weight at the marketing age, as those reared in continuous light (Classen et al., 1991; Buyse et al., 1994; Buys et al., 1998; Hassanzadeh et al., 2000, 2003, 2012, 2014). In the present study, although full compensatory growth was not achieved by chickens reared under dark conditions compared to their counterparts on 42 days of age, the difference (60 g) was not statistically significant. It seems that occasionally the management activities which are usually implemented to control metabolic disorders, e.g., heat stress at the farm level, are necessary to keep the profitability of broiler chicken farming, even by not being able to achieve the maximum growth potential of broiler chickens at the marketing age. Additionally, our data showed that exposing broiler chickens to acute heat stress but feeding them with a melatonin-supplemented diet or rearing them under the dark program has significantly beneficial effects on the hormonal activities that are involved in many biological functions and the mortality rate of birds. Whether the positive effect of the dark regime seen here can be attributed to itself or to the secretion of melatonin will need further studying.

Acknowledgements

This research was funded by the research committee of the University of Tehran, Faculty of Veterinary Medicine.

References

1. Abbas, A.O., Gehad, A.E., Hendricks, G.L., Gharib, H.B.A., Mushily, M.M. (2007) The effect of lighting program and melatonin on the alleviation of the negative impact of heat stress on the immune response in broiler chickens. Int J Poult Sci. 6: 651- 660.
2. Ahmad, T., Sarwar, M. (2006) Dietary electrolyte balance: Implications in heat stressed broilers. World's Poult Sci J. 62: 638-653.
3. Al-Masri, F. (2010) A comparative study on the influence of different lighting programs and anatomical parameters of cardiopulmonary systems on the incidence of ascites in broiler chickens. Ph.D thesis nr 399, Faculty of Veterinary Medicine, University of Tehran.
4. Ambriz-Tututi, M., Rocha-Gonzalez, HI., Cruz, S.L., Granados-Soto, V. (2009) Melatonin: a hormone that modulates pain. Life Sci. 84: 489-498.
5. Apeldoorn, E.J., Schrama, J.W., Mashaly, M.M., Parmentier, H.K. (1999) Effect of melatonin and lighting schedule on energy metabolism in broiler chickens. Poult Sci. 78: 223- 229.
6. Barlow-Walden, L.R., Reiter, R.J., Abe, M., Pablos, M., Menendez-Pelaez, A., Chen, L.D. (1995) Melatonin stimulates brain glutathione peroxidase activity. Neurochem Int. 26: 497-502.
7. Ben Nathan, D., Heller, E.D., Perek, M. (1976) The effect of short heat stress upon leucocyte count, plasma corticosterone level, plasma and leucocyte ascorbic acid content. Br Poult Sci. 17: 481-485.
8. Blair, R., Newberry, R.C., Gardiner, E.E. (1993) Effects of lighting pattern and dietary tryptophan supplementation on growth and mortality in broilers. Poult Sci. 72: 495-502.
9. Bowen, S.J., Washburn, K.W., Huston, T.M. (1984) Involvement of the thyroid gland in the response of the young chicken to heat stress. Poult Sci. 63: 66-69.
10. Brennan, C.P., Hendricks III., G.L., El-Sheikh, T.M., Mashaly, M. M. (2002) Melatonin and the enhancement of immune responses in immature male chickens. Poult Sci. 81: 371-375.
11. Buys, N., Buyse, J., Hassanzadeh, M., Decuypere, E. (1998) Intermittent lighting reduces the incidence of ascites in broilers: an interaction with protein content of feed on performance and the endocrine system. Poult Sci. 77: 54-61.
12. Buyse, J., Decuypere, E., Berghman, L., Ku¨hn, R.E., Vandesande, F. (1992) Effect of dietary protein content on episotic growth hormone secretion and on heat production of male broiler chickens. Br Poult Sci. 33: 1101-1109.
13. Buyse, J., Decuypere, E., Michels, H. (1994) intermittent lighting and broiler production. 1. Effect on female broiler performance. Arch fürGefl. 58: 69-74.
14. Calder, W., Schmidt-Nielsen, K. (1967) Temperature regulation and evaporation in the pigeon and the roadrunner. Am J Physiol. 213: 883-889.
15. Clark, W.D., Classen, H.L. (1995) The effects of continuously or diurnally fed melatonin on broiler performance and health. Poult Sci. 74: 1900-1904.
16. Classen, H.L., Riddell, C., Robinson, F.E. (1991) Effect of increasing photoperiod length

on performance and health of broiler chickens. Br Poult Sci. 32: 21-29.

17. Cooper, M.A., Washburn, K.W. (1998) The relationships of body temperature to weight gain, feed consumption and feed utilization in broilers under heat stress. Poult Sci. 77: 237-242.
18. Decuypere, E., Kühn, E.R. (1984) Alterations in thyroid hormone physiology induced by temperature and feeding in newly hatched chickens. Acta Physiol. 39: 380-391.
19. Decuypere, E., Scanes, C.G., Kuhn, E.R. (1983) Effects of glucocorticoids on circulating concentrations of thyroxine (T_4) and triiodothyronine (T_3) and on peripheral monodeiodination in pre- and post-hatching chickens. Horm Metab Res. 15: 233-236.
20. Decuypere, E., Darras, V.M., Vermijlen, K. Kuhn, E.R. (1989) Developmental changes in the corticosterone response to corticotrophin and in the adrenal corticosterone content of rapid and slow growing strains of chickens (*Gallus domesticus*). Br Poult Sci. 30: 699-709.
21. Decuypere, E., Vega, C., Bartha, T., Buyse, J., Zoons, J., Albers, G.A.A. (1994) Increased sensitivity to triiodothyronine (T3) of broiler lines with a high susceptibility for ascites. Br Poult Sci. 35: 287-297.
22. Deyhim, F., Teeter, R.G. (1991) Sodium and potassium chloride drinking water supplementation effects on acid-base balance and plasma corticosterone in broilers reared in thermoneutral and heat-distressed environment. Poult Sci. 70: 2551-2553.
23. Dröge, W. (2002) Aging-related changes in the thiol/disulfide redox state: implications for the use of thiol antioxidants. Exp Gerontol. 37: 1333-45.
24. Geraert, P.A., Padilha, J.C., Guillaumin, S. (1996) Metabolic and endocrine changes induced by chronic heat exposure in broiler chickens: biological and endocrinological variables. Br J Nutr. 75: 205-216.
25. Gharib, H.B.A., Desoky, A.A., El-Menawey, M.A., Abbas, A.O., Hendricks, G.L., Mashaly, M. (2008) The role of photoperiod and melatonin on alleviation of the negative impact of heat stress on broilers. Int J Poult Sci. 7: 749-756.
26. Halliwell, B.H., Gutteridge, J.M.C. (1989) Free Radicals in Biology and Medicine. (2nd ed.) Oxford, UK. Clarendon Press.
27. Hassanzadeh, M., Bozorgmeri, F.M.H., Akbari, A.R., Buyse, J., Decuypere, E. (2000) Effect of intermittent lighting schedules during the natural scotoperiod on T3-induced ascites in broiler chickens. Avian Pathol. 29: 433-439.
28. Hassanzadeh, M., Bozorgmehri, F.M.H., Buyse, J., Decuypere, E. (2003) The beneficial effects of alternative lighting schedules on the incidence of ascites and metabolic parameters of broiler chickens. Acta Vet Hung. 51: 513-520.
29. Hassanzadeh, M., Bozorgmeri fard, M.H., Buyse, J. Bruggeman, V., Decuypere, E. (2004) Effect of chronic hypoxia during the embryonic development on the physiological functioning and on hatching parameters related to ascites syndrome in broiler chickens. Avian pathol. 33: 558-564.
30. Hassanzadeh, M., Shojadoost, B., Feyzih, A., Buyse, J., Decuypere, E. (2005) Effect of intermittent lighting schedules at the young age of broiler chickens on the incidence of ascites and metabolic parameters. Arch Geflügelkd. 69: 57-61.
31. Hassanzadeh, M., Al-Masri, F., Maddadi, M.S., Shojaei, H., Eghbalian, A., Abbasi, S., Yousefi, K. (2012) Comparative study on the beneficial effects of different dark length schedules on the incidence of ascites and metabolic parameters in fast growing broiler chickens. Iran J Vet Med (University of Tehran). 6: 113- 121.
32. Hassanzadeh, M., Buyse, J., Toloei, T., Decuypere, E. (2014) Ascites syndrome in broiler chickens: A review on the aspect of endogenous and exogenous factors interactions. J Poult Sci. 51: 229-241.
33. Iqbal, A., Decuypere, E., Abd El Azim, A., Kuhn, E.R. (1990) Pre- and post-hatch high

temperature exposure affects the thyroid hormones and corticosterone response to acute heat stress in growing chickens (*Gallus domesticus*). J Therm Biol. 15: 149-153.
34. Julian, R.J. (2005) Production and growth related disorders and other metabolic disease of poultry-a review. Vet J. 169: 350-369.
35. Kusandi, E., Djulardi, A. (2011) Physiological dynamics of broilers at various environmental temperatures. Int J Poult Sci. 10: 19-22.
36. Lara, L.J., Rostagno, M.H. (2013) Impact of heat stress on poultry production. Animals. 3: 356-369.
37. Lin, H., Du, R., Zhang, Z.Y. (2000) The peroxidation in tissues of heat-stress broilers. Asian-Aust J Anim Sci. 13: 1373-1376.
38. Lin, H., Decuypere, E., Buyse, J. (2004a) Oxidative stress induced by corticosterone administration in broiler chickens (*Gallus gallus domesticus*) 1. Chronic exposure. Comp Biochem Physiol B. 139: 737-744.
39. Lin, H., Decuypere, E., Buyse, J. (2004b) Oxidative stress induced by corticosterone administration in broiler chickens (*Gallus gallus domesticus*) 2. Short-term effect. Comp Biochem Physiol B. 139: 745-751.
40. Lin, H., Jiao., Buyse, J., Decuypere, E. (2006a) Strategies for preventing heat stress in Poultry, World's Poult. Sci. J. 62: 71-89.
41. Lin, H., Decuypere, E., Buyse, J. (2006) Acute heat stress induces oxidative injury in broiler chickens. Comp Biochem Physiol A. 144: 11-17.
42. Mahmoud, K., Edens, F.W. (2003) Influence of selenium sources on age-related and mild heat stress-related changes of blood and liver glutathione redox cycle in broiler chickens (*Gallus domesticus*). Comp Biochem Physiol Part B. 136: 921-934.
43. May, J.D., Deaton, J.W., Reece, F.N., Branton, S.L. (1986) Effect of acclimation and heat stress on thyroid hormone concentration. Poultry Sci. 65: 1211-1213.
44. Naughton, M.P., Henderson, A., Mirabelli, M.C, Kaiser, R., Wilhelm, J.L., Kieszak, S.M. (2002) Heat-related mortality during a 1999 heat wave in Chicago. Am J Prev Med. 22: 221-227.
45. National Research Council. Subcommittee on Poultry, N. (1994) Nutrient requirements of poultry. National Academies Press. Washington, USA.
46. Osei, P., Robbins, K.R., Shirley, H.V. (1989) Effect of exogenous melatonin on growth and energy metabolism of chickens. Nutr Res. 9: 69-81.
47. Ozturk, G., Coskun, S., Erbas, G. (2002) Effect of melatonin treatment on serum and tissue zinc levels in rats. J Trace Elem Exp Med. 15: 1-8.
48. Pieri, C., Marra, M., Moroni, F. (1994) Melatonin: a peroxyl radical scavenger more effective than vitamin E. Life Sci. 55: 271-276.
49. Rasmussen, D.D., Marck, B.T., Boldt, B.M., Yellon, S.M., Matsumoto, A.M. (2003) Suppression of hypothalamic pro-opiomelanocortin (POMC) gene expression by daily melatonin supplementation in aging rats. J Pineal Res. 34: 127-33.
50. Sanotra, G., Damkjer, S., Lund, J., Vestergaard, K.S. (2002) Influence of light-dark schedules and stocking density on behaviour, risk of leg problems and occurrence of chronic fear in broilers. Br Poult Sci. 43: 344-354.
51. Sahin, N., Onderci, M., Sahin, K., Smith, M.O. (2003) Melatonin supplementation can ameliorate the detrimental effects of heat stress on performance and carcass traits of Japanese quail. Biol Trace Elem Res. 96: 169-172.
52. Siegel, H.S. (1995) Stress, strain, and resistance. Br Poult Sci. 36: 3-22.
53. Star, L., Decuypere, E., Parmentier, H.K., Kemp, B. (2008) Effect of single or combined climatic and hygienic stress in four layer lines: 2. Endocrine and oxidative stress responses. Poult Sci. 87: 1031-1038.
54. Stub, C., Vestegaard, K.S. (2001) Influence of zinc bacitracin, light regimen and dustbathing on the health and welfare of broiler chickens. Br Poult Sci. 42: 564-568.

55. Yahav, S., Hurwitz, H. (1996) Induction of thermotolerance in male broiler chickens by temperature conditioning at an early age. Poult Sci. 75: 402-406.
56. Yahav, S., McMurtry, J.P. (2001) Thermotolerance acquisition in broiler chickens by temperature conditioning early in life—the effect of timing and ambient temperature. Poult Sci. 80: 1662-1666.

Efficacy of *Echinacea purpurea* and protexin on systemic and mucosal immune response to Newcastle diseases virus vaccination (VG/GA strain) in commercial turkey poults

Tolouei, T.[1], Hassanzadeh, M.[1*], Nikbakht, Gh.[2], Alkaragoly, H.[2], Rezaei Far, A.[1], Ghahri, H.[3]

[1]*Department of Avian Diseases, Faculty of Veterinary Medicine, University of Tehran, Tehran, Iran*

[2]*Department of Microbiology and Immunology, Faculty of Veterinary Medicine, University of Tehran, Tehran, Iran*

[3]*Department of Poultry Sciences, Faculty of Veterinary Medicine, Islamic Azad University, Urmia Branch, Urmia, Iran*

Key words:

Echinacea purpurea, immunological parameters, probiotic, turkey, VG/GA vaccine

Correspondence

Hassanzadeh, M.

Department of Avian Diseases, Faculty of Veterinary Medicine, University of Tehran, Tehran, Iran

Email: mhzadeh@ut.ac.ir

Abstract:

BACKGROUND: It is important to understand the efficacy of immunoregulatory materials, herbal remedies or probiotics, in different parts of immune system following vaccination with different tropism. **OBJECTIVES:** Aim of this study was to evaluate the effect of *Echinacea purpurea* and a probiotic (protexin) on systemic and mucosal immune response in turkey. **METHODS:** A total of 288 1-day-old male turkey poults were randomized into 6 groups as follow: Group T1: Turkeys received *Echinacea purpurea* at the rate of 1 ml /1 liter water and Newcastle disease virus (NDV) vaccine, Group T2: Turkeys received probiotic at the rate of 1 g /1 liter water and NDV vaccine, Group T3: Positive control, turkey received NDV vaccine without any additives. Group T4: Turkeys received *Echinacea purpurea* at the rate of 1 ml /1 liter water without NDV vaccine. Group T5: Turkeys received probiotic at the rate of 1 g /1 liter water without NDV vaccine, Group T6: Negative control group, neither vaccinated against NDV vaccine nor given additives. At age of 10 and 20 days, poults were vaccinated with Villegas-Glisson/University of Georgia (VG/GA) strain of Newcastle disease vaccine by eye dropper method. For systemic and mucosal antibody analyses, blood samples and tracheal lavages were collected at different ages. The titers of antibody against NDV were measured using ELISA and HI tests. **RESULTS:** Addition of Echinacea to the water increased the systemic IgG, IgA and HI compared to the positive control group. Protexin supplementation to the water of T2 turkeys increased serum IgG and both total and specific IgA compared to the T3 group turkeys. Generally, turkeys that were supplemented with probiotic had higher specific and total tracheal IgA antibody levels than the other vaccinated groups. Among vaccinated turkeys only T1 group showed significantly higher HI antibody titers on day 42. **CONCLUSIONS:** Results indicated that systemic and mucosal immunity of turkeys following vaccination against Newcastle disease (ND) could be improved by supplementation of Echinacea and probiotic. The effect of *Echinacea purpurea* on systemic immunity of turkeys seemed more pronounced than on mucosal immunity; further, the effect of probiotic on mucosal immunity was more obvious.

Introduction

Nowadays, turkeys are raised under intensive production systems in densely populated colonies or flocks to achieve high levels of economic efficiency. In this intensive rearing process, turkeys may get stress from various factors such as overcrowding, unfavorable ambient temperature, feed-intake and vaccination. The application of herbal supplements such as *Echinacea purpurea* (EP) and probiotic could boost immunological reactivity, which contributes to better health and minimizes the stresses in turkeys.

Echinacea purpurea is one of the most important medical herbs. Its root and subterranean stem are widely used around the world to treat common cold and other infectious disorders with the claim of having para immunity-inducing and non-specific immune responses stimulating effects. All kinds of EP contain similar main ingredients including caffeic acid derivatives, alkamides, flavonoids, essential oils, and polyacetylenes (Manayi et al., 2015). The EP has been proven to show good immunoregulation, anti-inflammation and antioxidant capacity (Lee et al., 2009, 2012) with no hypersensitivity or other side effects (Saunders et al., 2007). A recent review showed that Echinacea treatment resulted in an increase of various cytokines, lymphocytes, and phagocytosis activity (Bauer, 2002; Fonseca et al., 2015). Studies with Echinacea to improve animal husbandry are rare. Kuhn et al. (2005) reported an immune stimulating effect in sows by a repeated 5 days of application of Echinacea juice.

Probiotics are defined as feed additives containing live microorganisms. Administration of probiotics has improved growth performance and feed efficiency (Getachew, 2016) and also stimulated the production of natural antibodies in chickens (Wondmeneh, et al., 2015). Actually, probiotics act by different means including adherence to the binding sites of the intestinal epithelium, competition with pathogenic bacteria and stimulus to the immune system (Menten, 2002). Balanced microbiota and a concomitant modulation of the host immune system are potential health-promoting probiotic effects. The use of protective probiotic cultures in poultry farming may serve as a useful strategy to improve food product safety right from the beginning of the food chain and thus may serve to protect consumer health (Seifert et al., 2011).

The importance of antibodies in the defense mechanism against viral infection has been emphasized by many studies (Scott, 2004). It appears that local immunity acts as a barrier at surfaces where primary viral infections occur, thereby interfering with further spread of the virus (Jayawardane and Spradbrow, 1995). Birds have a well-developed mucosal immune system and its characteristics include local production and secretion of IgA antibodies and traffic of IgA producing plasma cells (Al-Garib et al., 2003). The IgA class predominates and is detectable in tears, saliva, tracheal, intestinal washings and bile. The intranasal or eye drop vaccination with NDV induces antigen specific- IgA which can be detected in tears and tracheal washings (Ganapathy et al., 2005).

In the present study, the tropism of vaccine virus in turkey poults was used with the follow up of the local and systemic immunity measurements. To this aim, tracheal lavages were obtained in order to measure the level of IgA titer induced by specific

VG/GA strain vaccination.

The VG/GA strain of NDV isolated from the intestine of healthy turkeys is proposed to replicate both in the respiratory and intestinal tract, with preference for the intestine (Perozo et al., 2008). Most of the commercially available lentogenic vaccines are able to induce antibodies against NDV, however, systemic humoral immune response measured as the presence of specific NDV antibodies in serum is not enough for protection (Kapczynski et al., 2013; Reynolds and Maraqa, 2000). It has been established that the mucosal immunity represented by immunoglobulin A (IgA) production plays an important role in the development of protection in chickens vaccinated against NDV (Reynolds and Maraqa, 2000; Scott, 2004). We believe that it could be the same in turkeys. Therefore, in the present study, the mucosal and systemic humoral immune responses of male turkey poults were measured when they were vaccinated by VG/GA strain and also treated with *Echinacea purpurea* and probiotic to possibly enhance immune response of turkeys following NDV vaccination.

Materials and Methods

Experimental design and birds: A total of 288 1-day-old turkey poults of premium strain were obtained from a commercial hatchery (ZarinJooje) and kept for 42 days in the experimental rooms, in the Research Center, Faculty of Veterinary Medicine, University of Tehran, located in Karaj.

The poults were raised in concrete floor pens covered with 8 cm of clean pine wood shavings, and each pen was equipped with one tube feeder and one automatic drinker. Throughout the study, the turkeys were grown following standard temperature regimens, which were gradually decreased from 38 to 23°C. Turkeys were maintained on a 16L: 8D schedule and allowed to consume feed and water ad libitum. Air temperature was controlled according to Aviagen recommendations. A completely randomized experimental design was used, and poults were randomized into six groups, with four replicates per treatment and 12 poults (tom) per replicate as follows: Group T1: Turkeys received *Echinacea purpurea* at the rate of 1 ml/1 liter water and Newcastle disease virus (NDV) vaccine, Group T2: Turkeys received probiotic at the rate of 1 g/1 liter water and NDV vaccine, Group T3: Positive control, turkeys received NDV vaccine without any additives. Group T4: Turkeys received *Echinacea purpurea* at the rate of 1 ml/1 liter water without NDV vaccine. Group T5: Turkeys received probiotic at the rate of 1 g/1 liter water without NDV vaccine, Group T6: Negative control group, neither vaccinated against NDV vaccine nor given additives. Diets were fed in pellet form. The basal control diet was formulated and compounded to meet the nutritional requirements of commercial turkey, according to Aviagen manual. The juice of *Echinacea purpurea* (EP) and Protexin were treated intermittently which was supplied on days 1-3 of age and repeated three times on days 8-9, 18-19 and finally days 30-31 of the rearing period.

In this study a commercial probiotic (Protexin®) was used. Protexin is a highly concentrated pre-mix containing seven strains of bacteria (*Lactobacillus plantarum*, *Lactobacillus delbrueckii* subsp. Bulgaricus, *Lactobacillus acidophilus*, *Lactobacillus rhamnosus*, *Bifidobacterium bifidum*, *Streptococcus salivarius* subsp. Thermophilus,

Enterococcus faecium) and two yeasts (Aspergillus oryza, Candida pintolopesii). The juice of EP which was used in this trial contained caffeic acid derivatives, alkamides, flavonoids, polyacetylenes, mannos, glucomannan, arachidonic acid, and acetylated glucomannan. For preparation of EP juice, briefly, aloe vera leaves were obtained from Pars Immen Darou Co. They were washed with distilled water and sterilized with 70% ethyl alcohol. The gel was drained out. Then, leaf gel was dried at 80°C for 48 h and was powdered. 30 g of the powder was soaked in 200 ml of ethanol for 24 h, filtered and evaporated to dry. The obtained extract was dissolved in distilled water.

Vaccination and serology: Newcastle disease vaccine used in this study was a freeze-dried live vaccine against Newcastle disease produced by Merial Animal Health Limited (Lyon, France). The vaccine contained ND viruses of the VG/GA strain (lineage IIvirus), a lentogenic and naturally occurring strain in turkeys. Each dose (1 m) was determined via viral titration to contain 106.5 EID50 (50 percent Embryo Infectious Dose). At the age of 10 and 20 days, all poults were vaccinated with Avinew® Newcastle disease vaccine by eye dropper except for negative control group according to the recommendation of the manufacturer.

Systemic humoral immune response: On 10, 20, 28, 35 and 42 days of age, twelve turkeys from each experimental group were bled. Serum samples were taken, frozen and used for titration of antibody against NDV by Haemagglutination-inhibition (HI) test. Measurement of serum IgA and IgG was performed by Elisa method using a commercial ND Elisa kit (Flock check; IDEXX, Maine, USA).

Total and NDV-specific IgA detections: On 21, 22 and 23 days post hatch, six turkeys per group were selected to obtain tracheal lavages. Briefly, turkeys were killed humanely using a carbon dioxide chamber, the trachea was dissected out immediately after death for the collection of tracheal secretion. They were washed internally by flushing through 1.5 ml PBS 10 times (tracheal washings) and cut longitudinally, then transversely to give 4 pieces, each of which was gently scraped on its internal surface with a scalpel (tracheal scrapings). The scrapings were collected into a total of 2 ml PBS. At all stages great care was taken to avoid contamination with blood. Samples were placed in sterile containers and processed fresh. NDV-specific IgA levels in tracheal lavages were assayed two times using an indirect ELISA as described previously (Raj and Jones, 1996), except that the coating antigen used was the VG/GA strain of NDV and the chicken IgA binding to the coating antigen was detected with horse radish peroxidase (HRP)-labeled goat anti-chicken IgG (AbDSerotec, Oxford, UK).

To estimate the total (unspecific) IgA production in the respiratory mucosa, direct total IgA ELISA was performed. Microtiter plates were coated with 100 µl of serially diluted tracheal lavages. Overnight plates were washed with PBST and blocked with 100 µl of PBS-Blotto for 2 h at room temperature. Plates were washed three times with PBST before adding 100 µl of (1:10000) diluted conjugate and HRP-labeled goat anti-chicken IgA (AbDSerotec, Oxford, UK). Absorbance at 450 nm was measured using a microplate reader (Stat FAX 2000, Awareness Technology, Inc., USA).

Statistical analysis: Statistical analysis was performed using the "General linear model procedure" (SAS Institute Inc., 2008). If a significant overall effect ($p<0.05$) was found, treatment means were compared using the Scheffe test.

Results

Serum antibody response: The effects of *Echinacea purpurea* and probiotic treatments on specific serum IgG, IgA and HI antibodies production against NDV in turkeys are presented in Figs. 1-3. In the present study, vaccinated turkeys showed significantly ($p<0.0001$) higher titers of serum IgG, IgA and HI against NDV when compared to those of the non-vaccinated turkeys in all ages, except on day 20 that T3 group (positive control) turkeys showed significantly lower specific serum IgA titer (Fig. 2).

Addition of *Echinacea purpurea* to the water of T1 turkeys increased the IgG antibody titer production compared to the positive control turkeys from day 20 to day 42. EP increased the specific serum IgA titer of T1 turkeys compared to that of the positive control (T3), however, the difference was significant on 20, 28 and 35 days of age ($p<0.01$).

Among the vaccinated turkeys, addition of *Echinacea purpurea* to the water of T1 group turkeys influenced HI antibody titers compared to the T3 turkeys, however, the difference was only significant on day 42 of age ($p<0.01$) (Fig. 3).

Overall, Protexin supplementation to the water of T2 turkeys increased serum IgG antibody against NDV compared to the T3 group, however, the difference was only significant on day 28 ($p<0.05$) (Fig. 1). Protexin treated turkeys showed significantly higher specific serum IgA antibody titers (Fig. 2) against NDV compared to the T3 group turkeys on days 20, 28 and 35 of

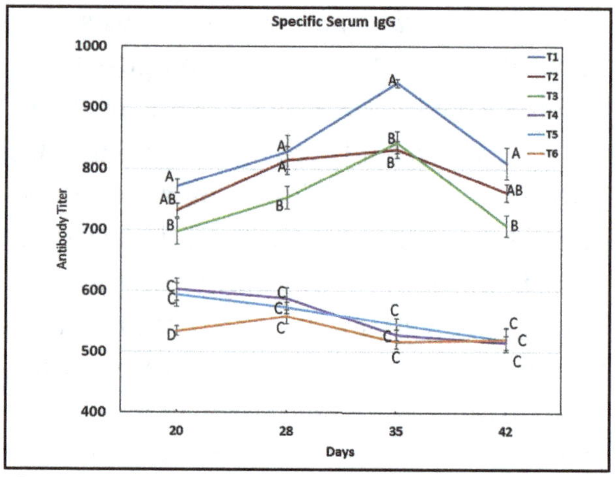

Figure 1. Effect of *Echinacea purpurea* and Protexin on specific serum IgG antibody titers against NDV vaccination turkey poults (12 samples/group) from 20 to 42 days of age. Values within an age with no common letters differ significantly. T1: Turkeys received NDV vaccine and *Echinacea purpurea*; T2: Turkeys received NDV vaccine and probiotic; T3: Turkeys received NDV vaccine without additives; T4: Turkeys received *Echinacea purpurea* without vaccination; T5: Turkeys received probiotic without vaccination; T6: Turkeys received no vaccine and no additives.

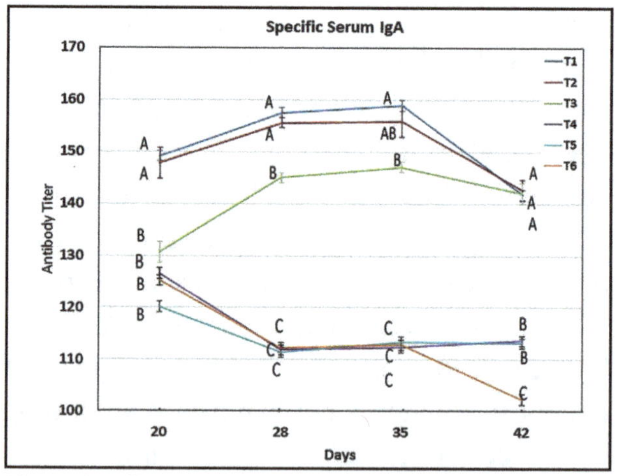

Figure 2. Effect of *Echinacea purpurea* and Protexin on specific serum IgA antibody titers against NDV vaccination turkey poults (12 samples/group) from 20 to 42 days of age. Values within an age with no common letters differ significantly. T1: Turkeys received NDV vaccine and *Echinacea purpurea*; T2: Turkeys received NDV vaccine and probiotic; T3: Turkeys received NDV vaccine without additives; T4: Turkeys received *Echinacea purpurea* without vaccination; T5: Turkeys received probiotic without vaccination; T6: Turkeys received no vaccine and no additives.

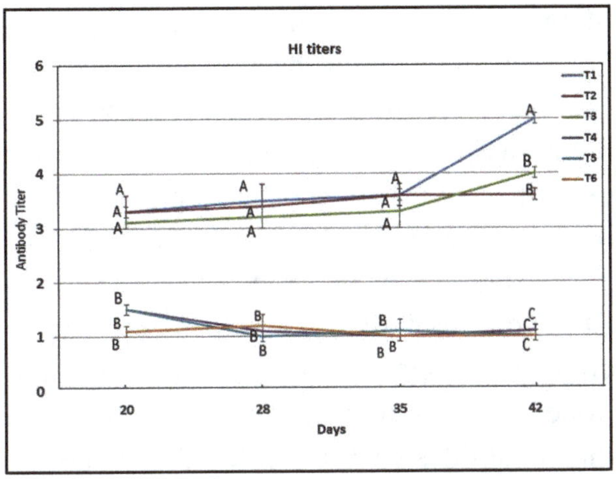

Figure 3. Effect of *Echinacea purpurea* and Protexin on HI antibody titers against NDV vaccination turkey poults (12 samples/group) from 20 to 42 days of age. Values within an age with no common letters differ significantly. T1: Turkeys received NDV vaccine and *Echinacea purpurea*; T2: Turkeys received NDV vaccine and probiotic; T3: Turkeys received NDV vaccine without additives; T4: Turkeys received *Echinacea purpurea* without vaccination; T5: Turkeys received probiotic without vaccination; T6: Turkeys received no vaccine and no additives.

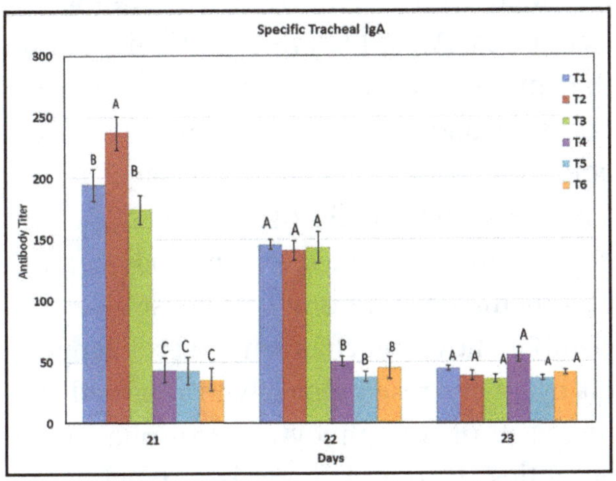

Figure 4. Effect of *Echinacea purpurea* and Protexin on specific tracheal IgA antibody titers against NDV vaccination turkey poults (6 samples/group) from 20 to 42 days of age. Values within an age with no common letters differ significantly. T1: Turkeys received NDV vaccine and *Echinacea purpurea*; T2: Turkeys received NDV vaccine and probiotic; T3: Turkeys received NDV vaccine without additives; T4: Turkeys received *Echinacea purpurea* without vaccination; T5: Turkeys received probiotic without vaccination; T6: Turkeys received no vaccine and no additives.

age ($p<0.001$). Between two groups of vaccinated (T2 and T3) turkeys, Protexin supplementation had no significant effect on HI titers ($p>0.05$) (Fig. 3).

Throughout the experimental period T1 group turkeys that received EP showed higher serum IgG titers against NDV than Protexin treated turkeys (T2), however, the difference was only significant on day 35 of age ($p<0.005$) (Fig. 1). No significant differences on serum IgA titer was found between the EP (T1) and the Protexin (T2) treated turkeys during the whole experimental period (Fig. 3). Comparing two vaccinated group turkeys (T1 and T2) it could be seen that HI titer of EP treated turkeys was only significantly higher than the Protexin supplemented on day 42 of age ($p<0.005$) (Fig. 3).

Mucosal antibody response: The results of specific and total tracheal IgA titers against NDV in turkeys are shown in Figs. 4 and 5. Specific tracheal IgA titers against NDV were significantly increased in vaccinated turkeys compared to those of the non-vaccinated group turkeys on days 21 and 22 of age ($p<0.0001$), however, it was not observed on day 23. On day 21, specific tracheal IgA titer tended to be significant ($p<0.06$) which was higher in protexin treated turkeys (T2) compared to the EP treated (T1) and even with the positive control (T3) group (Fig. 4). EP or Protexin did not show significant effect on specific tracheal IgA titers on days 22 and 23 of age ($p>0.05$). On day 23 of age, almost the same specific IgA titers were observed between vaccinated and non-vaccinated turkeys.

Total tracheal IgA titers against NDV were significantly higher in three groups of vaccinated turkeys in comparison with those of the non-vaccinated turkeys on days 21 and 22 of age ($p<0.0001$) (Fig. 5). However, on day 23 the picture was different

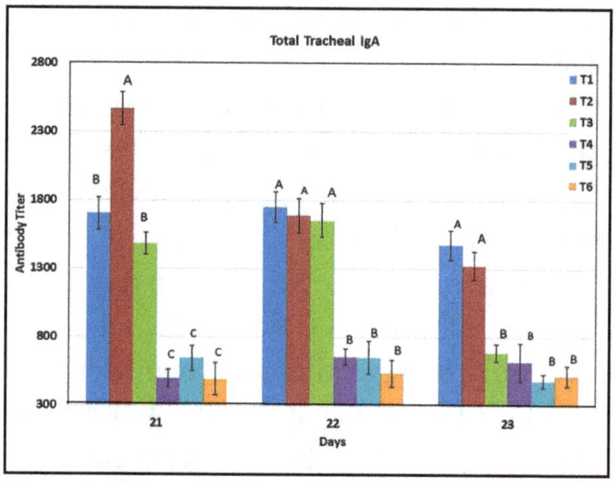

Figure 5. Effect of *Echinacea purpurea* and Protexin on total tracheal IgA antibody titers against NDV vaccination turkey poults (6 samples/group) from 20 to 42 days of age. Values within an age with no common letters differ significantly. T1: Turkeys received NDV vaccine and *Echinacea purpurea*; T2: Turkeys received NDV vaccine and probiotic; T3: Turkeys received NDV vaccine without additives; T4: Turkeys received *Echinacea purpurea* without vaccination; T5: Turkeys received probiotic without vaccination; T6: Turkeys received no vaccine and no additives.

among the three vaccinated groups of turkeys. In this age, EP (T1) and protexin (T2) treated turkeys presented significantly higher total tracheal IgA titers compared to the positive control (T3) group ($p<0.01$) (Fig. 5). On day 21, the turkeys supplemented with Protexin (T2) had significantly higher total tracheal IgA levels compared to those of the T1 and T3 groups ($p<0.0001$).

Discussion

The current study was the first report on the effect of EP and a probiotic like Protexin on systemic and local immunity of turkey poults, when birds received the VG/GA strain vaccine against NDV. In the present study, the vaccinated turkeys which consumed EP showed higher serum and mucosal antibody responses. However, regarding our results, it seems that efficiency of EP was more pronounced on the serum specific IgG and IgA titers than probiotic. The effect of probiotic on specific and total tracheal IgA was much better than EP.

It has been shown that Echinacea treatment has resulted in an increase of various cytokines, lymphocytes, and phagocytosis activity (Bauer, 2002; Fonseca et al., 2015). This effect might be related to alkamids in EP. The role of alkamides as an active principle of Echinacea has already been mentioned by Cruz et al. (2014). Authors argued that alkamides were considered as a class of cannabinomimetics and therefore a possible mode of action to modulate immune functions. Additionally, Cundell et al. (2003) found a significant increase in lymphocytes in rats when they were fed with dried Echinacea preparations for one week. Habibian Dehkordi et al. (2011) found a stimulation of the phagocytic response in chickens provided with ground root preparations of Echinacea. Also, the effect of Echinacea on the immune system is suggested by various substances such as derivate of caffeic acid (cichoric acid) and polysaccharides. The phagocytic cells of the innate system act within the context of antibody- and B cell-mediated immunity (Davison et al., 2008). These mechanisms were supported by many researchers who reported that increase of lymphocytes and phagocytic activities were a characteristic reaction associated with efficacy of Echinacea (Habibian Dehkordi et al., 2011; Barrett, 2003, Cundell et al., 2003). Moreover, Park et al, (2016) reported that stimulation of both humoral and cell mediated immunity through the enhanced production of natural interferons/cytokines increased macrophage, lymphocyte and natural killer (NK) cell activity, up-regulated oxidative burst in heterophils and also increased IgG, IgM and IgA. Based on this information it could be suggested that the improvement of systemic and mucosal antibodies observed in the present study could also be related to increase in activity of different kinds of immune cells by consumption of EP in turkeys.

It has been well documented that intermittent application of EP in humans has a significant effect on immunity, because immunity over stimulation was eliminated. Furthermore, the interval between applications was also recommended two to three times during the application (Jurcic et al., 1989). In the present study, the juice of EP was supplemented intermittently for a limited period of time on days 1-3, 8-9, 18-19 and 30-31 of the rearing period. This might have been potentiated to increase the humoral immune response of turkeys, especially serum IgG concentration. The benefits of such model treatment have already been studied in some other animals, e.g. layers, sows and piglets (Schranner et al., 1989; Kuhn et al., 2005; Abdel-Fattah et al., 2008; Bohmer et al., 2008).

According to our data, probiotic supplementation showed a slight increase in specific serum IgG, however, it significantly affected specific serum IgA when compared to the results of the control positive (T3) group turkeys. Furthermore, the effect of probiotic supplementation on mucosal antibodies was clearer, especially on day 21 of age, when compared to the effect of EP treated group.

Talazadeh et al. (2016) pointed that the direct effect of probiotic on increase in immune activity might be related to stimulation of the lymphatic tissue, whereas the indirect effect may occur via changing the microbial population of the lumen of gastrointestinal tract. Mehdizadeh Taklimi, et al. (2012) pointed out that the bursa of probiotic-treated chickens showed an increase in the number of follicles with high plasma cell reaction in the medulla. Similarly, increase in the weight of the thymus might be due to the effect of probiotic bacteria on functional activities of the immune system responses; this could result in increase in the number of lymphocytes in the primary lymphoid organs, as feeding of broilers with probiotic increased relative weights of spleen (Guimarães et al., 2014). Brisbin et al., (2011) suggested that some of these effects were mediated by cytokines secreted by immune system cells stimulated with probiotic bacteria.

Ao et al. (2013) indicated that defense cells in the gut-associated lymphoid tissue (GALT) could detect the presence of microbes by recognizing molecules unique to microorganisms then could increase the number of different lymphocytes and/or leukocytes in the GALT and in peripheral blood. In agreement with all of these researchers we could conclude that stimulating of such different defense cells, e.g. B and T lymphocytes or tissues like bursa or thymus, could directly modulate systemic and mucosal immune responses (Toloei et al., 2010; Ghahri et al., 2010).

The main site of the mucosal immune system in the respiratory tract is referred to as bronchus-associated lymphoid tissue (BALT), with the immune-associated cells including mast cells, goblet cells and secretory IgA (sIgA)-positive cells that are involved in many processes to prevent pathogen invasion (De Geus et al., 2012). Active replication in the mucosa induces virus protein production and local antigen presentation through MHC class I and II molecules stimulating a T-dependent B-cell response at the site of infection in the form of IgA-producing plasma cells in the respiratory trachea (Al-Garib et al., 2003).

Our results showed that the production of total and specific tracheal IgA increased in the treated groups which received vaccine in comparison with the control groups. The level of both total and specific tracheal IgA responses increased from 24 to 72 hours in the vaccinated turkeys and the highest level of antibody was observed at 24 and 48 hours after vaccination. These findings are very important because specific IgA plays a major role in protecting mucosal surfaces against colonization and possible invasion of pathogenic microorganisms (Corthesy and Kraehenbuhl, 1999).

Also, our results demonstrated that the level of the total and specific tracheal IgA following vaccination decreased shortly in few days. This might be because of fast clearance of VG/GA from the respiratory tract after vaccination (Perozo et al., 2008). Based on how fast the VG/GA is cleared from respiratory tract after priming the mucosal immune response, the mucosal IgA production in the respiratory and the levels of protection afforded by single or multiple doses of the vaccine, initial vaccination with the VG/GA strain may be advantageous for the integrity of the respiratory mucosa in young chickens when multiple vaccination and field exposure are expected (Perozo et al., 2008).

It is concluded that the systemic and mucosal immunity of turkeys following vaccination against NDV could be improved by supplementation of *Echinacea purpurea* and probiotic. It seems the effect of *Echinacea purpurea* on systemic immunity of turkeys is much better than on mucosal immunity. The effect of probiotic on mucosal immunity of tracheal was observed much clearer. So far, there are no studies available on the exact mode of action on activating the specific immune systems by Echinacea components or even probiotic. It is possible that the presence of pathogen associated molecular patterns, which are recognized by toll-like receptors and other pattern recognition receptors, could contribute to affect the specific immune system. This effect of Echinacea to stimulate adaptive immune function needs further researches.

Acknowledgements

This research was supported by the Research Committee of the University of Tehran, Faculty of Veterinary Medicine. The authors also would like to thank Zarin Jooje Shomal Company for delivery of turkey chickens.

References

Abdel-Fattah, S.A., El-Sanhoury, MH., El-Mednay, N.M., Abdel-Azeem, F. (2008) Thyroid activity, some blood constituents, organs morphology and performance of broiler chicks fed supplemental organic acids. Int J Poult Sci. 7: 215-222.

Al-Garib, S.O., Gruys, E., Gielkens, A.L., Koch, G. (2003) Detection of antibody-forming cells directed against Newcastle disease virus and their immunoglobulin class by double immunoenzymehisto chemistry. Avian Dis. 47: 453-457.

Ao, Z., Choct, M. (2013) Oligosaccharides affect performance and gut development of broiler chickens. Asian-Australas J Anim Sci. 26: 116-121.

Barrett, B. (2003) Medicinal properties of Echinacea: a critical review. Phytomedicine 10: 66-86.

Bauer, R. (2002) NeueErkenntnissezurWirkung und Wirksamkeit von *Echinacea pur-*

purea-Preßsaftzubereitungen. Wien Med Wochenschr. 15: 407-411.

Bohmer, M.B., Salisch, H., Paulicks, B.R., Roth, F.X. (2008) *Echinacea purpurea* as a potential immunostimulatory feed additive in laying hens and fattening pigs by intermittent application. Livest Sci. 122: 81-85.

Brisbin, J.T, Gong, J., Orouji, S., Esufali, J., Mallick, A., Parvizi, P., Patricia, E. (2011) Oral treatment of chickens with lactobacilli Influences elicitation of immune responses, Clin Vaccine Immunol. 18: 1447-1455.

Corthesy, B., Kraehenbuhl, J.P. (1999) Antibody-mediated protection of mucosal surfaces. Curr Trop Microbiol. 236: 93-111.

Cruz, I., Cheetham, J.J., Arnason, J.T., Yack, J.E., Smith, M.L. (2014) Alkamides from Echinacea disrupt the fungal cell wall-membrane complex. Phytomedicine. 21: 435-442.

Cundell, D.R., Matrone, M.A., Rarjaczak, P., Pierce, J.D. (2003) The effect of aerial parts of Echinacea on the circulating white cell levels and selected immune function of the aging male Spague-Dawley rat. Int Immunopharmacol. 3: 1041-1048.

Davison, F., Kaspers, B., Schat, K.A. (2008) Avian immunology. Elsevier Ltd. London, UK.

De Geus, E.D., Jansen, C.A., Vervelde, L. (2012) Uptake of particulate antigens in a non-mammalian lung: phenotypic and functional characterization of avian respiratory phagocytes using bacterial or viral antigens. J Immunol. 188: 4516-26.

Fonseca, N.F, Papanicolaou, G., Lin, H., Lau, C.B.S., Kennelly, E.J., Cassileth, B.R., Cunningham-Rundles, S. (2015) *Echinacea purpurea* (L.) Moench modulates human T-cell cytokine response. Int Immunopharmacol. 19: 94-102.

Ganapathy, K., Cargill, P., Montiel, E., Jones, R.C. (2005) Interaction between live avian pneumovirus and Newcastle disease virus-vaccines in specific pathogen free chickens. Avian Pathol. 34: 297-302.

Getachew, T. (2016) A Review on Effects of Probiotic Supplementation in Poultry Performance and Cholesterol Levels of Egg and Meat J World Poult Res. 6: 31-36.

Ghahri, H., Toloei, T., Habibi, M. (2010) Efficacy of esterified glucomannan, sodium bentonite and humic acid to counteract experimental aflatoxicosis on antibody titers against Newcastle disease in broilers. Afr J Biotechnol. 9: 4127-4131.

Guimarães, J.B., Dos Santos, É.C., Souza Dias, E., Bertechini, A.G., Da Silva Ávila, C.L., Silva Dias, F. (2014) Performance and meat quality of broiler chickens that are fed diets supplemented with *Agaricus brasiliensis* mushrooms. Trop Anim Health Prod. 46: 1509-1514.

Habibian Dehkordi, S., Fallah, V., Habibian Dehkordi, S.H. (2011) Enhancement of broiler performance and immune response by *Echinacea purpurea* supplemented in diet. Afr J Biotechnol. 10: 11280-11286.

Jayawardane, G.W., Spradbrow, P.B. (1995) Mucosal immunity in chickens vaccinated with the V4 strain of Newcastle disease virus. Vet Microbiol. 46: 69-77.

Jurcic, K., Melchart, D., Holzmann, M., Martin, P.L., Bauer, R., Doenecke, A., Wagner, H. (1989) Zwei Probandenstudienzur Stimulierung der Granulozyten phagozytose durch Echinacea-Extrakt-haltige Präparate. Z. Phytother. 10: 67-70.

Kapczynski, D.R., Afonso, C.L., Miller, P.J. (2013) Immune responses of poultry to Newcastle disease virus. Dev Comp Immunol. 41: 447-453.

Kuhn, G., Ender, K., Thomann, R., Tuchscherer, M., Tuchscherer, A., Stabenow, B., Krüger, M., Schrödl, W. (2005) Einsatz von Echinacea-Extraktbeitragenden und säugenden-

Sauen. Arch Tierz Dummerstorf. 48: 270-282.

Lee, T.T., Chen, C.L., Shieh Z.H., Lin, J.C., Yu, B. (2009) Study on antioxidant activity of *Echinacea purpurea* L. extracts and its impact on cell viability. Afr J Biotechnol. 8: 5097-5105.

Lee, T.T., Chen, C.L., Wang, C.C., Yu, B. (2012) Growth performance and antioxidant capacity of broilers supplemented with *Echinacea purpurea* L. in the diet. Appl Poult Res. 21: 484-491.

Manayi, A., Vazirian, M., Saeidnia, S. (2015) *Echinacea purpurea*: Pharmacology, phytochemistry and analysis methods. Pharmacogn Rev. 9: 63-72.

Mehdizadeh Taklimi, S.M.S., Lotfollahian, H., Zarea Shahne, A., Mirzaei, F., Alinejad, A. (2012) Study on efficacy of probiotic in broiler chickens diet. Agr Sci. 3: 5-8.

Menten, J. F. M. (2002) Probióticos, prebióticos e aditivosfitogênicosnanutrição de aves. In: 2° SimpósiosobreIngredientesnaAlimentação Animal, Uberlândia, Minas Gerais. Brasil. p. 251-276.

Park, Y.H., Hamidon, F., Rajangan, C., Soh, K.P., Gan, C.Y., Lim, T.S., Abdullah, W.N.W., Liong, M.T. (2016) Application of Probiotics for the Production of Safe and High-quality Poultry Meat. Korean J Food Sci Anim Resour. 36: 567-576.

Perozo, F., Villegas, P., Dolz, R., Afonso, C.L., Purvis, L.B. (2008) The VG/GA strain of Newcastle disease virus: mucosal immunity, protection against lethal challenge and molecular analysis. Avian Pathol. 37: 237-245

Raj, G.D., Jones, R.C. (1996) Local antibody production in the oviduct and gut of hens infected with a variant strain of infectious bronchitis virus. Vet Immunol Immunopathol. 53: 147-161.

Reynolds, D.L. Maraqa, A.D. (2000) Protective immunity against Newcastle disease: the role of cell-mediated immunity. Avian Dis. 44: 145-154.

Saunders, P.R., Smith, F., Schusky, R.W. (2007) *Echinacea purpurea* L. in children: safety, tolerability, compliance, and clinical effectiveness in upper respiratory tract infections. Can J Physiol Pharmacol. 85: 1195-1199.

Schranner, I., Wurdinger, M., Klumpp, N., Losche, U., Okpanyi, S.N. (1989) Influence of medicinal complex drug (Influex) and *Echinacea angustifolia* extract on avian humoral immune reactions. J Vet Med B. 36: 353-364.

Scott, T.R. (2004) Our current understanding of humoral immunity of poultry. Poult Sci. 83: 574-579.

Seifert, S., Fritz, C., Carlini, N., Barth, S.W., Franz, C.M.A.P., Watzl, B. (2011) Modulation of innate and adaptive immunity by the probiotic *Bifidobacterium longum* PCB133 in turkeys. Poult Sci. 90: 2275-2280.

Talazadeh, F., Mayahi, M., Zeinali, S. (2016) The effect of Aquablend Avian probiotic® including Lactobacillus, Streptococcus and Bifidobacterium on systemic antibody response against Newcastle and Influenza disease vaccine in broiler chickens. Int J Enteric Pathog. 4: e35689.

Toloei, T., Ghahri, H., Talebi, A. (2010) Efficacy of mannanoligosaccharides and humateon immune response to Avian Influenza (H9) diseasevaccination in broiler chickens. Vet Res Commun. 34: 709-717.

Wondmeneh, E., Arendonk, J.A.M., der Waaij, E.H., Ducro, B.J., Parmentier, H.K. (2015) High natural antibody titers of indigenous chickens are related with increased hazard in confinement. Poult Sci. 94: 1493-1498.

Mechanical behavior measurement of the sheep small intestine using experimental tests

Rassoli, A., Fatouraee, N.*

Biological Fluid Dynamics Laboratory, Biomechanics Department, Biomedical Engineering Faculty, Amirkabir University of Technology, Tehran, Iran

Key words:
anisotropic constitutive model, fung-type model, nonlinear tissue, modify Mooney-Rivlin model, strain-energy function

Correspondence
Fatouraee, N.
Biological Fluid Dynamics Laboratory, Biomechanics Department, Biomedical Engineering Faculty, Amirkabir University of Technology, Tehran, Iran

Email: Nasser@aut.ac.ir

Abstract:

BACKGROUND: There is no consistent data on the mechanical properties of sheep intestine. **OBJECTIVES:** We performed a series of biaxial strain measurement experiments and extracted the constitutive model to describe the mechanical characteristics of the sheep intestinal tissue. **METHODS:** Eleven specimens were obtained freshly from sacrificed sheep and the planar biaxial tests were performed on the tissue specimens by applying simultaneous loads along the circumfer-ential and longitudinal directions. Then the measured data were fitted into the anisotropic four-parameter Fung-type model and also to the modified Mooney-Rivlin model. **RESULTS:** The specimens showed some degree of anisotropy; the stiffer direction is not gener-ally predictable. Some of the specimens were stiffer in the circumferential direction, and the others in the longitudinal direction. However, the average results state the circumferential di-rection as the stiffer orientation. **CONCLUSIONS:** It can be concluded that sheep intestine be-haves normally as a nonlinear anisotropic tissue which is well-characterized by the modified Mooney-Rivlin model.

Introduction

From the anatomical view, the small intestine consists of three adjacent segments; duodenum, jejunum and ileum. The wall of these segments has a multi-layered structure; the four layers are asserosa, muscolaris, submucosa and mucosa. The mechanical p roperties of the small intestine are mainly dominated by the submucosa and the muscular layers, while the other layers contribution is negligible (Egorov et al., 2002).

To estimate intestine mechanical properties, researchers performed uniaxial tensile tests on human intestine and proposed that the mechanical properties of intestine in axial and transversal directions are different (Egorov et al., 2002). The inflation tests have also been applied to porcine intestine (Slatkin, 1999), human duodenum (Frøkjaer et al., 2006) and pig small intestine (Liao et al., 2010). Although the uniaxial tensile test data were presented comprehensively, they are inadequate to determine the mechanical properties, such as nonlinear and anisotropic responses. Moreover, the inflation tests lack the adaptability of a planar test in addition to the fact that the sample sizes in these tests are dependent on the pressure and size of the nozzle (Chong et al., 2005). Meanwhile biaxial planar test is a proper alternative for approaching a better view on the mechanics of soft tissues. Despite the fact that the researchers performed planar biaxial tensile tests on porcine duodenum, jejunum, and ileum and used anisotropic four-parameter Fung-type model and isotropic models in the Neo-Hookean and Mooney-Rivlin forms to describe them (Bellini et al., 2011), there is still a need for an anisotropic model of intestine for a reliable FE analysis in a standard software package. To the authors' knowledge, the anisotropic Fung-type model cannot be used in so many FE packages (e.g. a FSI procedure in a commercial finite-element package named ADINA).

Since the sheep intestine acts similar to human intestine in some diseases (Munday et al., 2006) the goal of this study was to develop an anisotropic constitutive model for the small intestine wall of sheep. By this aim, planar biaxial tests were performed on specimens by loadings applied along the circumferential and longitudinal directions. Then the data of the experimental tests were modeled by the anisotropic four-parameter Fung-type model and the anisotropic modified Mooney- Rivlin Model.

Materials and Methods

Sample preparation: Eleven intestine samples extracted from 6 healthy sheep were used in this study. All the sheep were in the range of 2-4 years old. Tissues were cleaned and stored in physiological 0.9% saline. Tests were completed within 8 hours after extraction. The specimen thicknesses were measured with a micrometer. Deviation of thickness was negligible, so average thickness was used in formulations. The specimens were cut along the longitudinal axis and shaped into squares of 18 mm sides which suits our biaxial test requirements.

Biaxial mechanical characterization: A planar biaxial test device with strain measurement capability was utilized to obtain stress/strain correlation along the longitudinal and circumferential axes of the specimens (Figure 1). In order to preserve the mechanical properties, samples were kept wet at temperature of 37◦C by use of a temperature controlled water bath. The clamps of the system were able to directly hold samples with dimensions ≥15×15 mm2 without damaging the tissue. After placement of the specimens on the device, they were preloaded with 0.01 N loading along both axes in order to obtain meaningful measurements. The loadings were applied with the rate of 0.02 mm/s through four microstepper motors in both

directions and the tensile forces were measured by two UMAA 2 kgf load cells. For the purpose of deformation measurement of the tissue, a USB digital microscope camera was used (300X zoom, 30 Hz and resolution of 480×640). The data of digital microscope camera were processed with

ImageJ package to obtain stretch in each direction. Due to small dimensions of samples there was no way to use ink markers in stretch (displacement) measurement. Initial distance between the ends of each clamp was considered as the reference measure of sample length in both directions.

The stress-strain curve for each specimen was obtained in two axes (the (11) corresponding to the circumferential direction and the (22) to the longitudinal direction). The experimental stresses for the samples were computed as follows:

(1) $\sigma_{11}^{exp}=\lambda_1(F_{11}/l_2t)$

(2) $\sigma_{22}^{exp}=\lambda_2(F_{22}/l_1t)$

where λ_1 and λ_2 are the stretch ratios, F_{11} and F_{22} are the forces measured by the load cells, t is the thickness of the samples, and l1 and l2 are the unloaded widths of the samples in the two directions.

Constitutive model: In this study, small intestine was modeled as an incompressible, homogeneous and hyperelastic material. These assumptions confirm the existence of a strain energy function W which is the criterion for the stored energy in the materials as a result of the deformation. By use of the strain energy function, the stresses can be computed from the strains as follows (Sun et al., 2003; Humphrey et al.,1990; Humphrey et al.,1990):

(3) $S_{ij}=PC^{-1}+2(\partial w/\partial C_{ij})=PC^{-1}+(\partial w/\partial E_{ij})$ (I,j=1,2,3)

(4) $C_{ij}=F_{ij}^{T}F_{ij}$

(5) $E_{ij}=(1/2)(C_{ij}-I_{ij})$

where S_{ij} is the second Piola-Kirchhoff stress tensor, p is the Lagrange multiplier introduced to enforce incompressibility, C_{ij} is the right Cauchy-Green deformation tensor, Eij is the Green-Lagrange strain tensor, Iij is the identity unit tensor and F_{ij} is the deformation gradient tensor which can be described as $F=\partial x/\partial x'$ in which x' and x are the position of material point in the reference and current configuration, respectively.

The Cauchy stress tensor σij is calculated as follows:

(6) $\sigma_{ij}=PI+2F_{ij}(\partial w/\partial C_{ij})F_{ij}^{T}=PI+F_{ij}(\partial w/\partial E_{ij})F_{ij}^{T}$

According to the strain energy function and investigating the hyperelastic models (Fung et al.,1979; Holzapfel et al., 200; Holzapfel et al.,1996; Holzapfel et al., 2004; Holzapfel et al., 2005) two appropriate constitutive models were chosen to express the mechanical properties of the intestine, as these models have been used previously for other soft tissues.

The first model utilized was a Fung-type model (Fung, 1991) which is able to describe the anisotropic behavior of tissue. In the Fung model, the strain energy density is given by:

(7) $W(Q)=0.5c(e^{Q}-1)$

where $Q(E)={}_{a1}E_{11}^{2}+{}_{a2}E_{22}^{2}+2_{a3}E_{11}E_{22}$, and c, a1, a2 and a3 are constitutive parameters.

The Cauchy stress components in the two directions were then calculated as follows:

(8) $\sigma_{11}=\{0.5c\lambda_1^{2}[a_1(\lambda_1^{2}-1)+a_3(\lambda_2^{2}-1)]*\text{-}\exp((1/4)[a_1(\lambda_1^{2}-1)^{2}+a_2(\lambda_1^{1}-1)^{2}+2a_3(\lambda_1^{2}-1)\ (\lambda_2^{2}-1)]\}$

(9) $\sigma_{22}=\{0.5c\lambda_2^{2}[a_2(\lambda_2^{2}-1)+a_3(\lambda_1^{2}-1)]*\exp((1/4)[a_1(\lambda_1^{2}-1)^{2}+a_2(\lambda_2^{2}-1)^{2}+2a_3(\lambda_1^{2}-1)(\lambda_2^{2}-1)]\}$

The second model was the modified Mooney-Rivlin model which shows anisotropic behavior of the tissues and can also be implemented into many standard FE packages. The strain energy density

Function of this model is given by:

(10) $W=C_1(I_1-3)+D_1[\exp(D_2(I_1-3))-1]+(k_1/2k_2)[\exp[k_2(I_4-1)^{2}-1]]$

where $I_1=\lambda_1^{2}+\lambda_2^{2}+(\lambda_1\lambda_2)^{-2}$ and $I_4=C_{ij}(n_c)_i(n_c)_i$, n_c is the circumferential direction of the tissue and c_1, D_1, D_2, k_1 and k_2 are the model parameters (Holzapfel et al., 2004; Bathe, 1996; Bathe, 2007).

According to the strain energy function, Cauchy stresses in the two axes are as follows:

(11) $\sigma_{11}=(2(\lambda_1^{2}-\lambda_3^{2})(C_1+D_1*D_2*\exp(\lambda_1^{2}+\lambda_2^{2}+\lambda_3^{2}-3)))\ (2*k_1*\lambda_1^{2}(\lambda_1^{2}-1)\exp(k2(\lambda_1 2-1)^{2}))$

(12) $\sigma_{22}=(2(\lambda_2^{2}-\lambda_3^{2})(C_1+D_1*D_2*\exp(\lambda_1^{2}+\lambda_2^{2}+\lambda_3^{2}-3)))$

Experimental data then were fitted to Cauchy stress of each model by using genetic algorithms and the parameters of constitutive models were obtained for each data set.

Then the anisotropy is calculated by using the Fung model parameters as follows:

(13) $\text{Anisotropy}=\min[(a_1+a_3)/(a_2+a_3),(a_2+a_3)/(a_1+a_3)]$

Statistical analysis: The results of the experimental tests were presented as average ± SD. The two-tailed paired t-test was used to compare collagen fibre orientation along the axes. Significance was set at $p<0.05$.

Results

After the specimens are placed in the biaxial device, a minimal force has to be applied to obtain a perfectly planar position. So preload of 0.01 N was applied along both axes to record meaningful measurements. Since it was not possible to protect the samples from dehydration, some specimens did not provide any acceptable data for us to report. It should be carefully noted that in thc calculation of stresses from force data, the average thicknesses for every sample are used. Naturally, this assumption may lead to additional error sources in the estimation of the constitutive

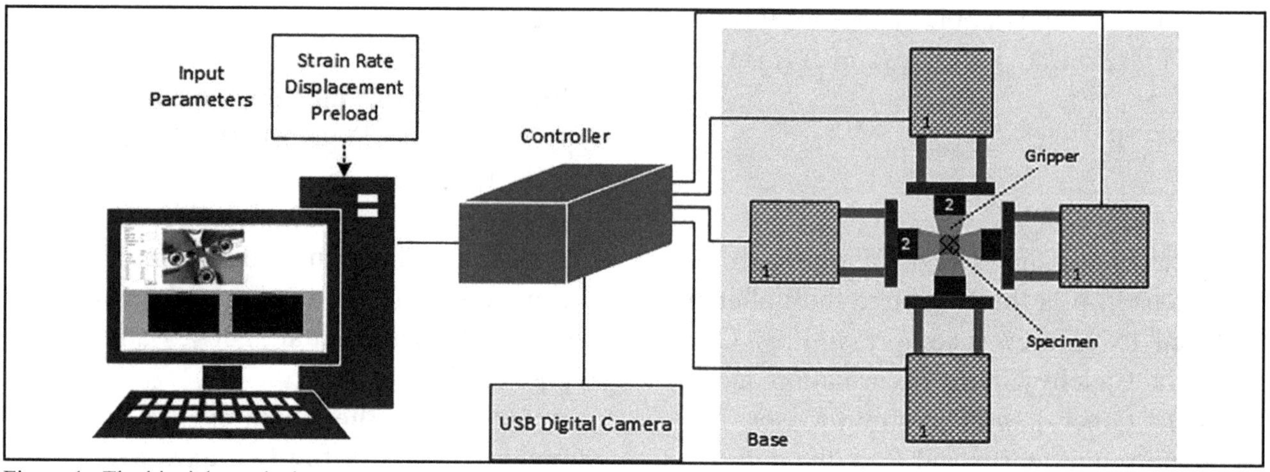

Figure 1. The biaxial test device.

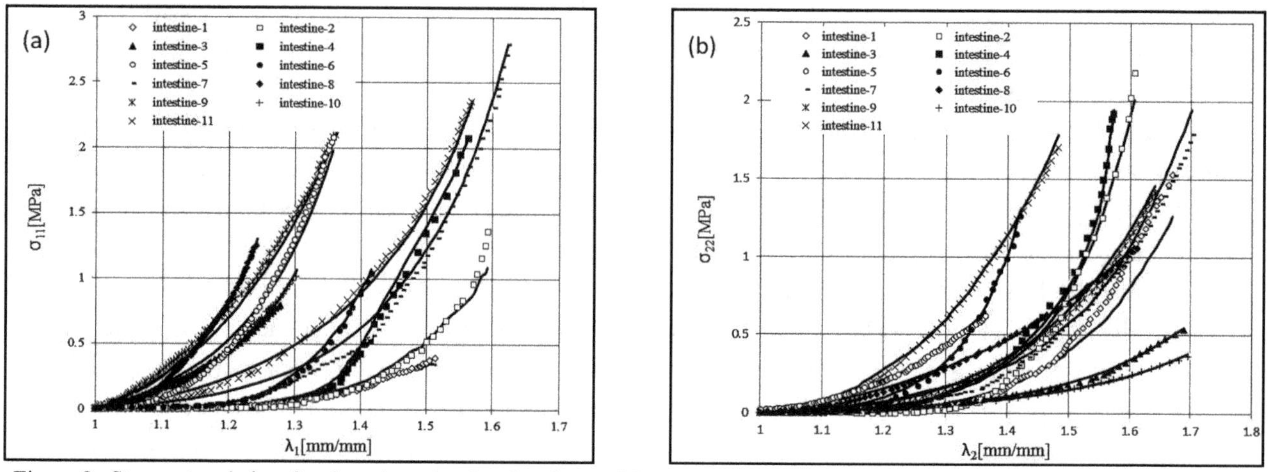

Figure 2. Stress-stretch data for sheep intestine fitted to the modified Mooney-Rivlin model. The left hand plots (a) show the stresses and stretches in the circumferential (11) direction while the right hand plots (b) show the stresses and stretches in the longitudinal (22) direction. Fitted modified Mooney-Rivlin models (solid lines) were superimposed over the raw data.

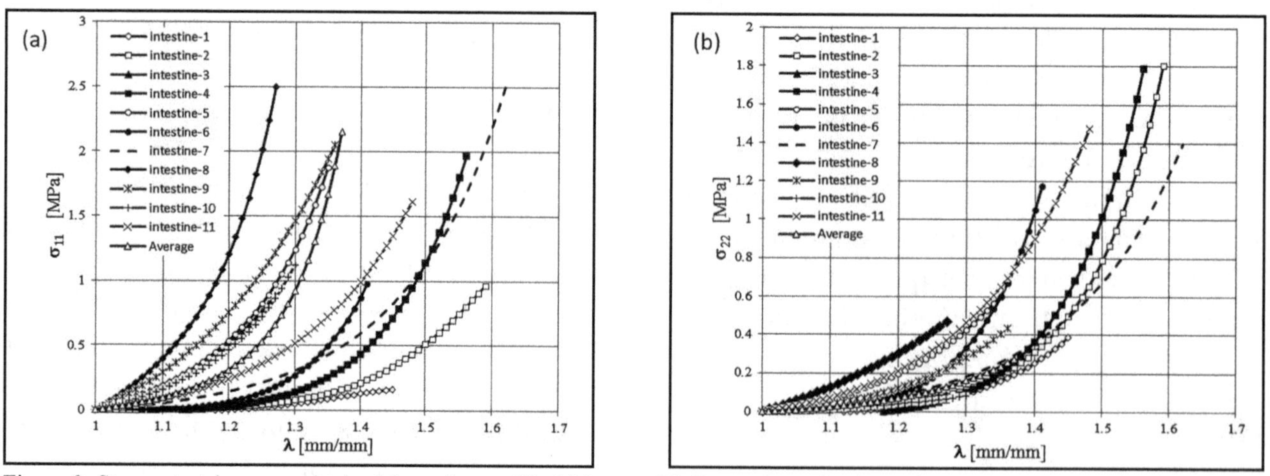

Figure 3. Stress-stretch curves obtained from the modified Mooney-Rivlin constants in circumferential (a) and axial (b) direc-tions ($\lambda 1 = \lambda 2 = \lambda$).

parameters. Average thickness of specimens was considered 0.7 mm. The plausible specimens exhibited stress-stretch curves which were derived from the Eqs. (1) and (2) which state that the experimental data were well-fitted to the Fung and modified Mooney-Rivlin

Table 1. Parameters for the two constitutive models.

Fung						
	c(MPa)	a1	a2	a3	Anisotropy	rms(MPa)
intestine-1	0.085	0.686	1.67	0.054	0.43	0.084
intestine-2	0.061	1.36	2.095	0.032	0.65	0.069
intestine-3	0.429	2.543	0.269	0.03	0.12	0.047
intestine-4	0.083	1.88	1.94	0.053	0.96	0.116
intestine-5	0.828	1.94	0.605	0.028	0.32	0.093
intestine-6	0.085	2.63	3.31	0.014	0.79	0.049
intestine-7	0.432	0.915	0.524	0.03	0.59	0.093
intestine-8	0.453	2.467	0.639	0.43	0.37	0.170
intestine-9	1.549	1.19	0.25	0.0076	0.22	0.082
intestine-10	0.644	1.897	0.126	0.027	0.08	0.019
intestine-11	0.812	0.815	0.804	0.05	0.98	0.112
Average	0.295	2.175	0.396	0.313	0.29	0.020
Modified Mooney-Rivlin						
	c1 (MPa)	D1 (MPa)	D2	k1 (MPa)	k2	rms(MPa)
intestine-1	-0.096	0.116	0.61	-0.099	1.3	0.066
intestine-2	-0.01	0.019	1.099	-0.01	1.02	0.088
intestine-3	-0.001	0.0595	0.6	0.33	0.52	0.015
intestine-4	-0.090	0.0422	0.99	0.014	0.3	0.049
intestine-5	0.001	0.2	0.64	0.22	0.97	0.079
intestine-6	-0.05	0.035	1.33	-0.016	1.2	0.03
intestine-7	-0.002	0.093	0.62	0.042	0.43	0.094
intestine-8	0.002	0.964	0.28	0.48	2.02	0.044
intestine-9	-0.07	0.241	0.54	0.49	0.07	0.032
intestine-10	0.008	0.042	0.57	0.27	1.06	0.017
intestine-11	-0.06	0.348	0.54	0.02	0.21	0.047
Average	0.0048	0.049	0.786	0.13	1.92	0.015

constitutive equations. According to calculated RMS error (Table1), the modified Mooney-Rivlin model approximately provides the best qualitative fit to the data. Figure 2 shows the stretch-stress curves obtained from the biaxial mechanical testing of all specimens in the circumferential (2-a) and in the axial (2-b) directions that were fitted to the constitutive modified Mooney-Rivlin model. It cannot be stated that the circumferential direction is consistently the stiffer (or less stiff) direction. But on average, the specimens act stiffer in the circumferential direction rather than the axial direction. Simultaneous loading in these two orthogonal directions also allowed us to conclude that the mechanical response in one direction is influenced by the characteristics in the other direction.

Detailed information on average model coefficients and anisotropy values are provided in Table 1. By using these material constants, stretch-stress curves were extracted and plotted in Figure 3. The mean biaxial stretch-stress curve for intestine was also obtained from the average modified Mooney-Rivlin

constants mentioned in Table 1 and plotted in Figure 3 as well.

Discussion

This study provides a complete set of experimental planar biaxial data for sheep intestine fitted to the Fung-type anisotropic model and the modified Mooney-Rivlin constitutive model to describe its mechanical characteristics.

The nonlinear thick-walled tubular theory (modified Mooney-Rivlin model) which could be used for FE analysis developed in this article, seems to be a realistic starting point in the simulation of intestine. These constitutive models demonstrated mechanical anisotropy and nonlinearity of the tissues and the data (Table 1) present some degree of anisotropy for intestine wall. Stiffer behavior in the longitudinal direction was mentioned in previous research from uniaxial tensile tests as well (Chong et al.,2005). Inflation tests on porcine small bowel (Hoeg et al.,2000) also showed stiffer characteristics in the circumferential direction. Indeed, it cannot be stated that the longitudinal direction is consistently the stiffer (or less stiff) direction. But on average, the specimens act stiffer in the circumferential direction rather than the axial direction. Overall variability in the direction of relative stiffness is in agreement with previous findings (Bellini et al., 2011; Terry et al., 2010). In Fung model the elevated values of parameter a1 than a2 (Tables 1) may be imparted by a preferred collagen fibre orientation along the circumferential axis, as certified for the extracellular matrix component of intestine tissue (Sokolis et all,2012).

All of the models presented in this study are nonlinear and anisotropic; in particular, the modified Mooney-Rivlin model is an anisotropic model which can be used for numerical analysis. Although the two models considered in this paper are phenomenological, they may be helpful as a research reference, offering good descriptive capability.

Conclusion: In this study the mechanical properties of sheep intestine have been determined by using biaxial mechanical device. The obtained stretch-stress curves from the experimental data were fitted to the four-parameter Fung-type model as well as the modified Mooney-Rivlin model, and the anisotropy values of the samples were calculated by the constitutive parameters. The samples showed some degree of the anisotropy. The curves, on average, also showed stiffer behavior in the circumferential direction than the longitudinal direction. To conclude, this paper can be the best reference for the mechanical investigations of sheep intestine tissue.

Acknowledgments

The authors would like to thank Malikeh Nabaei for their excellent assistance throughout this project.

References

1. Bathe, K.J. (1996) Finite Element Procedures, Englewood Cliffs. NJ: Prentice-Hall.
2. Bathe, K.J. (2007) Theory and Modeling Guide, Watertown, MA: ADINA and ADINA-F, ADINA R&D, Inc, Vol. I and II.
3. Bellini, C., Glass, P., Sitti, M., Di Martino, E.S. (2011) Biaxial mechanical modeling of the small intestine. J Mech Behav Biomed Mater. p.1727-1740.
4. Chong, C., Hung, H., Steinhart, A., Trexler, J.(2005) Design of a Biaxial Test Device for Compliant Tissue. Worcester Polytechnic Institute. 4: 3-44.
5. Egorov, V., Schastlivtsev, I., Prut, E., Baranov, A., Turusov, R.(2002) Mechanical properties of the human gastrointesti-nal tract. J Biomech. 35: 1417-1425.
6. Frøkjaer, J.B., Andersen, S.D., Drewes, A.M., Gregersen, H.(2006) Ultrasound-determined geometric and biomechanical properties of the human duodenum. Dig Dis Sci. 51: 1662-1669.
7. Fung, Y.C., Fronek, K., Patitucci, P. (1979) Pseudoelasticity of arteries and the choice of its mathematical expression. Am J Physiol. 237: 620-631.
8. Fung, Y.C. (1991) What are the residual stresses doing in our blood vessels?. Ann Biomed

Eng. 19: 237-249.

9. Liao, D., Zhao, J., Gregersen, H. (2010) 3D mechanical properties of the partially obstructed guinea pig small intestine. J Biomech. 43: 2079-2086.
10. Munday, J.S, Brennan, M.M, Jaber, A.M, kiupel, M. (2006) Ovine intestinal adenocarcinomas: histologic and phenotypic comparison with human colon cancer. J Comp Med (Memphis). 56: 136-41.
11. Holzapfel, G.A., Eberlein, R., Wriggers, P., Weizsacker, H. (1996) Large strain analysis of soft biological membranes: Formulation and finite element analysis. Comput Method Appl M. 132: 45-61.
12. Holzapfel, G.A., Gasser, T.C., Ogden, R.W. (2000) A new constitutive framework for arterial wall mechanics and a comparative study of material models. J Elasticity. 61: 1-48.
13. Holzapfel, G.A., Gasser, T.C., Ogden, R.W. (2004) Comparison of a multi-layer structural model for arterial walls with a Fung-type model, and issues of material stability. J Biomech ENG-T Asme. 126: 264-275.
14. Holzapfel, G.A. (2005) Similarities between soft biological tissues and rubber like materials. In: Constitutive Models for Rubber IV, A.A. Balkema Publishers. P.-E., Keri, L. (eds.). Balkema, Leiden. The Netherlands. p. 607-617.
15. Holzapfel, G.A., Sommer, G., Regitnig, P. (2004) Anisotropic mechanical properties of tissue components in human ath-erosclerotic plaques. J Biomech ENG-T Asme. 126: 657-665.
16. Humphrey, J.D., Strumpf, R.K., Yin, F.C.P. (1990) Determination of a constitutive relation for passive myocardium: A New Functional Form. J Biomech ENG-T Asme. 112: 333-339.
17. Humphrey, J.D., Strumpf, R.K., Yin, F.C.P. (1990) Determination of a constitutive relation for passive myocardium: II. Parameter Estimation. J Biomech ENG-T Asme. 112: 340-346. [19] Slatkin.(1999) Modeling and experiments for a class of robotic endoscopes. Ph.D. Thesis California Institute of Technology.
18. Sun, W., Sacks, M.S., Scott, M.J. (2003) Numerical simulations of the planar biaxial mechanical behavior of biological materials. Bioengineering Conference, Florida. p. 1-2.
19. Terry, B.S., Lyle, A.B., Schoen, J.A., Rentschler, M.E. (2010) Preliminary mechanical characterization of the small bowel for in vivo mobility. ASME International Mechanical Engineering Congress and Exposition, Vancouver, British Columbia, Canada.
20. Sokolis, D.P. (2012) Multiaxial mechanical behaviour of the passive ureteral wall: experimental study and mathematical characterisation. Computer methods in biomechanics and biomedical engineering. 15: 1145-1156.

12

Effects of artichoke (*Cynara scolymus* L.) extract on antioxidant status in chicken thigh meat

Mirderikvandi, M.[1], Kiani, A.[1], Khaldari, M.[1], Alirezaei, M.[2*]

[1]*Animal Sciences Group, Faculty of Agriculture, Lorestan University, Khorram Abad, Iran*
[2]*Division of Biochemistry, School of Veterinary Medicine, Lorestan University, Khorram Abad, Iran*

Key words:
Artichoke extract, broiler chicken, glutathione peroxidase, lipid stability

Correspondence
Alirezaei, M.
Division of Biochemistry, School of Veterinary Medicine, Lorestan University, Khorram Abad, Iran

Email: alirezaei_m54@yahoo.com

Abstract:

BACKGROUND: Artichoke extract (AE), containing natural antioxidant compounds, can be considered as a good source of antioxidant potential. **OBJECTIVES:** The aim of this study was to evaluate antioxidant abilities of AE on broiler meat quality. **METHODS:** 200 Ross chicken broilers were divided into five equal groups and received 100, 200, 300, and 500 mg/liter of AE in drinking water and pure water in the control group, respectively. Antiradical activity and phenolic content of AE were determined by 1,1-diphenyl-2-picrylhydrazyl (DPPH) method and gallic acid measurement before adding extract into drinking water. The broilers received AE extract form 21-35 day of growing phase and the samples from thigh muscles were taken for biochemical analysis in the 42 day of the growing phase. **RESULTS:** Antiradical activity of AE was 35% and phenolic content was 3.3 g/100g of dry extract. Regarding antioxidant enzymes, such as glutathione peroxidase (GPx) and catalase (CAT), the AE with dosage of 200 mg/l indicated maximum antioxidant ability compared to the other groups ($p<0.05$). Supplementation of AE200 mg/l also demonstrated the lowest GPx and CAT activities, compared to the control and AE 300 mg/l groups ($p<0.05$). Regarding performance weight gain, average daily weight gain, percentage of weight gain in 21 to 35 as well as final weight were similar in control and AE-received groups and AE indicated similar effect for all the treatments. **CONCLUSIONS:** This study showed that administration of 200 mg/l AE in drinking water during growing phase decreased GPx and CAT activities in chicken meat presumably due to down-regulation of gene expression for antioxidant enzymes.

Introduction

It is well-known that lipid peroxidation is one of the main factors limiting the quality and acceptability of meat (Morrisseyet al., 1998). Usually, lipid peroxidation occurs when antioxidant defenses (non-enzymatic and enzymatic antioxidants) are overcome by peroxidation mechanisms and lipid peroxidation refers to oxidation of lipids in the presence of oxygen (Gutteridge, 1995). During the oxidation of lipids, unsaturated fatty acids are oxidized in presence of reactive free radicals, such as superoxide anion, hydroxyl radical, and hydrogen peroxide. Unsaturated fatty acids exposed to oxygen produce compounds, such as malondialdehyde (MDA), therefore, MDA has been widely used as an indicator of lipid peroxidation in meat (Alirezaei et al., 2012). The antioxidant system contains non-enzymatic and enzymatic antioxidants (Sies, 1997). Glutathione peroxidase (GPx), catalase (CAT), and superoxide dismutase (SOD) are enzymatic antioxidants. SOD converts superoxide anion into hydrogen peroxide (H2O2). Then, CAT removes hydrogen peroxide by converting it into water and oxygen. GPx also removes hydrogen peroxide by oxidizing the glutathione into its oxidized form (Gutteridge, 1995), and also converts H2O2 into water. Natural components including phenolic acids, flavonoids, polyphenols, retinoids, tocopherols, and ascorbic acid act as non-enzymatic antioxidant (Chu et al., 2000).

A number of byproducts as sources of natural antioxidant compounds have been studied, such as Oregano, Sage, and Rosemary on meat quality of broilers (Bustoglou et al., 2002; Lopez-Bote et al., 1998). Artichoke (Cynarascolymus L.), as a rich source of non-enzymatic antioxidants, is a potential good source of antioxidant activity since it contains poly phenolic compounds, with mono- and dicaffeoylquinic acids as the major chemical components (Table 1). The most well-known caffeoylquinic acid derivative identified in artichoke is cynarin. The other phenolics are the flavones apigenin and luteolin, and the anthocyanidinscyanidin, peonidin, and delphinidin have also been found in artichoke (Lattanzio et al., 2009).

The aim of the present study was to evaluate antioxidant effect of AE in drinking water on meat quality of broilers. This effect was evaluated by antioxidant enzyme activities, such as GPx and CAT and lipid peroxidation marker as shown by MDA content.

Materials and Methods

Birds and treatments: A total of 200 one-day-old broiler chickens (Ross) obtained from a commercial hatchery (Dorbal Company, Boroojerd, Iran) were used in the present study. The chickens received 5% sugar and lemon juice mixture for 15 hours as soon as they arrived to the hall. The chickens were fed and reared according to Ross guidelines with similar diets throughout the experiment. All chickens were fed pre-starter (0.0-10 days), starter (11-21 days), grower (22-35 days), and finisher (36-42 days) diets. The ingredients and nutrient contents of the diets are shown in Table 2. The chickens had freely accessed to drinking water and exposed to 23 hours of light and 1 hour of darkness, daily. Vaccinations were performed against Newcastle and Bronchitis on the 4th and 18th days of the experiment. From day 21, chickens were randomly allocated into five treatments. Each treatment included 40 birds (male and female equally). AE obtained from Barij Essance Company (Kashan, Isfahan, Iran) (99% purity) was added to the chickens' drinking water from day 21 to day 35 of the experiment (Nateghi et al., 2013).

Drinking water was either with 100 (AE100), 200 (AE200), 300 (AE300), and 500 (AE500) mg per liter of AE or without AE (control group). At the end of the experiment (42 d), 40 chickens (8 chickens per each treatment) were randomly selected and slaughtered. Meat samples were taken from thigh muscles and were stored at -80°C for one month. Animal care, slaughter, and sampling methods used in the present study were approved by the Institutional Animal Care and Use Committee (IACUC) of Lorestan University.

Antiradical activity and phenol content determination: Radical scavenging activity of AE was determined using DPPH method according to Burits and Bucar (2000). In brief, different concentrations of ascorbic acid (0.0, 2, 4, 6, 8 and 10 μmol) were taken in different test tubes. The volume was adjusted to 100 μl by adding methanol. For drawing curve calibration, five ml of a 0.1 mM methanolic solution of DPPH was added to the standard tubes and shaken vigorously. The tubes were incubated at 27°C for 30 min. Similarly for AE samples, 50 μl and five ml of a 0.1 mM methanolic solution of DPPH were mixed and shaken vigorously. The control was prepared as above without addition of AE extract. The absorbance of the standards and AE samples (three samples) were measured at 517 nm by a spectrophotometer (52000 UV Model; WPA; Cambridge, UK). Radical scavenging activity was expressed as the percentage of inhibition and was calculated using the following formula:

% Radical scavenging activity = (Control Absorbance - Sample Absorbance/Control Absorbance) ×100.

The concentration of phenolic compounds in AE extract was determined according to the Singh et al. (2002). The AE (1 g) was dissolved in 100 ml distilled water (w/v). Then 20 μl of the dissolved AE were mixed with 1.58 ml water and 100 μl of Folin-Ciocalteu reagent as well as 300 μl of sodium carbonate solution (7%). The mixture were held for 30 min at the dark condition in room temperature. The absorbance was measured at 765 nm by a spectrophotometer. The estimation of phenolic compounds in AE was determined in triplicate and the results were averaged. Results were expressed as gallic acid equivalents. The free radical scavenging potential of Artichoke extract (AE) was 35% and the phenolic content of AE was 3.3 ± 0.2 g per 100 g of dry extract.

Muscle preparation for protein measurement, MDA detection and enzyme assay: Thigh samples were thawed and manually homogenized via liquid nitrogen in cold phosphate buffer (pH 7.4, 0.1 M) containing 5mM EDTA , the debris removed by centrifugation at 5000g for 10 min (Centrifuge 5415 R; Rotofix 32 A, Germany) (Alirezaei et al., 2012). Supernatants were recovered and used for measurement of protein, antioxidant enzyme activities and MDA concentration.

Protein measurement: Protein content of the tissue homogenates was determined using the colorimetric method of Lowry with bovine serum albumin as a standard (Lowry et al., 1951).

Measurement of glutathione peroxidase (GPx) activity: The activity of Glutathione peroxidase (GPx) was evaluated with Randox®GPx detection kit according to the manufacturer's instructions as described previously (Alirezaei et al., 2012). GPx catalyzes the oxidation of glutathione (GSH) by cumene hydroperoxide. In the presence of glutathione reductase (GR) and NADPH, the oxidized glutathione (GSSG) is immediately converted to the reduced form with a concomitant oxidation of NADPH to NADP+. The decrease in absorbance was measured spectrophotometrically against blank at 340 nm (52000 UV Model; WPA; Cambridge, UK). One unit (U) of GPx was defined as l μmol of oxidized NADPH per min per milligram of tissue protein. The GPx activity was expressed as unit per milligram of tissue protein (unit/mg protein).

Measurement of catalase (CAT) activity: Tissue catalase activity was assayed using the method described by Cliaborne (1986) and reported by Alirezaei et al. (2012). In brief, 900 μl of potassium phosphate (5 mM), 50 μl H2O2 (19 mM), and 50μl of homogenized tissue were added into a tube. The reaction was initiated by adding H2O2 and absorbance change was measured at 240 nm for 30 seconds (52000 UV Model; WPA; Cambridge, UK). The molar extinction coefficient for H2O2 is 43.6/Mcm. The CAT activity unit (U) was defined as 1 μmol of H2O2 consumption per min per milligram of tissue protein (U/mg protein).

Measurement of MDA content: The amount of lipid peroxidation was indicated by the content of thiobarbituric acid reactive substances (TBARS) in the homogenates. Tissue MDA was determined by following production of thiobarbituric acid reactive substances as described previously (Subbarao et al., 1990). In short, 40 μl of supernatant was added to 40 μl of 0.9% NaCl and 40 μl of deionized H2O, resulting in a total reaction volume of 120 μl. The reaction was incubated at 37°C for 20 min and stopped by the addition of 600 μl of cold 0.8 mol/l hydrochloride acid, containing 12.5% trichloroacetic acid. Following the addition of 780 μl of 1% TBA, the reaction was boiled for 20 min and cooled at 4°C for 1 hour. In order to measure the amount of TBARS produced by the homogenate, the cooled reaction was spun at 1500 g in a microcentrifuge for 20 min and the absorbance of the supernatant was spectrophotometrically read at 532 nm, using an extinction coefficient of 1.56×105/mol cm (52000 UV Model; WPA; Cambridge, UK). The blanks for all of the TBARS assays contained an additional 40 μl of 0.9% NaCl, instead of homogenate as just described. MDA results were expressed as nmol per milligram of tissue protein (nmol/mg protein).

Statistical analysis: This experiment was conducted in a complete randomized block design. The data obtained from the experiment were statistically analyzed using GLM procedure by SAS software (SAS, 2003). Significant differences among the control and treatment groups were compared using Duncan's multiple range tests with a 5% probability (Duncan, 1955). REG procedure was used to make a correlation between AE and content of TBARS (r= - 0.14, p= 0.37).

Results

Effect of AE on GPx and CAT activities in broiler thigh muscles was shown in Figures 1 and 2, respectively. The results showed that AE significantly decreased the GPx activity in AE100, AE200, and AE500 mg/l, compared to control group ($p<0.05$). In respect to antioxidant enzymes, such as GPx and CAT, the AE with dosage 200 mg/l indicated maximum antioxidant ability compared to the other groups. AE 200 mg/lalso demonstrated the lowest GPx and CAT activities when compared to the control and AE 300 mg/lgroups ($p<0.05$).

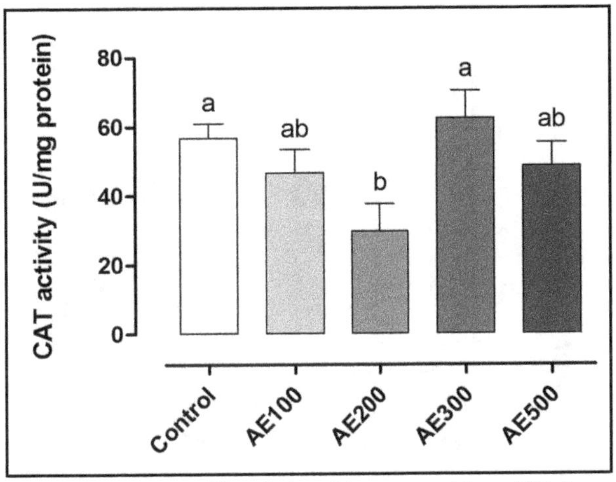

Figure 1. Means ± SD of glutathione peroxidase (GPx) activity in broiler thigh meat in control, AE 100 (100 mg/l), AE 200 (200 mg/l), AE 300 (300 mg/l) and AE 500 (500 mg/l) of Artichoke extract in liter drinking water. a,b means with different superscripts differ significantly ($p<0.05$). AE decreased significantly GPx activity in dosages 100, 200 and 500 mg/l in comparison with control group ($p<0.05$).

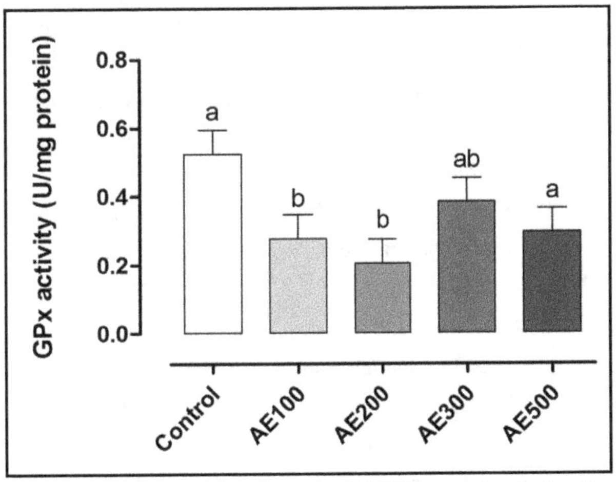

Figure 2. Means ± SD of catalase (CAT) activity in broiler thigh meat in control, AE 100 (100 mg/l), AE 100 (100 mg/l), AE 200 (200 mg/l), AE 300 (300 mg/l) and AE 500 (500 mg/l) of Artichoke extract in liter drinking water. a,b means with different superscripts differ significantly ($p<0.05$). AE 200mg/l demonstrated the lowest CAT activity. AE decreased significantly CAT activity in AE200 when compared with control, AE300 and AE500 groups ($p<0.05$).

Supplementation of 100-500 mg/l of AE decreased MDA concentration as a lipid peroxidation marker (Fig. 3). Although the AE-treated groups indicated lower lipid peroxidation marker than the control group, the difference tendency was decreased ($p=0.08$).

Water Consumption was similar in control and AE-treated groups ($p>0.05$), the extract

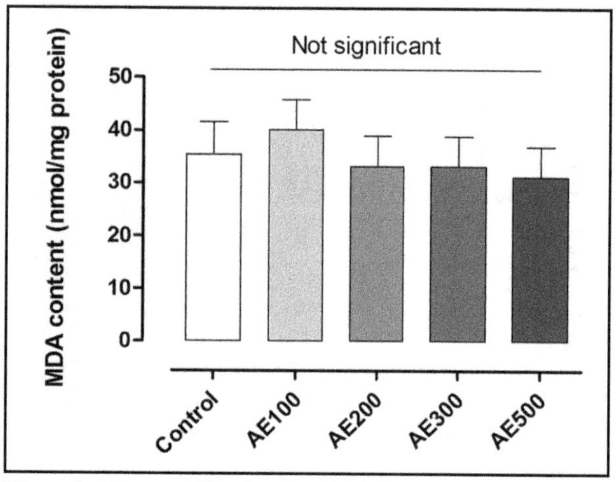

Figure 3. Means ± SD of malondialdehyde (MDA) content in broiler thigh meat in control, AE 100 (100 mg/l), AE 200 (200 mg/l), AE 300 (300 mg/l) and AE 500 (500 mg/l) of Artichoke extract in liter drinking water. There was not significant differences among control and AE-treated groups (p>0.05).

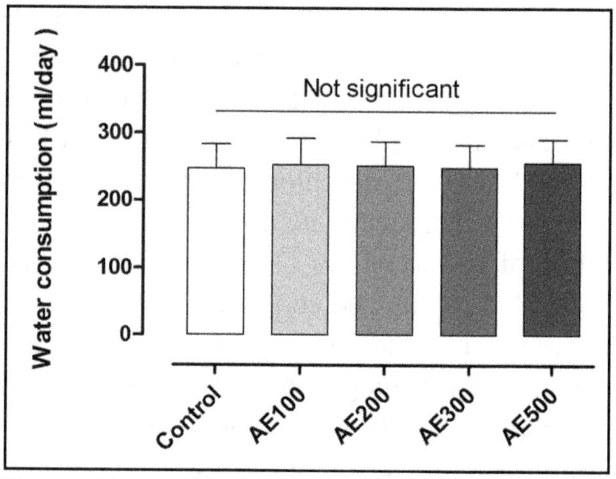

Figure 4. Means ± SD of water consumption (ml/day/chicken) in 21 to 35 d of growing phase in control, AE 100 (100 mg/l), AE 200 (200 mg/l), AE 300 (3 00 mg/l) and AE 500 (500 mg/l) of Artichoke extract in liter of drinking water. There was not significant differences among control and AE-treated groups (p>0.05).

Table 1. Mono and dicaffeoylquinic acids in 100 gram of Artichoke extract. (*) It was taken with permission from Lattanzio et al., 1978; J Food Chem., 24:37-50.

Caffeoylquinic acid derivatives*	mg/100 g dry weight AE
1-o-Caffeoylquinic acid	38.14
3-o- Caffeoylquinic acid	47.22
4-o-Caffeoylquinic acid	267.02
5-o-Caffeoylquinic acid	1544.91

1,3-o-Dicaffeoylquinic acid	61.24
1,4-o-Dicaffeoylquinic acid	142.91
4,5-o-Dicaffeoylquinic acid	224.56
3,5-o-Dicaffeoylquinic acid	347.05
1,5-o-Dicaffeoylquinic acid	837.01
3,4-o-Dicaffeoylquinic acid	428.71

had no effect on water consumption in broilers (Fig. 4).

Regarding growth performance, weight gain, average daily weight gain, percentage of weight gain in 21 to 35 d as well as final weight were similar in control and AE-treated groups (p>0.05), and AE indicated similar effect for all the treatments (Table 3).

Discussion

In the present study, the free radical scavenging potential of AE was 35%. In this regard, Wang et al. (2003) reported a wide range of relative activities toward DPPH (8.3- 49.7%), which were correlated with their polyphenol contents (1.7-9.86%) of the different artichoke samples. Moreover, Llorach et al. (2002) showed a relatively high free radical scavenging activity and capacity to inhibit lipid peroxidation in artichoke byproducts. The phenolic values estimated for the edible portion of artichoke give a range of 31-58 mg/g dry matter (Lattanzio and Sumere van, 1987). Our results showed that phenolic content of AE was 3.3 ± 0.2 g per 100 g of dry extract. In this regard, Schutz et al. (2004) reported that AE had 1.2 g phenolic contents per 100 g dry matter.

Thus, in the present study, AE had relatively high content of phenolic compounds compared to the previous reports. Phenolic compounds are the secondary metabolites and one of the best sources of natural antioxidants (Balasundram et al., 2006). Cynarin is the main phenolic compound in artichoke (Llorach et al., 2002). Other flavonoids, such as the flavones (apigenin and luteolin) and anthocyanidins (cyanidin, peonidin, and delphinidin) have been found in Artichoke (Lattanzio et al., 2009). The scavenging activity against ROS and antiradical activity of Artichoke was lin-

Table 2. Ingredient composition (%) and nutrient content of the chicken's diet (0-42 day). (1) One Kg Concentrate = Carbonate Calcium 174.06 g, Dicalcium phosphate 313.63 g, DL-Methionine 49.26 g, L-Lysine 21.35 g, Vitamin premix 41.05 g, Mineral premix 41.05 g, Salt 57.47 g, Soybean powder 240.56 g, Antioxidant 41.05 g, Colin colorid 20.53 g.

	Pre-starter (0-10 d)	Starter (11-21 d)	Grower (22-35 d)	Finisher (36-42 d)
Corn (%)	45.3	47.9	46.7	47.8
Soybean meal (44% CP)	34.8	33.9	26.9	23.6
Wheat (%)	7	12	20	22
Maize Gluten meal (%)	6	-	-	-
Concentrate1	6.9	6.2	6.4	6.6
Calculated composition				
ME (Mcal/kg)	2.96	2.88	2.95	2.99
Crude protein (%)	24.3	21.2	18.8	17.6
Calcium (%)	1.10	1.00	1.00	1.00
Available phosphorus (%)	0.55	0.50	0.50	0.50
Sodium (%)	0.22	0.21	0.18	0.18
Lysine (%)	1.29	1.09	0.95	0.88
Methionine (%)	0.59	0.51	0.45	0.43
Met+Cys (%)	0.93	0.80	0.72	0.68
Linoleic acid (%)	1.27	1.30	1.29	1.30
Tryptophan (%)	0.24	0.23	0.20	0.18

Table 3. The Effect of Artichoke Extract (AE) on Weight Gain, Average Daily Gain and Weight Gain (%) in 21-35 d in broiler chickens. There were not significant differences among the groups for weight gain, average daily weight gain, percent of weight gain in 21-35 days and final weight of the treatments (p>0.05).

Treatment	Period	Control	AE 100	AE 200	AE 300	AE 500	SEM	p-Value
Intel Weight (g)		47.190	46.610	45.160	45.360	45.970	0.34	0.29
Weight Gain (g)	1 to 21 (Starter)	638.14	649.94	654.14	656.32	662.08	4.37	0.54
	21 to 42 (Grower)	1505.23	1485.28	1468.05	1503.23	1462.05	9.43	0.51
	1 to 42 (Total)	2143.36	2135.22	2122.19	2159.54	2124.13	9.50	0.76
	21 to 35 (Experimental Period)	744.73	721.93	740.00	722.88	712.13	5.60	0.33
Average Daily Gain (g)	1 to 21 (Starter)	30.38	30.94	31.14	31.25	31.52	0.21	0.54
	21 to 42 (Grower)	71.677	70.727	69.907	71.582	69.621	0.45	0.51
	1 to 42 (Total)	51.032	50.838	50.528	51.417	50.574	0.23	0.76
	21 to 35 (Experimental Period)	53.195	51.566	52.857	51.634	50.866	0.40	0.33
Weight Gain (%) 21-35	Total Weight	34.75	33.82	34.89	33.47	33.53	0.69	0.46
	Final Weight	34.003	33.103	34.163	32.791	32.829	0.68	0.47
Final Weight (g)		2190.55	2181.83	2167.35	2204.90	2170.10	9.54	0.76

early correlated to its phenolic concentration (Llorach et al., 2002). In fact, AE is known as a natural non-enzymatic antioxidant (Balasundram et al, 2006) because of its high phenolic contents.

As previously mentioned, for evaluation of the effects of AE on antioxidant status and meat quality, some antioxidant enzymes and the concentration of MDA as a lipid peroxidation marker were measured. GPx and CAT are two key antioxidant enzymes that can decompose hydrogen peroxide to water (Kheradmand et al., 2010). With respect to antioxidant enzyme activities, our results showed a significant decrease in GPx and CAT activates in AE 200 mg/l-treated broilers. In this regards,

Bobek et al. (1998) performed a hypercholesterolemic study in which rats were fed with a diet supplemented with tomato, apple, or grape pomaces. In all of the supplemented diets, decreases were observed in SOD, CAT, and GPx enzymes (range 36-56%). Dietary supplementation with thyme oil and thymol, rich in antioxidant terpenoids, also prevented the age-induced decline of GPx activity in rat brain (Youdim and Deans, 2000).

Moreover, Breinholt et al. (1999) observed activity of GPx and Glutathione reductase (GR) decrease after gavage administration of natural flavonoids to rats. Experimental administration of low molecular weight antioxidant (such as poly phenolic components) has also been shown to cause compensatory changes in enzymatic antioxidant defenses (Sohal and Allen, 1986). In this setting, Masella et al. (2005) have expressed that "Antioxidant Responsive Elements (AREs) are present in the promoter regions of many of the genes inducible by oxidative and chemical stresses". Thus, it appears that in the present study, consumption of AE (as source of phenolic compounds) was able to decrease activity of the GPx and CAT by the compensatory mechanism via AREs. This effect presumably is due to quenching of free radicals by phenolic compounds in AE-treated broilers compared to the control group (Chu et al., 2000).

It is well-known that superoxide radicals and peroxides are continuously produced within the cell by various subcellular reactions. The first defense of the cell to protect against oxidation is non-enzymatic antioxidants (Sies, 1997). If the non-enzymatic antioxidants are not adequate to cope with continuously produced free radicals in the cells, then enzymatic antioxidant comes through. Therefore, reduction in GPx activity in 100 and 200 mg /l AE-treated groups probably occurs due to high content of phenolic compound in these groups. Generally, compounds like flavonoides and vitamin C destroy free radicals and trap ROS (Chu et al., 2000). Considering that AE is rich in flavonoides and vitamin C, AE might reduce the concentration of ROS in the thigh meat. Reduction in ROS consequently postpones the need for enzymatic antioxidants (i.e. GPx and CAT). On the other hand, the AE may cause a decrease in GPx activity by down regulation of gene expression in the thigh muscles during growing period in broiler chickens. Although we were not able to measure gene-expression of antioxidant enzymes, a previous report indicated a decrease in GPx activity by non-enzymatic antioxidants in broiler muscles and a negative relationship between GPx activity and tissue α-tocopherol levels and a positive relationship between MDA and antioxidant enzyme activity has been observed by Maraschiello et al. (1999).

Regarding lipid peroxidation, MDA concentration decreased with AE treatments, however, the differences between groups were not significant. In this regards, Dobbau et al. (2014) demonstrated that the supplementation of Artichoke brackets did not induce any effect on MDA content in rabbit meat. Moreover, Llorch et al. (2002) reported that the extracts from artichoke by-products showed a high capacity to inhibit linoleic acid (LA) peroxidation and prevented lipid peroxidation. The MDA results, probably due to small sample size of broilers or less specific TBA method, is unable to determine differences among the groups as significant.

Herein, weight gain, average daily weight gain; percentage of weight gain in 21 to 35 d as well as final weight were similar in control and AE-treated groups. In this regard, Yildiz et al. (2006) concluded that the supplementation of Jerusalem artichoke as an inulin source with or without Vetch had no adverse effect on laying hen performance. Findings of the current study are in agreement with those of Dora et al (2005), which reported that treatment using Echinacea cob produced a significantly lower body weight compared to the control group, and was contrary to those reported by Lee et al. (2004), in which dietary additions of cinnamon to broiler diet improved weight gain. It seems, our results are correct since, AE dose not induce diet consumption or feed conversion ratio to enhance weight gain in the broilers.

Taken together, it seems that administration of 200 mg/l AE in drinking water during growing phase decreases GPx and CAT activities in chicken meat, presumably due to down-regulation of gene expression for antioxidant enzymes. However, further studies should be performed to evaluate antioxidant properties of AE with large sample size of broilers and more specific methods, such as Vyncke (1975), for evaluation of lipid peroxidation in meat of broilers.

Acknowledgements

We are most grateful to Dr. Rasoulian in Razi Herbal Medicines Research Center, Lorestan University of Medical Sciences for his kindly cooperation.

References

1. Alirezaei, M., Reza Gheisari, H., Reza Ranjbar, V., Hajibemani, A. (2012) Betaine: a promising antioxidant agent for enhancement of broiler meat quality. J Br Poult Sci. 53: 699-707.
2. Balasundram, N., Sundram, K., Samman, S. (2006) Phenolic compounds in plants and agri-industrial by-products: antioxidant activity, occurrence, and potential uses. J Food Chem. 99: 191-203.
3. Bobek, P., Ozdín, L., Hromadova, M. (1998) The effect of dried tomato, grape and apple pomace on the cholesterol metabolism and antioxidative enzymatic system in rats with hypercholesterolemia. Food/ Nahrung. 42: 317-320.
4. Botsoglou, N.A., Fletouris, D.J., Florou-Paneri, P., Christaki, E., Soais, A.B. (2002) Inhibition of lipid oxidation in long-term frozen stored chicken meat by dietary oregano essential oil and α-tocopheryl acetate supplementation. J Food Res. 36: 2007-2013.
5. Brand-williams, W., Cuvelier, M.E., Berset, C. (1995) Use of free radical method t evaluate antioxidant activity. Lebensm Wiss Technol. 28: 25-30.
6. Breinholt, V., Lauridsen, S.T., Dragsted, L.O. (1999) Differential effects of dietary flavonoids on drug metabolizing and antioxidant enzymes in female rat. Xenobiotica. 29: 1227-1240.
7. Burits, M., Bucar, F. (2000) Antioxidant activity of Nigella sativa essential oil. Phytother Res. 14: 323-328.
8. Chu, Y.H., Chang, C.L., Hsu, H.F. (2000) Flavonoid content of several vegetables and their antioxidant activity. J Agric Food Chem. 45: 2374-2378.
9. Claibrone, A. (1985) Catalase activity. In: Handbook of the Methods for Oxygen Radical Research. Greenwald, R.A. (ed.) (2nd ed.) CRC Press. Boca Raton. p. 283-284.
10. Dabbou, S., Gasco, L., Gai, F., Zoccarato, I., Rotolo, L., DabbouFekih, S., Peiretti, P.G. (2014) Dried artichoke bracts in rabbits nutrition: effects on the carcass characteristics, meat quality and fatty-acid composition. Animal. 8: 1547-1553.
11. Dora, A., Roth-Maier, B., Bohmer, M., Maab, N., Damme K., Paulicks, M.B.R. (2005) Efficiency of Echinacea purpureaon performance of broilers and layers. Eur J Poult Sci. 69: 123-127.
12. Duncan, D.B. (1955) Multiple range and multiple F test. Biometrics. 11: 1-42.
13. Gutteridge, J.M. (1995) Lipid peroxidation and antioxidants as biomarkers of tissue damage. Clin Chem. 41: 1819-1828.
14. Jacob, R.A. (1995) The integrated antioxidant system. Nutr Res. 15: 755-766.
15. Jimenez-Escrig, A., Dragsted, L.O., Daneshvar, B., Pulido, R., Saura-Calixto, F. (2003) In vitro antioxidant activities of edible artichoke (*Cynara scolymus* L.) and effect on biomarkers of antioxidants in rats. J Agric Food Chem. 51: 5540-5545.
16. Kheradmand, A., Alirezaei, M., Birjandi, M.

(2010) Ghrelinpromotes antioxidant enzyme activity and reduces lipidperoxidation in the rat ovary. Regul Pept. 162: 84-89.
17. Lattanzio, V., Kroon, P.A., Linsalata, V., Cardinali, A. (2009) Globe artichoke: a functional food and source of nutraceutical ingredients. J Func Foods. 1: 131-144.
18. Lattanzio, V., Sumere van, C.F. (1987) Changes in phenolic compounds during the development and cold storage of artichoke (*Cynara scolymus* L.) heads. J Food Chem. 24: 37-50.
19. Lee, K.W., Everts, H., Kappert, H.J., Beynen, A.C. (2004) Growth performance of broiler chickens fed a carboxymethyl cellulose containing diet with supplemental carvacrol and/or cinnamaldehyde. Int J Poult Sci. 3: 619-622.
20. Llorach, R., Espin, J., Tomas-Barberan, F.A.,-Ferreres, F. (2002) Artichoke (*Cynara scolymus* L.) byproducts as a potential source of health-promoting antioxidant phenolics. J Agric Food Chem. 50: 3458-3464.
21. Lopez-bote, C.J., Gray, J.I., Gomaa, E.A., Flegal, C.J. (1998) Effect of dietary administration of oil extracts from rosemary and sage on lipid oxidation in broiler meat. J Br Poult Sci. 39: 235-240.
22. Lowry, O.H., Rosebrough, N.J., Farr, A.L., Randall, R.J. (1951) Protein measurments with the folin phenol reagent. J Biol Chem. 193: 265-275.
23. Maraschiello, C., Sarraga, C., Garcia Regueiro, J.A. (1999) Glutathione peroxidase activity, TBARS, and alfa-tocopherol in meat from chickens fed different diets. J Agric Food Chem. 47: 867-873.
24. Masella, R., Benedetto, R.D., Varì, R., Filesi, C., Giovannini, C. (2005) Novel mechanisms of natural antioxidant compounds in biological systems: involvement of glutathione and glutathione-related enzymes. J Nutr Biochem. 16: 577-586.
25. Morrissey, P.A., Sheehy, P.J.A., Galvin, K., Kerry, J.P., Buckley, D.K. (1998) Lipid stability in meat and meat products. J Meat Sci. 49: S73-S86.
26. Nateghi, R., Samadi, F., Ganji, F., Zerehdaran, S. (2013) Hepatoprotective effects of *Cynara scolymus* L. extract on CCl4 induced liver injury in broiler chickens. Int J Agric Sci. 3: 678-688.
27. Schutz, K., Kammere, D., Carle, R., Schieber, A. (2004) Identification and quantification of caffeoylquinic acids and flavonoids from artichoke (*Cynara scolymus* L.) heads, juice, and pomace by HPLC-DAD-ESI/MS(n). J Agric Food Chem. 52: 4090-4096.
28. Sies, H. (1997) Oxidative stress: oxidants and antioxidants. J Exp Phy. 82: 291-295.
29. Singh, R.P., Murthy, K.N., Jayaprakasha, G.K. (2002) Studies on the antioxidant activity of pomegranate peel and seed extracts using in vitro models. J Agric Food Chem. 50: 81-86.
30. Sohal, R.S., Allen, R.G. (1986) Relationship between oxygen metabolism, aging and development. Adv Free Radical Biol Med. 2: 117-160.
31. Subbarao, K.V., Richardson, J.S., Ang, L.C. (1990) Autopsy samples of Alzheimer's cortex show increased peroxidation in vitro. J Neurochem. 55: 342-345.
32. Vyncke, W. (1975) Evaluation of the direct thiobarbituric acid extraction method for determining oxidative rancidity in mackerel (*Scomber scombrus* L.). Fette Seifen Anstrichmittel. 77: 239-240.
33. Wang, M., Simon, J.E., Aviles, I.F., He, K., Zheng, Q.Y., Tadmor, Y. (2003) Analysis of antioxidative phenolic compounds in artichoke (*Cynara scolymus* L.). J Agric Food Chem. 51: 601-608.
34. Yildiz, G., Sacakli, P., Gungor, T. (2006) The effect of dietary Jerusalem artichoke (*Helianthus tuberosus* L.) on performance, egg quality characteristics and egg cholesterol content in laying hens. J Poult Sci. 51: 349-354.
35. Youdim, K.A., Deans, S.G. (2000) Effect of thyme oil and thymol dietary supplementation on the antioxidant status and fatty acid composition of the ageing rat brain. Br J Nutr. 83: 87-93.

13

Effect of *Lipia citridora* leaves powder on growth performance, carcass traits, blood metabolites and meat quality of broilers

Mehrparvar, M.[1], Mazhari, M.[1*], Esmaeilipour, O.[1], Sami, M.[2]

[1]*Department of Animal Sciences, Faculty of Agriculture, University of Jiroft, Kerman, Iran*

[2]*Department of Food Hygiene, Faculty of Veterinary Medicine, Shahid Bahonar University, Kerman, Iran*

Key words:
broiler, blood metabolites, growth performance, *Lipia citridora*, meat quality

Correspondence
Mazhari, M.
Department of Animal Sciences, Faculty of Agriculture, University of Jiroft, Kerman, Iran

Email: mozhgan.mazhari@gmail.com

Abstract:

BACKGROUND: Since the prohibition of antibiotic growth promoter in poultry ration by the European Union, poultry producers have been trying to replace them by other growth promoters like medicinal herbs. *Lipia citridora* is a medicinal herb enriched by several powerful phenolic compounds and with antioxidant and antimicrobial properties which lead to enhancing appetite and growth performance of broiler. **OBJECTIVES:** The aim of this study was to investigate the effect of *Lipia citridora* leaves powder (LCLP) on growth performance, carcass traits, blood metabolites, and meat quality of broilers. **METHODS:** The experiment was carried out with 160 one-day-old male Ross 308 broiler chickens in a completely randomized design. The chicks were allocated to four diets including basal diet and treatment diets which were supplemented with 3 levels of LCLP (0.25, 0.5 and 1.0% of diet) in 16-floor pens with 10 chickens each. At the end of the experiment, 2 chicks/pen were selected and the assigned parameters were evaluated. **RESULTS:** All levels of LCLP improved ($p<0.01$) feed intake, body weight gain and feed conversion ratio in all periods except for starter phase. Also, 1% LCLP improved FI (1.49%), BWG (4.20%) and FCR (2.59%) compared to control group during the whole period. Birds fed herbal additive had a significantly higher relative weight of carcass, breast, bursa of fabricius and spleen in 1% LCLP group compared with the control group. Addition of 1% of LCLP decreased ($p<0.05$) LDL (15.85%), cholesterol (8.73%), triglyceride (8.82%), and increased ($p<0.01$) white blood cells (8.04). Meat quality enhanced via an intense reduction ($p<0.01$) in thiobarbituric acid (50.15%) and cooking loss (14.16%). **CONCLUSIONS:** Our finding showed that the highest level of LCLP in this study (1%) performed the best as improved growth performance, ameliorated serum lipids, increased white blood cells and enhanced the meat quality.

Introduction

Increasing growth performance in broilers needs more research trials on nutrition requirements. In this line the growth promoters are the main purpose of nutrition studies. Antibiotic growth promoters (AGP) have been used for reducing the spread of diseases and as growth promoter to enhance broiler performance. However, many AGP have already been restricted by animal farms in the European Union and some parts of Asia because of their residual effects on poultry products and harmful effects on human health (Lillehoj and Lee, 2012). Consequently, nutritionists and production managers have to find alternatives that have potential to alleviate the problems related to AGP. Therefore, herbal additives including herbs, spices and various plant extracts have received increased attention as possible AGP replacements due to their effects on microflora. Scientific evidence suggests that these herbal additives have appetite and digestion stimulating properties and promote the growth of beneficial bacteria and inhibit the growth of unfavorable bacteria in the gut (Windicsh et al., 2008).

Lippia citriodora with the common names of lemon verbena and lemon beebrush, is a species of flowering plant in the verbena family Verbenaceae. *Lippia citriodora* (LC) is a perennial shrub or sub-shrub with pointed and slightly rough to touch leaves and emits a powerful scent reminiscent of lemon when bruised. *Lippia citriodora* leaves are used to add a lemony flavor in many culinary purposes such as fish and poultry dishes, vegetable marinades, salad dressings, jams, puddings, and beverages. It is also used to make herbal teas and refreshing sorbets (Funes et al., 2009). Therefore, LC products and their compounds can be considered in the food category. This plant is mainly used as a spice and as a medicinal plant. This medicinal herb has already proven its antimicrobial effect and stimulating growth performance in lambs (Casamassima et al., 2013). It has been reported that the most phenolic compounds in this herb include Apigenin, 7-glucuronide, Luteolin-7-diglucuronide, Verbascoside, Isoverbascoside, and Martinoside, of whichthe major one is Verbascoside (Bilia et al., 2008). Verbascoside has a high potency of antioxidant, is antibacterial and antitumor and promotes the growth performance. *Lippia citriodora* contains mucilage, tannin and flavonoids as well, and is alkaloids-free (Bilia et al., 2008). There are not enough findings about using this herb in broiler ration, thus, the aim of this study was to evaluate the effect of *Lippia citriodora* leaves powder on growth performance, carcass traits, blood metabolites and meat quality of broilers.

Materials and Methods

Birds, diets and management: The experimental protocols were approved by the Animal Care Committee of University of Jiroft, Iran. A total number of 160 day-old male Ross 308 broiler chicks (average weight of 45 g) were obtained from Mahan commercial hatchery (Mahan, Kerman, Iran). The birds were fed to match the requirements recommended by the Ross 308 recommendations (Aviagen, 2007) during the starter (1-10 d), grower (11-25 d) and finisher (26-42 d) periods (Table 1). During the whole experiment the chicks were allocated to four diets including control (basal) diet and treatment diets which were supplemented with 3 levels of *Lippia citriodora* leaves powder (0.25, 0.5 and 1.0%) in 16-floor pens with 10 chickens each in a completely randomized design. *Lippia citriodora* leaves were prepared from university farm (University of Jiroft, Jiroft, Iran), rinsed and chopped by hand and then dried at room temperature. It was added to each treatment diet daily. All diets were provided isocaloric and isonitrogenous. No antimicrobials or anticoccidials were added into the diets. Each pen was equipped with a feeding trough and nipple drinkers and birds had free access to feed and water. The pen (1×1.5 m2) floor was covered with wood-shaving litter. Broilers were vaccinated against common diseases of the area based on Jiroft University Veterinary Protocol. Birds received 24 h light in first week of age and were then subjected to 23-h light: 1-h darkness until 42 d of age. Temperature was initially set at 32°C for the first 3 d of age and decreased by 3°C per week. The humidity was 50-60% during the experiment.

Sample collection and measurements: Body weight gain of birds was measured per pen at the end of each period. Feed intake of the birds was measured on a pen basis for the same periods. Mortality and the weight of birds that died or were culled during the trial were recorded. Feed conversion ratio was calculated for these periods. At day 42 of age, two birds per replicate whose weight were close to the average weight of each pen, were selected and killed by cervical dislocation, and blood samples were collected from the brachial vein in two tubes to obtain serum and plasma. One tube of blood samples was immediately centrifuged at 1000 × g for 15 min at 4 °C for analyzing serum glucose, total cholesterol, triglyceride, HDL, LDL by an autoanalyser using the protocol provided by the kit manufacturer (Zist-Shimi, Tehran, Iran). Heparin-containing tubes were used to avoid blood clot formation. Blood smears were prepared on slides and painted by Gimsa method. The white blood cells (WBC) and red blood cells (RBC) counts and the hemoglobin (Hb) values were determined by SysmexK-1000 apparatus (Japan).

The blood-collected birds mentioned above were considered to determine the carcass traits. Carcass yield was determined as the carcass weight in relation to live BW and expressed as percentage of BW, whereas other carcass cuts including breast, leg, liver, Bursa fabricius, spleen and ventral fat were expressed as percentage of carcass weight.

Muscle from the right side of breast was used to determine objective thiobarbituric acid, water-holding capacity, cooking loss, drip loss and pH.

The concentration of thiobarbituric acid (TBA) in the sausage was measured photometrically according to Bruna et al., (2001). One gram of the sausage homogenate was minced in 10 ml of TBA (20%) for 2 min. After the addition of 0.5 ml of butylated hydroxytoluene (0.19 M) and centrifugation for 6 min at 3,000 × g (Hermle Z383 K, Hermle GmbH, Wehingen, Germany), the solution was filtered through filter paper (MN 613, Macherey-Nagel GmbH, Dueren, Germany). To 0.7 mL of the filtrate, the same volume of TBA (0.02 M) was added and heated for 30 min at 100°C (LAT GmbH, Garbsen, Germany). After cooling for 10 min, the TBA concentration was determined at 532 nm (Helios β, Unicam Chromatography GmbH, Kassel, Germany). All experiments were performed in triplicate, and results were expressed as micrograms of malondialdehyde per gram of sample.

For measuring Water-holding capacity, one gram of minced breast meat sample was placed on a round plastic plate with small holes. The plate with meat sample on it was then fitted into a 2-mL plastic tube. This tube was centrifuged at 920 × g for 10 min. The released water content was measured and calculated as a percentage of the initial weight (Castellini et al., 2002).

To obtain Cooking loss, one fillet from each whole breast was individually weighed and cooked in a convection oven on aluminum trays at 180°C until the core temperature reached 80°C. The fillet was then allowed to equilibrate to room temperature and reweighed, and cooking loss was determined as the percentage of weight lost by the sample (Bertrama et al., 2003).

For determining drip loss, breast fillet was individually weighed, sealed in plastic bags, stored at 4°C for 24 h, and then reweighed (Saenmahayak et al., 2010).

The pH value was determined at 24 h (ultimate pH) postmortem in the breast muscle at a 2-cm depth (Jaturasitha et al., 2008), using a portable pH meter (IQ150, IQ Scientific Instruments Inc., Carlsbad, CA) equipped with a stainless electrode (pH57-SS).

Statistical analysis: Prior to analysis, all percentage data were normalized by subjecting to arc sine transformation. As the pen represented the experimental unit, the effect of LCLP on performance, carcass traits, serum parameters, immunity and meat quality of broilers was statistically analyzed in a completely randomized design using the GLM procedure of SAS 9.1 (2001). Treatment means were compared using Tukey's multiple range test.

Results

Growth performance: The effect of *Lippia citriodora* leaves powder (LCLP) on feed intake (FI), body weight gain (BWG) and feed conversion ratio (FCR) of broilers at different periods is shown in Table 2. Dietary supplementation of LCLP increased ($p<0.01$) FI and BWG during the grower, finisher and whole periods compared with the control group. Also, 1% LCLP improved FI (1.49%), BWG (4.20%) and FCR (2.59%) compared to control group during the whole period ($p<0.01$). However, none of the three levels of LCLP had significant effect on performance during the starter period.

Carcass traits: Birds fed different levels of LCLP had a significantly heavier relative weight of carcass and breast, spleen and bursa of fabricius, whereas significant difference was not detected on relative weight of thigh, liver and abdominal fat by treatments in this study (Table 3).

Serum metabolites: Serum glucose level was not affected in birds fed LCLP in this study (Table 4), but by increasing the level of LCLP in diet the hypo-effect of this herb on serum lipids was more pronounced. All levels of LCLP decreased ($p<0.05$) cholesterol, triglyceride and LDL, compared to the control group. Adding LCLP to the diet increased ($p<0.01$) white blood cells, while red blood cells counts, hemocrite and hemoglobin values were not changed among the control and treatment groups.

Meat quality: The effect of LCLP on meat quality of broilers at 42 d of age is shown in Tables 5. Data showed when LCLP was introduced into the diet, the meat quality was improved ($p<0.05$) via an intense reduction ($p<0.01$) in TBA and cooking loss. Although meat quality was enhanced ($p>0.05$) in terms of increase in water holding capacity (WHC) and pH and decrease in drip loss, these changes were not significant.

Discussion

Growth performance: According to our

Table 1. Composition of starter, grower, and finisher diets. [1]Vitamin mix provided the following per kilogram of diet: vitamin A (trans-retinyl acetate), 9,000 IU; vitamin D3 (cholecalciferol), 215 IU; vitamin E (DL-α-tocopheryl acetate), 18 IU; vitamin K (menadione), 2 mg; thiamine, 18 mg; riboflavin, 6.6 mg; pyridoxine, 3 mg; vitamin B12 (cyanocobalamin), 0.015 mg; niacin, 10 mg; pantothenic acid (D-calcium pantothenate), 4.8 mg; folic acid, 1 mg; biotin, 0.15 mg; choline chloride, 500 mg; ethoxyquin (antioxidant), 1 mg. [2]Mineral mix provided the following per kilogram of diet: Fe, 50 mg; Mn, 100 mg; Zn, 7.84 mg; Cu, 10 mg; I, 1 mg; Se, 0.2 mg.

Ingredient (%)	Starter (1-10 d)	Grower (11-25)	Finisher (26-42)
Corn	53.38	54.81	60.63
Soybean meal	38.45	36.23	30.85
Vegetable oil	3.49	5.00	4.85
Limestone	1.54	1.35	1.30
Dicalcium Phosphate	1.64	1.29	1.21
Vitamin mix1	0.25	0.25	0.25
Mineral mix2	0.25	0.25	0.25
Salt (NaCl)	0.29	0.29	0.29
L-Lysine	0.33	0.23	0.13
DL-Methionine	0.39	0.29	0.25
Calculated nutrients			
ME (kcal/kg)	3025	3150	3200
Crude protein (%)	22	21	19
Lysine (%)	1.43	1.30	1.09
Methionine+Cystine (%)	1.07	0.95	0.86
Threonine (%)	0.94	0.90	0.85
Calcium (%)	1.05	0.90	0.85
Available phosphorus (%)	0.50	0.45	0.42

Table 2. The effect of *Lipia citridora* leaves powder (LCLP) on performance of broilers at different periods.1FI = feed intake, BWG = body weight gain and FCR = feed conversion ratio. Means within the same column with uncommon superscript differ significantly (p<0.05).

	Treatments					
Parameters	Control	0.25% LCLP	0.5% LCLP	1% LCLP	SEM	p-Value
FI (g/b)1						
1-10 d	189.6	191.4	191.6	191.9	1.43	0.68
11-25 d	760.6	771.1	765.9	761.1	5.39	0.50
26-42 d	2071.8^{b}	2100.5^{ab}	2105.9^{a}	2115.3^{a}	7.89	0.01
Overall	3127.6^{b}	3170.0^{a}	3169.8^{a}	3174.1^{a}	8.02	0.004
BWG (g/b)1						
0-10 d	143.8	144.5	145.4	145.5	1.17	0.73
11-25 d	428.6^{b}	440.7^{a}	441.4^{a}	450.6^{a}	2.43	0.0003
26-42 d	1124.3^{b}	1155.0^{a}	1160.9^{a}	1171.9^{a}	6.01	0.0008
Overall	1760.4^{c}	1805.3^{b}	1812.9^{ab}	1834.3^{a}	6.63	0.0001
FCR1						
0-10 d	1.33	1.32	1.32	1.32	0.008	0.89
11-25 d	1.77^{a}	1.75^{a}	1.74^{ab}	1.69^{b}	0.01	0.006
26-42 d	1.84^{a}	1.82^{b}	1.81^{b}	1.80^{b}	0.005	0.002
Overall	1.78^{a}	1.76^{ab}	1.75^{bc}	1.73^{c}	0.005	0.0004

data, addition of *Lipia citridora* leaves powder (LCLP) improved growth performance

Table 3. The effect of *Lipia citridora* leaves powder (LCLP) on relative weight of carcass (relative weight: g/100 g of live weight), and carcass cuts (relative weight: g/100 g of carcass weight) of broilers at 42 d of age. [a,b]Means within the same column with uncommon superscript differ significantly (p<0.05).

	Treatments					
Parameters	Control	0.25% LCLP	0.5% LCLP	1% LCLP	SEM	p-Value
Carcass	83.72^{b}	84.62^{ab}	85.10^{ab}	86.45^{a}	0.523	0.02
Breast	26.54^{b}	26.76^{b}	27.68^{a}	27.96^{a}	0.195	0.0005
Thigh	23.38	23.54	23.82	23.89	0.509	0.87
Liver	2.58	2.74	2.77	2.76	0.118	0.66
Spleen	0.050^{b}	0.059^{ab}	0.069^{ab}	0.076^{a}	0.005	0.027
Bursa	0.11^{b}	0.13^{ab}	0.13^{ab}	0.14^{a}	0.005	0.014
Abdominal fat	1.47	1.42	1.37	1.31	0.078	0.56

Table 4. The effect of *Lipia citridora* leaves powder (LCLP) on Blood parameters (mg/dl) of broilers at 42 d of age. 1HDL: High Density Lipoprotein; LDL: Low Density Lipoprotein. 2WBC: White Blood Cells; RBC: Red Blood Cells. Hb: Hemoglobin. HCT: Hematocrit. Means within the same column with uncommon superscript differ significantly (p<0.05).

	Treatments					
Parameters	Control	0.25% LCLP	0.5% LCLP	1% LCLP	SEM	p-Value
Serum metabolites						
Glucose (mg/dl)	208.00	204.50	203.25	202.75	1.990	0.28
Triglyceride(mg/dl)	110.50^{a}	104.50^{ab}	102.75^{ab}	100.75^{b}	2.010	0.03
Cholesterol (mg/dl)	114.50^{a}	110.25^{ab}	105.50^{b}	104.50^{b}	1.840	0.008
HDL1 (mg/dl)	72.50	73.75	75.75	76.50	1.550	0.330
LDL1 (mg/dl)	20.50^{a}	18.25^{b}	18.00^{b}	17.25^{b}	0.420	0.0009
Blood cells2						
WBC ($\times 10^3/\mu l$)	21.55c	22.44^{b}	23.15^{ab}	23.28^{a}	0.191	0.0001
RBC ($\times 10^6/\mu l$)	2.20	2.24	2.26	2.26	0.030	0.690
Hb (g/dl)	9.32	9.40	9.60	9.62	0.130	0.340
HCT (%)	33042	33.55	35.60	35.82	0.62	0.06

during the grower, finisher and whole periods; just there was not an improvement at starter period. The best growth performance was observed by addition of 0.5 and 1% LCLP. In a study by Rafiee et al. (2016), using 0.5 and 1% *Lipia citridora* in broiler ration from 25 to 42 days of age and in heat stress condition resulted in increasing average weight gain and feed intake by 5.81 and 3.29%, and reducing feed conversion ratio by 2.59% by 1% *Lipia citridora* compared to control group. In line with our study, Casamassima et al. (2013) investigated the influence of 2.5 and 5 mg/kg *Lipia citridora* extract on lambs and showed that both levels of extract increased FI and average daily gain and decreased FCR. In another experiment the levels of 5 and 10 mg/kg *Lipia citridora* extract on pigs was assessed and only the higher level improved FI, BWG and FCR as compared to the control group (Pastorelli et al., 2012). Administration of herbal additives to the poultry diets has a positive effect on the food flavor that results in a higher feed consumption by modulating appetite and secretion of gastrointestinal digestive enzymes in birds. Also, Casamassima et al. (2013) reported that the pure extract of phenylpropanoid at the rate of 1 and 2 mg/kg increased weight gain of rats by 6.9 and 7.8%, respectively. Phenylpropanoids (especially verbascoside) are the main active components existing in *Lipia citridora* extract which act as a digestibil-

Table 5. The effect of *Lipia citridora* leaves powder (LCLP) on meat quality of broilers at 42 d of age. 1TBA: Thiobarbituric Acid, (μg MDA/g meat), MDA: Malondialdehyde; WHC: Water Holding Capacity. Means within the same column with uncommon superscript differ significantly (p<0.05).

	Treatments					
Parameters	Control	0.25% LCLP	0.5% LCLP	1% LCLP	SEM	P-Value
TBA1	0.27^{a}	0.17^{bc}	0.19^{b}	0.14^{c}	0.008	<0.0001
WHC1 (%)	74.33	74.93	75.12	77.30	0.900	0.16
Cooking loss (%)	35.85^{a}	32.65^{b}	30.80^{b}	30.77^{b}	0.750	0.001
Dripping loss (%)	44.00	41.50	39.75	40.50	1.830	0.420
pH	5.81	5.89	6.00	5.92	0.070	0.310

ity enhancer, balancing the gut microbial ecosystem and stimulating the secretion of endogenous digestive enzymes, and thus improving growth performance in poultry (Newall et al., 1996).

Carcass traits: Data showed that addition of LCLP increased the relative weight of carcass and breast. The higher breast yields of birds fed diet with 1% LCLP might be associated with higher activity of digestive enzymes and more efficient uptake of nutrients (specifically proteins) which led to better growth rate (Lewis et al., 2003). Parallel to our study, the relative weight of breast increased in broiler fed with 1% *Lipia citridora* (Rafiee et al., 2016). The results expressed that inclusion of LCLP to diet elevated the relative weight of spleen and bursa of fabricius in treated birds but the relative weight of abdominal fat (AF) did not change among treatments. Increased weight of these two lymphoid organs may indicate a higher immunity in *Lipia citridora*-treated birds which could be justified by the antimicrobial activity of phenylpropanoids and flavonoids in this herb. Demir et al. (2003) reported that herbal additives had no significant effect on relative weight of AF, but Kamisoyama et al. (2008) observed that 1 and 2% flavonoid oil suppressed the relative weight of AF in rats fed diet with high fat content. It was attributed to the increased activity of acetyl-CoA carboxylase and decreased activity of fatty acid synthase by flavonoid oil supplementation.

Serum metabolites: The present study revealed that the higher levels of LCLP were supplemented to the diets, a more hypocholesterolemic effect was seen in birds. Similar results were found in an investigation by Pastorelli et al. (2012) with pigs fed 5 and 10 mg/kg *Lipia citridora* extract. These authors suggested that feeding 10 mg/kg *Lipia citridora* extract suppressed serum LDL in pigs by 17%. One mechanism involved in the overall hypocholesterolemic effect of *Lipia citridora* supplementation might be attributed to the active components of this plant as the natural antioxidants. Phenolic compounds (flavonoids, tannins, phenolic acids, terpenes) are the molecules responsible for antioxidant activity of herbal additives. These components can adhere to LDL, inhibit the free radicals and in turn decrease cholesterol absorption to the blood (Lee et al., 2004). The other mechanism might be attributed to Verbascosides in *Lipia citridora* that are known to decrease cholesterol biosynthesis by inhibiting key enzymes, that is, 3-hydroxyl-3-methylglutaryl-coenzyme A reductase in poultry (Liu et al., 2003). Biochemical analysis of serum is very important for explanation of clinical findings. Biochemical analysis is used to support a diagnosis, to determine a cure for the disease, or to control the applied cure, to evaluate and to interpret the results of the research.

Serum Cholesterol, triglyceride and LDL levels showed a decreasing pattern when *Lipia citridora* was supplemented to the diet but glucose and HDL did not differ significantly. Pastorelli et al., (2012) showed decreasing serum LDL by 17% in pigs fed 10 mg/kg lemon verbena extract. Hypercholesterolemia is associated with an increased risk of coronary heart disease and one of the several efforts in lowering the blood cholesterol is supplementing animal and avian diets with medicinal plants or natural feed additives with Hypocholesterolemic activity (Rojhan, 2000). Adding LCLP to the diet increased white blood cells (WBC). It may be due to the effect of phenolic compounds of *Lipia citridora* on different parts of WBC, including lymphocytes. Rafiee et al. (2016) revealed that addition of *Lipia citridora* to broiler diets increased lymphocytes by 4.51% compared to control group. White blood cells also called leukocytes, are an important part of the immune system. These cells help fight infections by attacking bacteria, viruses, and germs that invade the body. Lee et al. (2004) concluded that the flavonoid-rich herbs resulted in improved immunity of birds due to their antimicrobial activity. Pastorelli et al. (2012) showed that the supplementation of 5 and 10 mg/kg *Lipia citridora* extract in broilers elevated the IgA and IgG. These results validate the responsibility of herbs that are rich in flavonoids such as *Lipia citridora* as antioxidants and may therefore enhance the immune functions.

Meat quality: Meat quality was improved in this study via decreasing ($p<0.05$) TBA and cooking loss and good modification ($p>0.05$) of WHC, drip loss and pH. Lipid peroxidation is an autocatalytic mechanism leading to oxidative destruction of cellular membranes. The destruction can lead to cell death and also to the production of toxic and reactive aldehyde metabolites, known as free radicals. Among these free radicals, malondialdehyde (MDA) is the most important and main final product of lipid peroxidation that has often been used for determining oxidative damage (Paradis et al., 1997). Overall, the amount of thiobarbituric acid (TBA) is considered as the indicator of MDA level. Medicinal herbs have strong antioxidant activity and active components of *Lipia citridora* are reported to inhibit lipid peroxidation (Casamassima et al., 2013). The results obtained in the present study imply that the active substances of the *Lipia citridora* may improve the antioxidative status of broilers due to the antioxidant property of Verbascoside by reducing the level of TBA. It was suggested that the high antioxidant activity of Verbascoside is due to the presence of phenolic OH groups which act as hydrogen donors to the proxy radicals produced during the first step in lipid oxidation, thus retarding the hydroxyl peroxide formation (Funes et al., 2009). Based on these findings, we state that *Lipia citridora* might play an important role as an exogenous antioxidant and could also be applicable as a protective agent against tissue damage. Several studies have been conducted on the improving effect of medicinal herbs on meat quality. The inclusion of Verbascoside to diets depressed the lipid peroxidation in muscles of rats significantly (Gao et al., 1999). Choiem Hwang (2005) demonstrated that medicinal plants elevated the antioxidant enzymes activity and reduced the MDA level in rats. Natural antioxidant-fed birds showed a lower meat oxidation degree than those that did not receive natural antioxidant in their diet (Sarraga and Regueiro, 1999). Considering that MDA is produced as a result of PUFA oxidation, Pallazo et al. (2015) reported that the intake of *Lipia citridora* resulted in a decrease in saturated fatty acids level and a higher level of PUFA in rabbit meat. No influence on carcass characteristics and the chemical composition of meat was observed. A positive effect on alpha-tocopherol tissue content and on thiobarbituric reactive substance (TBARS) values was observed in their study. These researches concluded that the *Lipia citridora* extract had the potential to improve rabbit meat without altering the chemical and physical characteristics of meat. The pH is an important index of meat quality. Decreased pH after slaughter is due to the proteins denaturation which results in lower WHC and lighter color meat (Briskey and Wismer-Pedersen, 1961). Jang et al. (2008) reported that a blend of herbal extracts increased pH of broiler meat and Mirshekar et al. (2009) showed a decrease on TBA of meat. The WHC of meat products is a very important quality attribute which has an influence on product yield, which in turn has economic implications, but is also important in terms of eating quality. A number of pre-and post-mortem factors influence the WHC of meat. Proteins denaturation and reduction of pH in meat cause the contraction of myofibrils of muscle and decrease the WHC and nutritive value of meat (Castellini et al., 2002). The other factor influencing the WHC is a proteolytic enzyme called μ-calpain which is activated after slaughter, resulting in higher WHC and which leads to meat tenderness. Although the oxidation and lower pH stop the activity of this enzyme, the medicinal herbs promote the proteolytic activity of μ-calpain and improve the meat quality (Huff-Lonergan and Lonergan, 2005). The more WHC there is in meat, the lower the occurrence of cooking loss and drip loss (Warris, 2000).

Conclusion: The results showed that the *Lipia citridora* supplementation served as a good growth promoter and immune enhancer in this study, since it improved growth performance, ameliorated serum lipids, increased white blood cells and enhanced the meat quality. The best results were observed by the highest level of *Lipia citridora* (1%), however, the results obtained in this study justify further research in this area.

Acknowledgements

The authors greatly acknowledge the financial support of University of Jiroft, Iran and the staff of the Animal Science Department for their technical assistance.

References

1. Aviagen. (2007) Ross 308: Broiler Nutrition Specification. Aviagen Inc., Huntsville, AL. USA.
2. Bertrama, H.C., Andersena, H.J., Korlssona, A.H. (2003) Prediction of technological quality (cooking loss) of pork based on fresh meat characteristics. Meat Sci. 65: 707-712.
3. Bilia, A.R., Giomi, M., Innocenti, M., Gallori, S., Vincieri, F.F. (2008) HPLCDAD-ESI-MS analysis of the constituents of aqueous preparations of verbena and lemon verbena and evaluation of the antioxidant activity. J Pharm Biomed Anal. 46: 463-470.
4. Briskey, E.J., Wismer-Pedersen, J. (1961) Biochemistry of pork muscle structure. Rate of anaerobic glycolysis and temperature change versus the apparent structure of

muscle tissue. J Food Sci. 26: 297-305.
5. Bruna, J.M., Ordonez, J.A., Fernandez, M., Herranz, B., dela Hoz, L. (2001) Microbial and physico-chemical changes during the ripening of dry fermented sausages superficially inoculated with or having added an intracellular cell-free extract of *Penicillium aurantiogriseum*. Meat Sci. 59: 87-96.
6. Casamassima, D., Palazzo, M., D'Alessandro, A.G., Colella, G.E., Vizzarri. F., Corino, C. (2013) The effects of lemon verbena (*Lippia citriodira*) verbascoside on the productive performance, plasma oxidative status, and some blood metabolites in suckling lambs. J Anim Feed Sci. 22: 204-212.
7. Castellini, C., Mugnai, C., Dal Bosco, A. (2002). Effect of organic production system on broiler carcass and meat quality. Meat Sci. 60: 219-225.
8. Choiem Hwang, J.K. (2005) Effect of some medicinal plants on plasma antioxidant system and lipid levels in rats. Phytother Res. 19: 382-395.
9. Demir, E., Sarica Ozcan, M.A., Suicmez, M. (2003) The use of natural feed additives as alternatives for an antibiotic growth promoter in broiler diets. Br Poult Sci. 44: 44-45.
10. Funes, L., Fernandez, A.S, Laporta, O., Pons, A., Roche, E., Segura, C.A., Fernandez, G.A. (2009) Correlation between plasma antioxidant capacity and verbascoside levels in rats after oral administration of lemon verbena extract. Food Chem. 17: 589-598.
11. Gao, J.J., Igalashi, K., Nukina, M. (1999) Radical scavenging activity of phenylpropanoid glycosides in *Caryopteris incana*. Biosci Biotechnol Biochem. 63: 983-988.
12. Huff-Lonergan, E., Lonergan, S.M. (2005) Mechanisms of water-holding capacity of meat: The role postmortem biochemical and structural changes. Meat Sci. 71: 194-204.
13. Jang, A., Liu, X.D., Shin, M.H., Lee, B.D., Lee, S.K., Lee, J.H., Jo, C. (2008) Antioxidative potential of raw breast meat from broiler chicks fed a dietary medicinal herb extract mix. Poult Sci. 87: 2382-2389.
14. Jaturasitha, S., Srikanchai, T., Kreuzer, M., Wicke, M. (2008) Differences in carcass and meat characteristics between chicken indigenous to northern Thailand (Black-Boned and Thai Native) and imported extensive breeds (Bresse and Rhode Island Red). Poult Sci. 87: 160-169.
15. Kamisoyama, H., Honda, K., Tominaga, Y., Yokota, S., Hasegawa, S. (2008) Investigation of the anti-obesity action of licorice flavonoid oil in diet-Induced obese rats. Biosci Biotechnol Biochem. 72: 3225-3231.
16. Lee, K.W., Everts, H., Beynen, A.C. (2004) Essential Oils in Broiler Nutrition. Int J Poult Sci. 3: 738-752.
17. Lewis, M.R., Rose, S.P., MaCkenzie, A.M., Tucker, L.A. (2003) Effects of dietary inclusion of plant extracts on the growth performance of male broiler chickens. Br Poult Sci. 44: 42-43.
18. Lillehoj, H.S., Lee, K.W. (2012) Immune modulation of innate immunity as alternatives-to-antibiotics strategies to mitigate the use of drugs in poultry production. Poult Sci. 91: 1286-1291.
19. Liu, M.J., Li, J.X., Guo, H.Z., Le,e K.M., Qin, L., Chan, K.M. (2003) The effects of verbascoside on plasma lipid peroxidation level and erythrocyte membrane fluidity during immobilization in rabbits: a time course study. Life Sci. 73: 883-892.
20. Mirshekar, R., Dastar, B., Shabanpour, B. (2009) Effect of Rosemary, Echinacea, Green tea Extracts and ascorbic acid on broiler meat quality. Pak J Biol Sci. 12: 1069-1074.
21. Newall, C.A., Anderson, L.A., Phillipson, J.D. (1996) Herbal Medicines -A Guide for

Healthcare Professionals. The Pharmaceutical Press, London, UK.

22. Palazzo, M., Vizzarri, F., Nardoia, M., Ratti, S., Pastorelli, G., Casamassima, D. (2015) Dietary *Lippia citriodora* extract in rabbit feeding: effects on quality of carcass and meat. Arch Anim Breed. 58: 355-364.
23. Paradis,V., Kollinger, M., Farbe, M., Holstage, A., Poynard, T., Bedossa, P. (1997) In situ detection of lipid peroxidation by-product in chronic liver diseases. Hepatology. 26: 135-143.
24. Pastorelli, G., Rossi, R., Corino, C. (2012) Influence of *Lippia citriodora* verbascoside on growth performance, antioxidant status, and serum immune globulins content in piglets. Czech J Anim Sci. 57: 312-322.
25. Rafiee, F., Mazhari, M., Ghoreishi, M., Esmaeilipour, O. (2016) Effect of lemon verbena powder and vitamin C on performance, and immunity of heat stressed broilers. J Anim Physiol Anim Nutr. doi: 10.1111/jpn.12457.
26. Rojhan, M. (2000) Medicine and medicinal cure. (1st ed.) Alavi Press. Tehran, Iran.
27. Saenmahayak, B., Bilgili, S.F., Hess, J.B., Singh, M. (2010) Live and processing performance of broiler chickens fed diets supplemented with complexed zinc. J Appl Poult Res. 19: 334-340.
28. Sarraga, C., Regueiro, J.A. (1999) Membrane lipid oxidation and proteolytic activity in thigh muscles from broilers fed different diets. Meat Sci. 52: 213-219.
29. Warris, P.D. (2000) Meat Science. An Introductory Text. CABI Pub. Inc. New York, USA.
30. Windisch, J., Schedle, W., Plitzner, C., Kroismayr, A. (2008) Use of phytogenic products as feed additives for swine and poultry. J Anim Sci. 86: 140-148.

14

Doppler echocardiographic findings in tissue engineered aortic valve in a sheep model

Mokhber Dezfouli, M.R.[1,4]**, Tavanaeimanesh, H.**[1,4*]**, Dehghan, M.M.**[2,4]**, Hayati, F.**[2]**, Sadeghian Chaleshtori, S.**[1,4]**, Akbarein, H.**[3]**, Pournaghi, P.**[5]

[1]*Department of Internal Medicine, Faculty of Veterinary Medicine, University of Tehran, Tehran, Iran*

[2]*Department of Surgery and Radiology, Faculty of Veterinary Medicine, University of Tehran, Tehran, Iran*

[3]*Department of Food Hygiene and Quality Control, Faculty of Veterinary Medicine, University of Tehran, Tehran, Iran*

[4]*Institute of Biomedical Research, Faculty of Veterinary Medicine, University of Tehran, Tehran, Iran*

[5]*Department of Biology, Payame Noor University, Tehran, Iran*

Key words:

echocardiography, heart, hemodynamic, tissue engineer, valve

Correspondence

Tavanaeimanesh, H.

Department of Internal Medicine, Faculty of Veterinary Medicine, University of Tehran, Tehran, Iran

Email: hamidtavana@ut.ac.ir

Abstract:

BACKGROUND: Heart valve diseases are considered a common disease in human and animals, and valve replacement is an option for treatment of valvular diseases. **OBJECTIVES:** In this study efficacy of a tissue engineered valve in thoracic aorta was evaluated with transthoracic echocardiography. **METHODS:** This study was undertaken on 6 male sheep. Echocardiography was performed on all sheep 24 hours before surgery and repeated 24 hours (D1), 2 weeks (W2) and 4 weeks (W4) after surgery. Right parasternal long axis view of left ventricular outflow tract (LVOT) was used to assess hemodynamic across new valve. **RESULTS:** Velocity time integral (VTI) significantly decreased from 18.98±2.88 before surgery to 12.55±2.48 one day after surgery (D1) ($p<0.05$). Mean Velocity (Vmean) decreased significantly from 52.56±12.01 to 39.72±12.30 at D1 ($p<0.05$). But maximum velocity (Vmax) was constant during study. There was not any statistical difference between mean Pressure gradient (Pgmean) or maximum pressure gradient (Pgmax) in comparison with pre-surgery and D1, W2 and W4. At D1, W2 and W4, time to peak (TTP) differed significantly from previous time. **CONCLUSIONS:** Our results demonstrated that this tissue engineered aortic valve (TEAV) could change some hemodynamic parameters, but heart could compensate some of them. Valve movement remained normal but the major complication was aneurism which seems to be the result of poor scaffold.

Introduction

Prosthetic valve (PV) replacement is a common procedure in patients with cardiac valve dysfunction. Valvular replacement is the most prevalent method of treating advanced cardiac valves dysfunction. Over 80 models of prosthetic valves have been introduced and applied since 1950 (Cebotari et al. 2002). PVs are mainly mechanical or bioprosthetic. Mechanical valves are the oldest and long-lasting prosthetic valves. Biological prostheses span a range from porcine or bovine trileaflet valves and homografts (processed human cadaveric valves (Tobias and Frank 2010). One of the main concerns about prosthetic valve dysfunction is their life threatening potential. Transthoracic echocardiography (TTE) is a noninvasive diagnostic method for PVs evaluation. The accuracy, noninvasive nature, broad availability, and absence of exposure to ionizing radiation have established echocardiography/Doppler as the standard for the clinical assessment of heart valve function (Bonow et al. 2006; Vahanian et al. 2012) including the assessment of hemodynamics after aortic valve replacement (Bach 2010). This enables immediate evaluation of replaced valve soon after surgery and provides critical and specific information about hemodynamic status of the valves. Color Doppler and spectral Doppler are the main echocardiographic procedures for hemodynamic assessment. Flow velocities across PVs and peak and mean gradients should be assessed by continuous wave Doppler (CWD) as in a native valve (Tobias and Frank 2010). PVs may cause obstruction, especially in patient-prosthetic mismatch which will cause functional obstruction despite its good mechanical performance (Rahimtoola 1978). Regurgitation is another complication after PVs replacement which is often difficult to assess particularly in mechanical prosthetics (Tobias and Frank 2010).

The purpose of this study was TTE evaluation of tissue engineered aortic valve (TEAV) placed in thoracic aorta of sheep model and assessment of post-operative hemodynamic values TEAV.

Materials and Methods

All of the procedures were performed in Critical Care Center of Experimental Medicine Institute of University of Tehran and approved by Research Council of Veterinary Faculty.

Animals: This study was undertaken on 6 male sheep between 45-55 kg in weight and 2-3 years of age. All sheep were considered normal on clinical examination.

Echocardiography: Echocardiography was performed 24 hours before surgery. Sheep were prepared for echocardiography by clipping the region between 3rd and 5th intercostal spaces, washing with surgical spirit and covering the clipped area with acoustic coupling gel. Echocardiography was done in standing position. For aortic valve evaluation echocardiography (Micro Maxx: SonoSite Inc, Bothell, WA, USA with a phase array transducer 1-5 MHz). was performed from right parasternal window and left ventricular outflow tract (LVOT) view was used for assessment of both native aortic valve and TEAV. To evaluate hemodynamic status, color Doppler and pulse wave Doppler were used. Gate was placed distal to the native valve and TEAV. Echocardiography was repeated using the same procedure at 24 hours, 2 and 4 weeks after surgery. Echocardiograph machine with a phase array transducer (1-5 MHz) was used. Velocity time integral (VTI), time to peak (TTP), mean and maximum velocity (V¬mean¬ and V¬max) and mean and maximum pressure gradient (PGmean and PGmax) were measured and data was compared statistically at the four mentioned times.

Statistical analysis. Repeated measures analysis and paired t test with 95% Confidence Interval were done by General Linear Model (GLM) procedure of the SPSS version 16.0. Data was expressed as Mean ± SE. A P-value of less than 0.05 was considered statistically significant.

Results

VTI significantly decreased from 18.98±2.88cm before surgery to 12.55±2.48cm one day after surgery (D1) ($p<0.05$). Two weeks after surgery (W2) this value increased and again 4 weeks after surgery (W4) decreased none of which was statistically significant (Table1).

The mean value of Vmax was constant

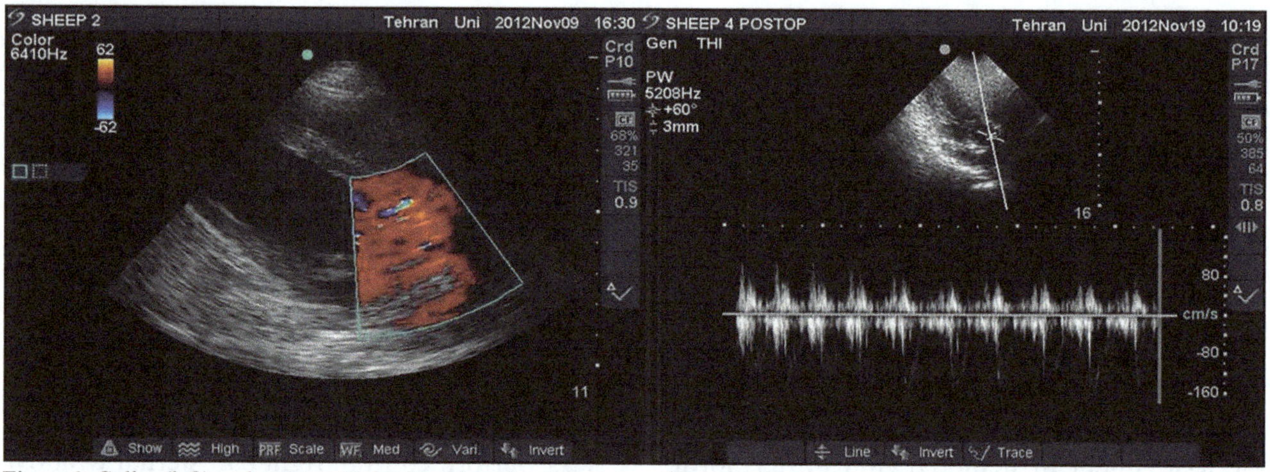

Figure 1. Collor (left) and spectral (right) Doppler of native aortic valve.

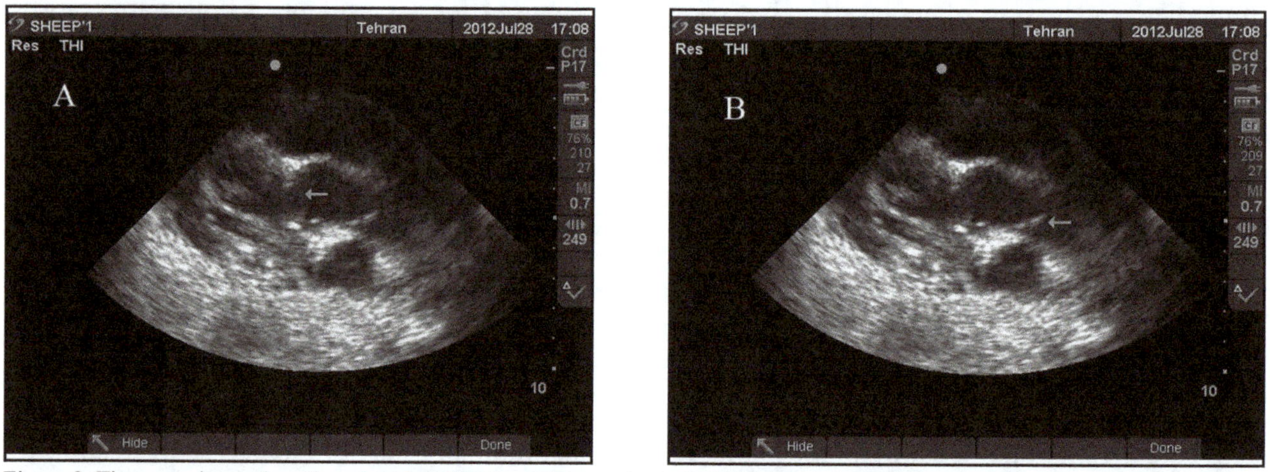

Figure 2. Tissue engineered aortic valve placed in thoracic aorta (arrow). A) Native valve B) Tissue engineered valve.

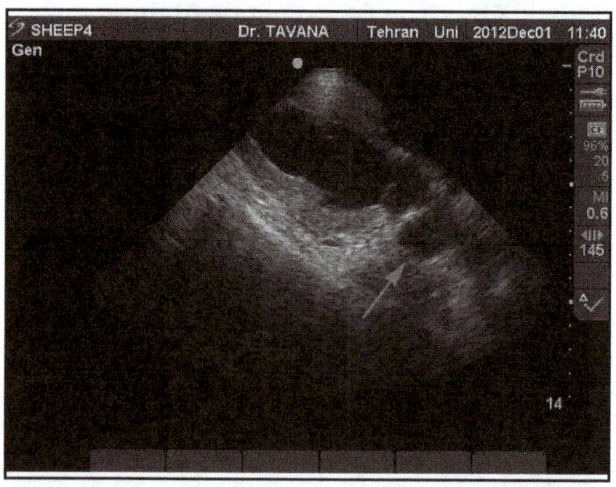

Figure 3. Aneurism 2 weeks after surgery in graft (arrow).

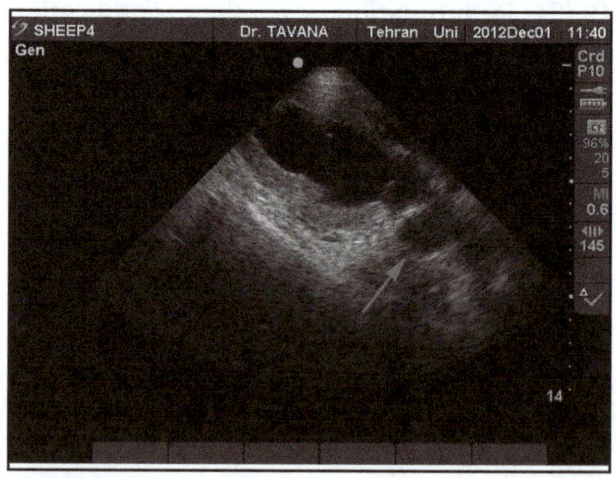

Figure 4. Aneurism 2 weeks after surgery in our graft which is shown on CT angiograph (arrow).

during the study and there were no significant changes at D1, W2 and W4 in comparison with previous time and pre-surgery. Vmean decreased significantly from 52.56±12.01cm/s to 39.72±12.30cm/s at D1 ($p<0.05$). At W2 and W4 the Vmean value increased to 41.26±8.78cm/s and 52.26±4.40cm/s respectively, that was not significantly different from

Table 1-Hemodynamic parameters before surgery, one day (D1), 2 weeks (W2) and 4 weeks (W4), after surgery. Data are shown as mean ± SE. § p<0.05 versus pre-surgery values. ‡ p<0.05 versus previous time. VTI, velocity time integral; Vmax, maximum velocity; Vmean, mean velocity; PGmax, maximum pressure gradient; PGmean, mean pressure gradient; TTP, time to peak.

	Before	D1	W2	W4
VTI (cm)	18.98±2.88	12.55±2.48 § ‡	16.23±3.60	14.50±2.30
V_{max} (cm/s)	103.56±11.80	98.02±14.71	94.46±12.07	100.12±5.58
PG_{max} (mmHg)	4.20±1.16	4.19±1.40	3.96±0.84	3.57±0.16
V_{mean} (cm/s)	52.56±12.01	39.72±12.30 § ‡	41.26±8.78	52.26±4.40
PG_{mean} (mmHg)	1.19±0.67	0.87±0.52	0.84±0.28	1.12±0.17
TTP (ms)	195.40±58.73	431±32.57 § ‡	128±28.53 ‡	138±37.07 ‡

pre-surgery time and their previous time.

PGmax had a decreasing trend, but there were not any statistical differences between specific times. PGmean had the same pattern as PGmax but at W4 its value increased from 0.84±0.28mmHg at W2 to 1.12±0.17mmHg which was not significant.

At D1, W2 and W4 TTP differed significantly from previous time. The value increased from 195.40±58.73ms (pre-surgery) to 431±32.57ms (D1) and decreased to 128±28.53ms at W2, it increased significantly again to 138±37.07ms at W4. Just at D1 was the TTP value significantly higher than pre-surgery time.

Color Doppler finding was normal in our study and there was not any stenosis or regurgitation along any valves (Figure 1). Valves movement was normal and their morphology was maintained during the study (Figure 2),the only abnormal finding was aneurism in our graft; After 2 weeks 3 sheep and after 4 weeks another 2 sheep showed aneurism in acellular grafts (Figure 3). Finally CT angiography was done to evaluate the aneurism (Figure 4).

Discussion

Previous studies focused on echocardiographic assessment of mechanical prosthetic valves (Vitarelli et al. 2004; Sadoshima et al. 1992) This study is the first one in veterinary medicine that has tried to evaluate the efficacy of TEAV placed in thoracic aorta. The aim of this case control study was evaluation of spectral Doppler parameters to determine the practicality of this type of valve.

The early postoperative echocardiography is important in predicting the late outcomes (Corti et al, 2001). During the first week and months of valve replacement significant reduction of left ventricular size and myocardial function improvement appears (Gaasch et al. 1983; Fioretti et al. 1985). The general principles for evaluating the prosthetic valve function are similar to those of native valve stenosis (Parnell and Swanevelder 2009; Quiñones et al. 2002). The best parameter for assessment of AV hemodynamic is transvalvular gradient (Bach 2010). Increase in gradient across the replaced valve represents valvular stenosis and, according to Bernoulli equation, pressure gradient is in relation to velocity. So, when a constant volume of blood flows through a narrowed valve its velocity must increase, and increasing pressure gradient is expected.

Bernoulli equation:ΔP=P1-P2=4(V_2^2-V_1^2)

The greater the obstruction the greater the pressure difference between chamber and receiving vessel and also the greater the velocity. The peak difference between pressures is the maximum gradient, and average difference over the duration of flow is the mean gradient. Gorlin equation PG and valve area have a relationship. For constant valve orifice area, PG increases in high flow state like pain, anxiety, fever or anemia (Bach 2010) and decreases in low flow state, like dehydration. Systemic hypertension in patient with aortic stenosis may lead to decreasing left ventricle output following reduction in transvalvular PG (Little et al. 2007; Bermejo 2005).

Gorlin equation: Aortic valve area= (cardiac output)/(systolic ejection period ×Heart rate×44.3√(mean gradient))

PGmax is less reliable in comparison with PGmean because it is highly dependent on left ventricle contractility and transvalvular flow. Severe aortic stenosis in a native valve is defined as flow velocity more than 4.5 m/sec, PGmean more than 50 mmHg and PGmax more than 80mmHg. However, in newly implanted prosthetic valve Vmax, PGmean and PGmax more than 3.5 m/sec, 30mmHg and 50 mmHg respectively would be considered significant (Parnell and Swanevelder 2009).

The aortic VTI is an echocardiographic tool used to estimate cardiac output (Pees et al. 2013) and is independent of body surface area, inversely related to heart rate and not sex related (Evangelista et al. 1996). VTI is directly proportional to stroke volume (Darke 1992, Hatle 1985) and is representative of the distance a volume of blood travels through inflow or outflow tracts.

This study showed that TEAV placed in thoracic aorta at D1 caused significant reduction in VTI and Vmean and increased in TTP. PGmax and PGmean were not significantly different from pre-surgery values. There was a significant difference in TTP at W2 and W4 in comparison with their previous time but there was not a statistical difference from pre-surgery values. According to our finding, surgery VTI decreased one day after surgery as a result of new obstacle in flow path, in fact, it was an outcome of diminished velocity, so blood traveled a lesser distance in comparison to pre-surgery time. But this condition alleviates after 2 and 4 weeks, and could be a compensatory response of left ventricle by increasing contractility. PG was constant during the study, meaning that our TEAV did not cause any stenosis in aorta. TTP increased significantly one day after surgery and undoubtedly was a subsequence of new obstacle in thoracic aorta that increased time span to reach the peak velocity; it decreased after 2 and 4 weeks, which could be the result of compensatory response of left ventricle by increasing contractility again.

Steinhoff used allogenic acellular valve in pulmonary artery of sheep model, the valves morphology remained normal in 5 sheep of a total 6 sheep, in echocardiography subvalvular calcification was seen in all sheep, and pulmonary regurgitation was seen only in one sheep (Steinhoff et al. 2000).

In another study valves produced from absorbable polymer were placed in 6 lambs. In echocardiography all valves were normal and there was no stenosis, thrombosis and aneurism, their movement was normal as well (Hoerstrup et al. 2000).

In another research a cellular valve was used in sheep model and all echocardiographic findings were normal after 7 and 10 days and 3 months after surgery (Elkins et al. 2001).

Conclusion: According to the mentioned results the TEAV used in this study was functional except aneurism that appeared after two weeks, probably it was a result of weak scaffold, and we recommend using a durable scaffold in next study to obtain better results.

Acknowledgments

We would like to show our gratitude to the Institute of biomedical research and also surgery department staff of faculty of veterinary medicine, university of Tehran, who provided insight and expertise to this research.

References

1. Bach, D.S. (2010) Echo/Doppler evaluation of hemodynamics after aortic valve replacement: principles of interrogation and evaluation of high gradients. JACC Cardiovasc Imaging. 3: 296-304.
2. Bermejo, J. (2005) The effects of hypertension

on aortic valve stenosis. Heart. 91: 280-282.

3. Bonow, R.O., Carabello, B.A., Chatterjee, K., de Leon, A.C., Jr,Faxon, D.P., Freed, M.D., Gaasch, W.H., Lytle, B.W., Nishimura, R.A., O'Gara, P.T., O'Rourke, R.A., Otto, C.M., Shah, P.M., Shanewise, J.S., Smith, S.C.Jr, Jacobs, A.K., Adams, C.D., Anderson, J.L., Antman, E.M., Fuster, V., Halperin, J.L., Hiratzka, L.F., Hunt, S.A., Lytle, B.W., Nishimura, R., Page, R.L., Riegel, B. (2006) ACC/AHA 2006 guidelines for the management of valvular heart disease: a report of the American College of Cardiology/American heart association task force on practice guidelines (writing committee to develop guidelines for the management of patients with valvular heart disease). J Am Coll Cardiol. 48: e1-e148.
4. Cebotari, S., Mertsching, H., Kallenbach, K., Kostin, S., Repin, O., Batrinac, A., Kleczka C, Ciubotaru, A., Haverich, A. (2002) Construction of autologous human heart valves based on an acellular allograft matrix. Circulation. 106: I-63-I-68.
5. Corti, R., Binggeli, C., Turina, M., Jenni, R., Lüscher, T.F., Turina, J. (2001) Predictors of long-term survival after valve replacement for chronic aortic regurgitation Is M-mode echocardiography sufficient?. Eur Heart J. 22: 866-873.
6. Darke, P.G.G. (1992) Doppler echocardiography. J Small Anim Pract. 33: 104-112.
7. Elkins, R.C., Dawson, P.E., Goldstein, S., Walsh, S.P., Black, K.S. (2001) Decellularized human valve allografts. Ann Thorac Surg. 71: S428-S432.
8. Evangelista, A., García del Castillo, H., González-Alujas, T., Brotons, C., García-Dorado, D., Soler-Soler, J. (1996) Normal values of valvular flow velocities determined by Doppler echocardiography: relations with heart rate and age. Rev Esp Cardiol. 49: 189-195.
9. Fioretti, P., Roelandt, J., Sclavo, M., Domenicucci, S., Haalebos, M., Bos, E., Hugenholtz, P.G. (1985) Postoperative regression of left ventricular dimensions in aortic insufficiency: a long-term echocardiographic study. J Am Coll Cardiol. 5: 856-861.
10. Gaasch, W.H., Carroll, J.D., Levine, H.J., Criscitiello, M.G. (1983) Chronic aortic regurgitation: prognostic value of left ventricular endsystolic dimension and end-diastolic radius/thickness ratio. J Am Coll Cardiol. 1: 775-782.
11. Hatle, L. (1985) Doppler ultrasound in cardiology. Physical Principles And Clinical Applications. (2nd ed.) Lippincott Williams and Wilkins. Philadelphia, USA.
12. Hoerstrup, S.P., Sodian, R., Daebritz, S., Wang, J., Bacha, E.A., Martin, D.P., Moran, A.M., Guleserian, K.J., Sperling, J.S., Kaushal, S., Vacanti, J.P., Schoen, F.J., Mayer, J.E. (2000) Functional living trileaflet heart valves grown in vitro. Circulation. 102: III44-49.
13. Little, S.H., Chan, K.L., Burwash, I.G. (2007) Impact of blood pressure on the doppler echocardiographic assessment of severity of aortic stenosis. Heart. 93: 848-855.
14. Parnell, A., Swanevelder, J., (2009) High transvalvular pressure gradients on intraoperative transesophageal echocardiography after aortic valve replacement: what does it mean?. HSR Proc Intensive Care Cardiovasc Anesth, 1: 7-18.
15. Pees, C., Glagau, E., Hauser, J., Michel-Behnke, I. (2013) Reference values of aortic flow velocity integral in 1193 healthy infants, children, and adolescents to quickly estimate cardiac stroke volume. Pediatr Cardiol. 34: 1194-1200.
16. Quiñones, M.A., Otto, C.M., Stoddard, M., Waggoner, A., Zoghbi, W.A. (2002) Recommendations for quantification of doppler echocardiography: a report from the doppler quantification task force of the nomenclature and standards committee of the American Society of Echocardiography. J Am Soc Echocardiogr. 15: 167-184.
17. Rahimtoola, S.H. (1978) The problem of valve prosthesis-patient mismatch. Circulation. 58: 20-24.
18. Sadoshima, J., Koyanagi, S., Sugimachi, M.,

Hirooka, Y., Takeshita, A. (1992) Evaluation of the severity of mitral regurgitation by transesophageal Doppler flow echocardiography. Am Heart J. 123: 1245-51.

19. Steinhoff, G., Stock, U., Karim, N., Mertsching, H., Timke, A., Meliss, R.R., Pethig, K., Haverich, A., Bader, A. (2000) Tissue engineering of pulmonary heart valves on allogenic acellular matrix conduits: in vivo restoration of valve tissue. Circulation. 102: III 50-III 55.
20. Tobias, P., Frank, A.F. (2010) Echocardiographic follow-up after heart valve replacement. Heart. 96: 75-85.
21. Vahanian, A., Alfieri, O., Andreotti, F., Antunes, M.J., Barón-Esquivias, G., Baumgartner, H., Borger, M.A., Carrel, T.P., De Bonis, M., Evangelista, A., Falk, V., Iung, B., Lancellotti, P., Pierard, L., Price, S., Schäfers, H.J., Schuler, G., Stepinska, J., Swedberg, K., Takkenberg, J., Von Oppell, U.O., Windecker, S., Zamorano, J.L., Zembala, M. (2012) Guidelines on the management of valvular heart disease (version 2012). Eur Heart J. 33: 2451-2496.
22. Vitarelli, A., Conde, Y., Cimino, E., Leone, T., D'Angeli, I., D'Orazio, S., Stellato, S. (2004) Assessment of severity of mechanical prosthetic mitral regurgitation by transoesophageal echocardiography. Heart. 90: 539-544.

Evaluation of cardiac troponin I (cTnI), creatine kinase (CK), aspartate aminotransferase (AST) and electrocardiography, in diagnosis of selenium deficiency in goat kids

Fakour, Sh.[1*], **Alimohammadzadeh, P.**[2], **Vaziry, A.**[3]

[1]*Department of Clinical Sciences, Faculty of Veterinary Medicine, Sanandaj Branch of Islamic Azad University, Sanandaj, Iran*

[2]*Young Research and Elite Club, Sanandaj Branch Islamic Azad University, Sanandaj, Iran*

[3]*Department of Clinical Sciences, Faculty of Agriculture, University of Kurdistan, Sanandaj, Iran*

Key words:
electrocardiography, enzyme, markhoz goat, selenium, troponin

Correspondence
Fakour, Sh.
Department of Clinical Sciences, Faculty of Veterinary Medicine, Sanandaj Branch of Islamic Azad University, Sanandaj, Iran

Email: Fakour@yahoo.com

Abstract:

BACKGROUND: Cardiac Troponin I (cTnI) is known as a cardiac biomarker in determining the myocardial damage of diseases which affect the heart muscle. **OBJECTIVES:** This study aims to evaluate the serum cTnI concentration in Markhoz Breed goats suffering selenium (Se) deficiency and its correlation with electrocardiographic parameters, and activity of creatine kinase (CK) and aspartate aminotransferase (AST) enzymes, as well as to determine the diagnostic value of troponin in that disease. **METHODS:** Blood samples of 94 goat kids of Markhoz breed with the age less than one month were taken, serum analyzed for the assessment of cTnI, CK and AST, and 2 ml blood was used for determination of selenium concentration. Electrocardiography was recorded from all kids by using base-apex lead. Kids were divided into two groups based on serum selenium concentration. **RESULTS:** The concentration of cTnI was significantly higher in deficient kids compared with the control group. Results indicated significant negative correlation between cTnI and selenium concentration. There was no significant correlation between cTnI and AST, CK in deficient kids. Results show no significant difference in concentration of AST and CK enzymes for two groups of deficient kids and control group. The presence of arrhythmia is significantly higher in deficient kids than control group. **CONCLUSIONS:** The results of this study showed that the measurement of serum cTnI concentration can be useful in diagnosis of kids suffering from Se deficiency. Also, ECG can be used in the diagnosis of arrhythmia in kids with Se deficiency.

Introduction

Nutritional muscular Dystrophy (NMD) is a peracute muscular degenerative disease to sub acute of skeletal and cardiac muscles which occurs in all farm animal species, but most commonly in young, rapidly growing calves, lambs, goat kids and foals born from dams that have been fed for long periods, usually during the winter months, on diets low in selenium and vitamin E (Radostits et al., 2014).

Selenium and vitamin E appear to be synergistic in preventing NMD. However, on the basis of prophylaxis and response to treatment, selenium deficiency appears to be more important (Smith, 2015).

Selenium and vitamin E both are involved in enzyme responses which control oxidative process in mammalian tissues by oxidation reduction reactions (Smith and Sherman, 2009).

Lack of vitamin E and selenium in body cause accumulation of toxic peroxides and loss of cell and tissue membranes and evident myopathy.

Muscle damage is associated with the increase of the release of lysosomal enzymes and myoglobin in the cell (Mostaghni et al., 2005).

Plasma Creatine kinase (CK) is most commonly used enzyme in laboratory and in the diagnosis of NMD. The enzyme is highly specific for cardiac and skeletal muscles and is released into the blood following unaccustomed exercise and myodegeneration. AST (Aspartate Aminotransferase) activity is also an indicator of muscle damage, but is not as reliable as the CK because increased AST level may also indicate liver damage. The magnitude of the increase in AST and CK is directly proportional to the extent of muscle damage. Both are elevated initially, an elevated AST and declining CK would suggest that muscle degeneration is no longer active (Radostits et al., 2014).

Today, Troponin I and Troponin T, as selective analytes of cardiac damage have been replaced for the above mentioned enzymes (Wells and Sleeper 2008).

Troponin is the biomarker of choice for the detection of cardiac injury. The 3-unit Troponin complex (Troponin I, T, and C) along with Tropomyosin is located on the actin filament and is essential for the calcium mediated regulation of skeletal and cardiac muscle contraction. Because the cardiac isoform of the Troponin C is shared by "slow-twitch" skeletal muscles, troponin C does not have cardiac specificity and thus is not used in assays for the diagnosis of cardiac injury. There is one cardiac Troponin I (cTnI) isoform in myocardial tissue.

Since the half-life of troponin and its complexes is about 2 hours, the prolonged window during which troponin levels are elevated allows for increased clinical detection of cardiac events and thus, functionally, greater clinical sensitivity (Babium et al., 2004,Uncogil et al.2004, Leonardi et al.2008).

Ataollahy et al. (2011) conducted the diagnostic value of cardiac troponin I compared with other indices of muscle damage such as aspartate aminotransferase, and creatine kinase in sheep with selenium deficiency in Khorasan Province. Tunca et al. (2008) reported that the increase of cardiac troponin I and decrease or lack of troponin I in tissues are widely associated with the severity of FMD and changes in myocardial degeneration. Mellor et al. (2006) for the first time, announced the increase of serum troponin concentrations for a period of 16 days as a diagnostic marker of severe heart muscle injury in connection with heat stress in dogs. Identifying the animals affected or in general understanding the epidemiology status of metabolic disease of selenium deficiency can be studied in any area with different ways, which include the measurement of the blood and hair selenium in animals, liver selenium in slaughterhouse animals, regional soil selenium, regional plant

Table 1. The mean ± SE of serum selenium, cTnI, CK and AST concentration in se-deficient and non- deficient goat kids. [a,b] Mean with different superscript on the same row are significantly different (p≤0.5).

	Se non-deficient group Number (%)		Se deficient group Number (%)	
Selenium (ppm)	60(63.8%)	0.13±0.18 [a]	34(36.2%)	0.033±0.14 [b]
Troponin (μg/L)	82(87.2%)	0.118±0.11 [a]	12(12.8%)	2.18±3.07 [b]
CK(IU/L)	35(37.2%)	145±42.8 [a]	59(62.8%)	3302±476 [a]
AST (IU/L)	73(77.7%)	142.8±122 [a]	21(22.23%)	1327±729 [a]

Table 2. relationship between changes of amount of cTnI, Se and the activities of AST and CK in goats. * Significant relationship ** No significant relationship.

	Correlation coefficient
cTnI and Se	-0.496*
cTnI and CK	0.150**
cTnI and AST	0607**

Table 3. The type and number of arrhythmia in Se-deficient and non- deficient goat kids.

Arrhythmia	Se-deficient group	Se- non deficient
Sinus tachycardia	20	35
Atrial premature	18	12
Sinus arrhythmia	13	4
Atrial fibrillation beat	8	1
AV block II	4	1
Sinus arrest	3	0
Ventricular premature beat	1	0
AV block III	1	0
Ventricular fibrillation	1	0

selenium or the measurement of muscular damages indices such as CK and AST. The aim of this study is assessment of serum concentration of cardiac troponin I in Markhoz breed goat kids with the deficiency of selenium and its relationship with electrocardiography parameters and activity of CK and AST enzymes, as well as determining the diagnostic value of troponin in the same disease.

Materials and Methods

In this study blood samples of 94 Markhoz goats of both sexes, female (n=37) and male (n=37), weight 5-10 kg, kept in Breeding Center of Markhoz Goats in Sanandaj (in thewest of Iran) with the age of less than one month old were taken randomly. Electrocardiography was also done, while previously coordinating and ensuring that no injection of selenium to pregnant ewes took place.

First, electrocardiogram was recorded in standing position from all goats, using electrocardiography device (model ECG2000 (Bionet) made in Korea) on base-apex lead. The paper speed was adjusted to 25 mm/sec and calibration was 10 mm/mV. Electrocardiograms were studied with respect to the presence of the arrhythmia and its type recognition. Then 5 ml blood sample were collected from jugular vein of all goats. 3 ml blood was added into the plain tube for serum harvesting. Plain tubes were centrifuged at 3500×g for 10 min followed by removal serum. The activities of AST, CK enzyme were measured by commercial kits of (Pars Azmoon, Tehran, Iran); using an autoanalyzer (Auto-chemistry Analyzer, model DIRUI, CS-T240, China) and concentration of cardiac troponin I was measured also using ELISA method by commercial kit (Monobind Inc, USA) and the results were determined, according to manufacturer's instructions. Mean concentrations for AST and CK in goat kids were 513 IU/L and 219 IU/L respectively (Smith, 2015).

2 ml of the remaining blood was used as whole blood for determining the selenium concentration using atomic absorption spec-

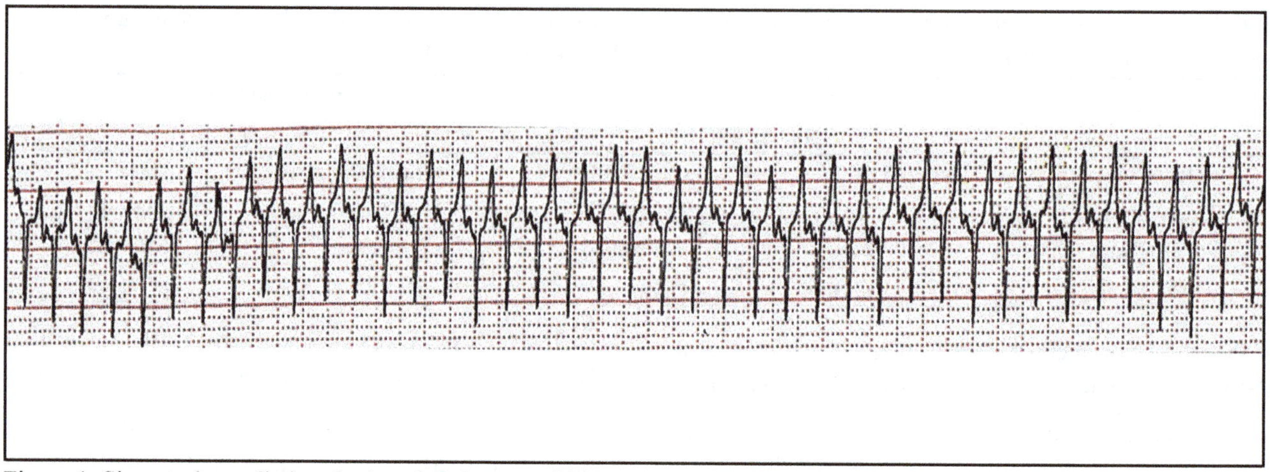

Figure 1. Sinus tachycardia in selenium deficient goat kids.

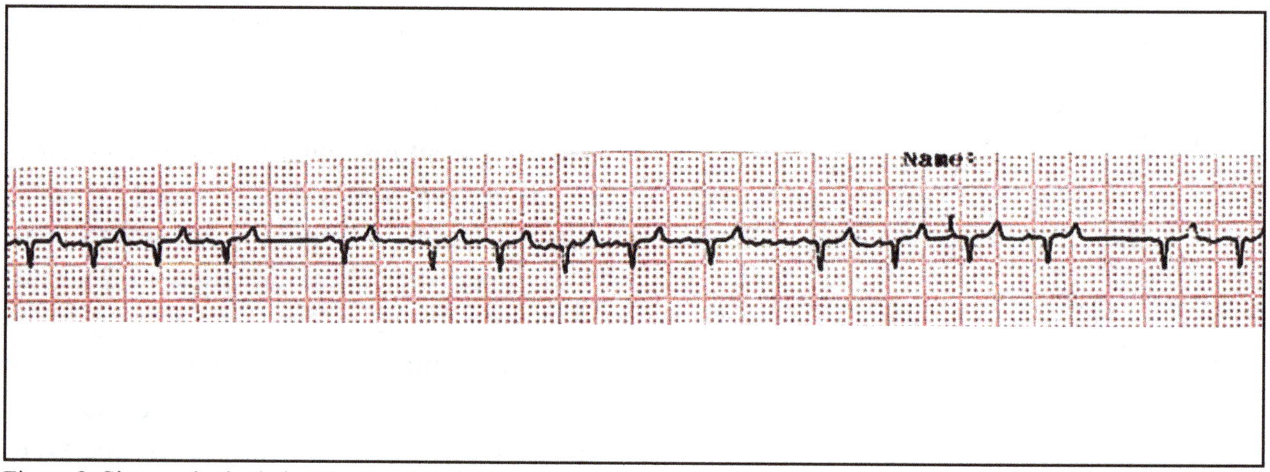

Figure 2. Sinus arrhythmia in selenium deficient goat kids.

trophotometry (Perkin-Elmer 2380, Britain, Model) with a wavelength of 196 nm.

Kid goats were divided into two groups based on serum selenium concentration: deficient kids with Se concentration of ≤ 0.05 ppm (n=34) and control kids (n=60) with Se concentration of higher value (Smith, 2015).

There are no reports indicating the normal value of cardiac troponin I (cTnI) in Markhoz breed goats and for the kids less than one month, hence, for determining this value, the level of serum (cTnI) concentration of 100 Markhoz breed goats with the age of less than one month and apparently healthy was measured by a method similar to that mentioned above during the present study. All sampled kids underwent clinical exam and 2 kids had WMD based on clinical signs, which was confirmed by necropsy, pathology, and serum Se concentration. The statistical analysis was conducted using SPSS for windows (release 16, SPSS Inc, Chicago, USA). Based on Kolmogorov-Smirnov normality test, parametric t-test, non- parametric Mann-Whitney U test, and correlation coefficient test were used to investigate significant difference between groups for measured analyses. For all comparisons $p \leq 0.05$ was considered as significant (Ataollahy et al., 2013).

Results

The results of selenium concentration for 94 kids with the age of less than one month

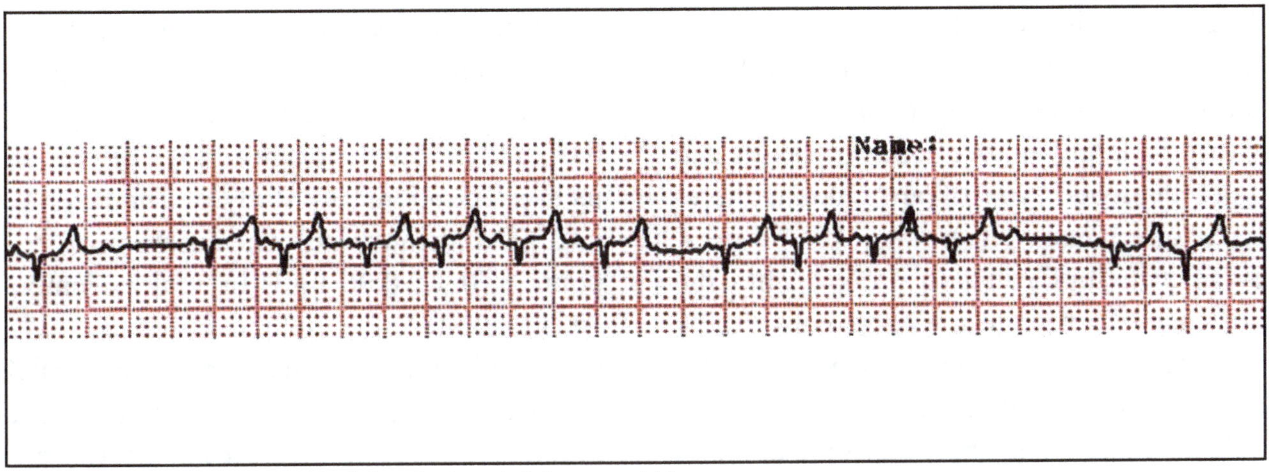

Figure 3. Second- degree AV block in selenium deficient goat kids.

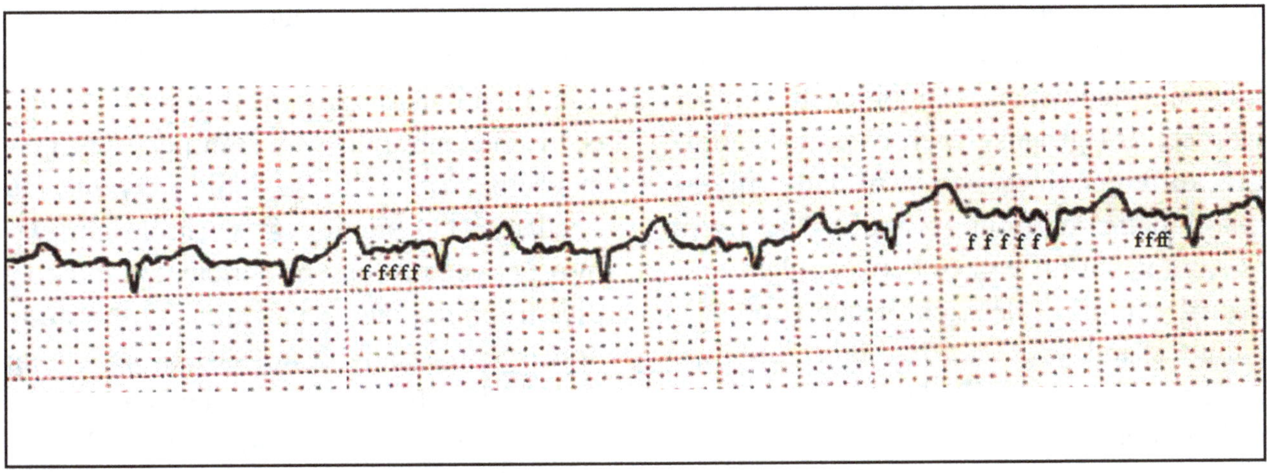

Figure 4. Atrial fibrillation in selenium deficient goat kids.

in both sexes are shown in Table 1. Accordingly, 94 goats were divided into two groups, one group with selenium deficiency (34 goats) and control group with normal selenium (60 goats).

As mentioned, due to the absence of report indicating the reference value of cTnI in goat kids aged less than one month of Markhoz breed, cTnI of 100 apparently healthy goats less than one month was measured and range of 0.0_ 0.47 µg/l was considered as reference value in the goats under study. Similar action was done in the study of Basbugan ct al. (2010).

The results of cTnI concentration for 94 goats are revealed in Table 1.

The results show that serum concentration of cTnI in the group with selenium deficiency was significantly higher than that of control groups ($p \leq 0.05$) and using the correlation coefficient statistical test reveals that there is a significant negative correlation between changes of amount of cardiac troponin I and selenium deficiency in Markhoz goats, $p \leq 0.05$.

The results of the AST and CK activities in 94 goats are shown in Table 1.

Using the correlation coefficient statistical test reveals that there is no significant relationship between changes in amount of cTnI and the activities of AST and CK in goats, ($p>0.05$) (Table 2). Also, the changes of the AST and CK activities in two groups of goats did not show significant differences ($p>0.05$).

The results obtained from the electrocardiography indicate that there is one or more types of arrhythmia in 94 goats. Table 3 shows the different types of arrhythmia.

Since a large number of sampled kids had more than one type of arrhythmia, therefore, for evaluating the diagnostic efficiency of arrhythmia in two groups, only the presence of arrhythmia without considering its type has been analyzed using correlation coefficient statistical test, and a significant relationship between the selenium deficiency and the presence of arrhythmia was observed ($p \leq 0.05$), it means that the presence of arrhythmias in the group with selenium deficiency is significantly higher than control groups. There was no significant difference between cTnI and arrhythmia in deficient group ($p > 0.05$). There was no significant difference between the types of arrhythmia in deficient group ($p > 0.05$). Numbers and types of arrhythmia are shown in Table 2. Figures 1-3 show three types of arrhythmias diagnosed in this study.

Discussion

Some researchers have reported that early diagnosis is important in WMD as appropriate treatment and prophylactic protocols are applied (Kozat et al., 2011). There are few reports concerning diagnostic value of cTnI in sheep and goats medicines (Ataollahy et al., 2013; Tharwat et al., 2013). To the authors' knowledge, none of the reports investigated Se deficiency in Markhoz breed goat's kids and no correlations were described between Se with cTnI, AST, CK, electrocardiography and its diagnostic value in field conditions. Ataollahy et al. (2013) described these correlations in lambs except electrocardiography. Concerning the reference value of cTnI, Basbugan et al. (2010) reported reference value of cTnI concentration in ruminants. According to their report, the mean of cTnI concentration in sheep was 0.0- 0.27 μg/l with no age and sex effects on its concentration. The study of Tunca et al. in 2009 indicates the concentration of troponin I (0.32±0.06 μg/l) in healthy lambs. As mentioned, due to the absence of reports indicating the reference value of cTnI in goat kids with the age of less than one month of Markhoz breed, cTnI of 100 apparently healthy goats less than one month was measured and range of 0.0_ 0.47 μg/l was considered as reference value in the goat kids under study. In this study, serum cTnI concentration was significantly higher in goat kids with Se deficiency, and the results reveal significant negative correlation between selenium deficiency and cardiac troponin, which is similar to the study done by Ataollahy et al. (2013), indicating that cardiac troponin I can be regarded as specific and sensitive marker in the field of determining the damage of cardiac muscle cells in white muscle disease in lambs. The concentration of cTnI in present study was close to Ataollahy et al.'s (2013) report, whereas it was lower than Tunca et al. (2009) and Basbugan et al.'s (2010) reports. Two reasons could be considered for this reference; firstly, acute form of disease was considered in these studies. In the present study, regarding the possibility of following up the animals under study, 3 goat kids of the group with selenium deficiency had the clinical symptoms related to selenium deficiency; after death, their blood selenium concentrations were proved by necropsy findings and histopathology. Secondly, difference in method of measurement of cTnI as suggested by Wells and Sleeper, (2008) must be considered (Ataollahy et al., 2013).

In addition to sheep and goats, various studies were performed in cattle concerning cTnI changes in cardiac and non-cardiac disorders. cTnI concentration in cows with idiopathic pericarditis is reported to be higher than in healthy cows (Gunes et al., 2008). Increased concentration of cTnI was reported significantly higher in calves with FMD compared to control (Koya et al., 2013). In another study, serum cTnI concentration as a Myocarditis marker was significantly higher in lambs with FMD (Aslani et al., 2013). In one study the diagnostic value of increases of troponin I and T concentration were confirmed in cattle with traumatic Reticulopritonitis (TRP) (Gunes et al., 2008). Although other researchers have reported significant increase of CK in the lambs with selenium deficiency (Abood et al., 2012; Kosat et al., 2011; Tunca et al., 2010). The results of this study reveal that there is no significant difference between selenium and CK activity for the group with selenium deficiency compared with the group with normal selenium. Our results were consistent with those of researchers (Ataollahy et al., 2013; Varga et al., 2009).

Two reasons for the results obtained in CK enzyme could be described; firstly, in the present study breed differences must be considered, secondly, increase of CK concentration in blood, following the skeletal muscles damages caused by trauma, injections, falls and transportation must be considered. Therefore, considering the age of the goat kids, the possibility of the appearance of such increase in both groups under study can be considered as another reason for statistical analysis in both groups.

In this study, between the group with selenium deficiency and AST activity no significant relationship was observed, which is consistent with the results of another study (Ataollahi et al., 2013). In yet another study considerable increases in activities of CK and AST in calf were reported which can be used as indicator of cardiac damage, but they are not specific and can also increase following skeletal muscle damage (Aslani et al., 2013). AST is also an indicator of muscle damage, but is not as reliable as the CK because increased AST levels may indicate liver damage (Radostits et al., 2014). AST enzyme exists in the mitochondria of almost all cells and also in plasma, and increase of this enzyme may be caused by injuries in skeletal and cardiac muscles in addition to liver injuries. CK is a more specific index for muscle damage compared to AST; however, AST is often used as a supplement for CK (Kaneko et al., 1997).

The results of this study show that there is significant difference between the presence of arrhythmia and selenium deficiency. Since the concentration of Troponin was more in the group with selenium deficiency compared to the group with normal selenium, it can be concluded that there was some degree of damage in cardiac muscular cells in group with selenium deficiency that appears as a disorder in electrical or mechanical activity of the heart, and this disorder has been revealed in arrhythmia. But no significant relationship is observed between types of arrhythmia and selenium deficiency. Varga et al. (2009) reported cTnI was significantly associated with left ventricular shortening fraction in cattle with monensin toxicosis, and increased heart rate, lengthening of the duration of QRS complex, prolongation of QT interval, low voltage R wave and IT segment elevation were observed, indicative of myocardial injury. In one study cardiac dysrhythmias and cTnI were evaluated in low and high yielding dairy cows, cardiac arrhythmias were detected in low yielding dairy cows, probably due to metabolic and electrolyte disorders (Jafary Dehkordi et al., 2014). Fartashvand et al. (2013) reported that serum concentration cTnI was significantly higher in cattle with theileriosis, but there were no pathologic arrhythmias detected in sick animals. This season could be a reason for this result; all cardiac arrhythmias are not caused by heart damage and can have multiple reasons, in addition a number of arrhythmias in ruminants (Markoz goat breed) are physiologic (Fakour et al., 2013), which could explain the non significance of the relationship of arrhythmias types and troponin concentrations in goats with selenium deficiency.

Considering the fact that one of the types of white muscle disease in young livestock is cardiac muscle dystrophy, the results of this study can indicate some degree of damage to cardiac muscular cells due to the selenium deficiency. Cardiac form of white muscle disease in young animals is acute with the appearance of the least clinical signs. The results of this study show that some degree of damage to cardiac muscular cells can be predicted before developing clinical and acute form, by measuring the cardiac troponin I. cTnI concentration of kids may be increased due to myocardium involvement caused by other cardiac and non-cardiac disorders (Ataollahy et al.2103). On the other hand, cTnI concentration was not increased in all Se deficiency groups, nevertheless our results reveal significant negative correlation between selenium concentration and cardiac troponin, as serum cTnI concentrations were also significantly higher in goat kids with Se deficiency. In conclusion the evaluation of Cardiac Troponin I would be useful for diagnosis of Se deficiency in goat kids at herd with better diagnostic efficiency than CK and AST. Also, ECG can be used in the diagnosis of arrhythmia in kids with Se deficiency.

Acknowledgments

The authors would like to state their appreciation to the honorable managers and personnel of the Center for Rearing and Breeding Markhoz Goats in Kurdistan Province for their kind cooperation.

References

Abood, H.K., Judi, A.M.H., AL-Ani, A.A. (2012) The effect of experimentally induced vitamin E and selenium deficiency on Creatine Kinase (CK) and Aspartate Amino transferase (AST) activities in Awassi ewes and their newborn lambs. Kufa J Vet Med Sci. 3: 80-86.

Aslani, M., Mohri, M., Movassaghy, A. (2013) Serum troponin I as an indicator of myocarditis in lambs affected with foot and mouth disease. Vet Res Forum. 4: 59-62.

Ataollahi, F., Mohri, M., Seifi, H.F. (2013) Diagnostic value of cardiac troponin I (cTnI), creatine kinase (CK), and aspartate amino transferase (AST) in selenium deficiency in lamb.Revue Méd Vét. 164: 207-211.

Babium, L., Jaffe, A.S. (2005) Troponin: The biomarker of choice for the detection of cardiac injury .Can Med Assoc J. 173: 1191_1202

Basbugan, Y., Agaoglu, Z., Yusksek. (2010) An investigation on serum troponin concentration in healthy ruminants. Kafkas Univ Vet Fak Derg. 16: 641-645.

Fakour, Sh., Mokhber Dezfuli, M.R., Nadalian, M.G., Rezakhani, A., LotfollahZadeh, S. (2013) Electrocardiographic parameters of

Markhoz goat usingbase apex lead and six standard limb leads. Iran J Vet Res. 14: 241-244.

Fartashvand, M., Nadalian, M.G., Sakha, M., Safi, S. (2013) Serum cardiac troponin I cattle with theileriosis. J Vet Intern Med. 27: 194-9

Gunes, V., Atalan, G., Citil, M., Erdogan, H.M. (2008) Use of cardiac troponin kits for the qualitative determination of myocardial cell damage due to the traumatic reticulo peritonitis in cattle. Vet Rec. 162: 514-517.

Jafary Dehkordi, A., mohebbi, A.N., Balali dehkordi, Sh. (2014) Evaluation of dysrhythmias and myocardial biomarkers in highand low-yielding dairy cows. Iran J Vet Med. 8: 101-109.

Kaneko, J. (1997) Clinical Biochemistry of Domestic Animals. (5th ed.) Akademic Press. San Diego, USA.

kayat, A., Kosat, S., Ozkan, C. (2013) Serum homocysteine levels in calves with foot and mouth disease. J Anim Vet Adv. 12: 1357-67.

Kosat, S., Altug, N., Yuksek, N., Oskan, C. (2011) Evaluation of the levels of homocysteine, troponin I, and nitric oxide in lambs with subclinical white muscle disease. Kafkas Univ Vet Fak Derg. 17: 441-444.

Leonardi, F., Passeri, B., Fusari, A. (2008) Cardiac troponin I (cTnI) concentration in an ovine model of myocardial ischemia. Res Vet Sci. 85: 141-144.

Mellor, PJ., Mellanby, RJ., Baiens, EA., Villiers, EJ., Hertbye, ME. (2006) High serum troponin I concentration as a marker of severe myocardial damage in a case of suspected exertional heatstoke in a dog. J Vet Cardiol. 8: 55_62

Mostaghni, K.H. (2005) Animal Farms in Deficiencies Nutritional and Diseases Metabolic. (2nd ed.). University of Shiraz, Shraz, Iran.

Radostits, O. M., Gay, C. C., K. Hinchcliff, W.,-Constable, P. D. (2014) Veterinary Medicine, Atextbook of the Diseases of Cattle, Horses, Sheep, Pigs and Goats. (10th ed.). Saunders Elseviere Company. London, UK.

Smith, B.P. (2015) Large Animal Internal Medicine, C.V. (5th ed.). Mosby Co.,St. Louis, USA.

Smith, M.C. Sherman, D.M. (2009) Goat Medicine. (2nd ed.). Wiliams and Wilkins, USA.

Tharwt, M., Al-sobaiyl, F., El-sayed, M. (2013) Cardiac troponin I in healthy new born goat kids and in goat kids with cardiac nutritional muscular dystrophy. ActaVet Hung. 61: 442-53.

Tunca, R., Sozmen, M., Erdogan, H., Citil, M., Uzlu, E. (2008) Determination of cardiac troponin I in the blood and heart of calves with foot - and - mouth disease. J Diagn Invest. 20: 589-605.

Tunca, R., Erdogan, M., Sozmen, M., Citil, M., Derim, A., Eriginsoy, S., Uzlu, E. (2009) Evaluation of cardiac troponin I and inducible nitric oxide synthetase expressions in lambs with white muscle disease. Turk J Vet Anim Sci. 33: 53-59.

Uncugil, F., Elmas, Q., Erbay, A.R., Duzoylum, A., Yucel, D. (2004) Nitric oxide metabolites and cardiac troponin I levels in cardiomyopathies. Turk J Biochem. 29: 199-203.

Varga, A., Shober, K.E., Holloman, C.H., Stromberg, P.C. (2009) Correlation of serum cardiac troponin I and myocardial damage in cattle with monensin toxicosis. J Vet Intern Med. 23: 1108–1116.

Wells, S., Sleeper, M. (2008) Cardiac troponin. J Vet Emerg Crit Care. 18: 235-45.

Identification of atypic and classic, mucinous and nonmucinous forms of ovine pulmonary adenocarcinoma (OPA) and TTF1 marker expression

Sasani, F.*, Khaki, F., Gharagouzloo, M.J.

Department of Pathology, Faculty of Veterinary Medicine, University of Tehran, Tehran, Iran

Key words:
Adenocarcinoma, ovine, pneumocyte, pulmonary, retrovirus

Correspondence
Sasani, F.
Department of Pathology, Faculty of Veterinary Medicine, University of Tehran, Tehran, Iran

Email: fsasani@ut.ac.ir

Abstract:

BACKGROUND: Ovine pulmonary adenocarcinoma (OPA) is a worldwide contagious bronchioalveolar carcinoma caused by infection of a beta retrovirus in sheep and less in goat. Neoplastic proliferation of type II pneumocytes and clara cells, produce papillary to acinar tumoral pattern with infiltration of macrophages, lymphocytes and plasma cells and interstitial fibrosis tissue. **OBJECTIVES:** This study was conducted to investigate the patterns of OPA and check the expression of TTF1. **METHODS:** A total of 7952 ovine lungs were studied for macroscopic and microscopic pathology examination and so, to check TTF1 marker. **RESULTS:** 25 cases were diagnosed as OPA and, based on macroscopic and histopathologic lesions, two different classifications were defined. Tumoral lesions were divided to classic (68%) and atypic (32%) forms of OPA based on growth pattern and progression and two other forms of mucinous (56%) and non-mucinous (44%) OPA based on histologic characterization of neoplastic secretory cells were descripted. 6 out of 8 examined cases for TTF1 marker staining, were positive and 2 cases were negative in immunohistochemical test. **CONCLUSIONS:** Two forms of classic and atypic lesions and so mucinous and non-mucinous forms were found. The classic form was more than the atypic and the mucinous form was more than non-mucinous lesions. TTF1 marker expression revealed the pulmonary origin of tumors.

Introduction

Ovine pulmonary adenocarcinoma (OPA) is a contagious retroviral bronchioalveolar carcinoma in sheep that is rarely observed in goats. It is a financially significant disease. More than 80% of the herd might be wasted at the first encounter with the virus and up to 20% of the herd might be infected on average. No effective treatment or vaccine is readily available to control and eradicate this disease. It is known as a worldwide disease with infectious origin. The etiology of this neoplasm is based on a beta retrovirus of retroviridae family. There is not any oncogenic agent in the virus and it has been shown that the envelope protein of the virus is enough to induce the tumor (Palmarini and Fan, 2001; Martineau et al., 2010; Jubb, Kennedy and Pulmer´s, 2007). The histological feature of this tumor is differentiated carcinoma in bronchioloaveolar tissue. Columnar or Cuboidal epithelial neoplastic cells cover the airways and lead to papillary or acinar structures. Alveolar walls in these neoplastic masses are covered by Columnar or Cuboidal epithelial neoplastic cells. These structures fill the alveolar spaces and obstruct their ways and alveoli surrounding neoplastic area. The adjacent alveoli show atelectasis. Macrophages are abundant in alveoli. There is interstitial fibrosis in severe cases. Neoplastic cells show type II pneumocyte phenotype including cytoplasmic lamellar bodies and surface microvilli. Less commonly, dense granules might be seen in these cells and phenotype indicates Clara cell structure. These specifications explain the form of bronchioloalveolar carcinoma tissue (Jubb, Kennedy and Pulmer´s, 2007 - Khodakaram-Tafti and Hematian 2011 - Martineau et al., 2010 - Beytut et al., 2009 - Bahari et al., 2016). Prevalence of the disease in slaughterhouses of sheep over three years old has been estimated about 3 percent in Chaharmahal and Bakhtiari Province (Kojouri, and Karimi, 2002). A study was conducted on tracing the virus in Fars Province by RT-PCR showed that the virus was detected in all infected lungs (Khodakaram-Tafti et al., 2009). Pulmonary adenomatosis has been detected in 4 goats in Khuzestan province microscopically and histopathologically (Sayyari and Mohamadian ,2012). Infection was highly prevalent in the northwest of Iran and controlling it seems very important (Rezazadeh et al., 2012).

Materials and Methods

The tissue specimens were collected for about one year, accidentally and weekly from one industrial slaughterhouse in Shahryar township of Tehran province. In this survey 7952 specimens of sheep lungs were studied. The lungs with macroscopic lesions which were suspected to be involved with adenocarcinomatous lesions accompanied by mediastinal lymph nodes were taken and fixed in 10% neutral buffered formalin solution. The tissues were passaged and imbedded in paraffin blocks, sectioned at 5 micron thickness and finally stained with hematoxylin and eosin method. 8 cases of tissues were chosen for immunoreactive staining of TTF1 marker by avidin-biotin-peroxidase complex method using the DAKO kit, to determine whether the tumor is primary or metastatic form of carcinoma in lung. Tissue sections were studied histopathologically by two pathologists for evaluation of nuclear expression of protein.

Results

Macroscopic Observations: From 7952 cases, 27 lung specimens had macroscopic appearance similar to that characteristic of pulmonary adenomatosis. By histological examination 25 cases were detected as adenocarcinoma bronchioalveolar structure. There were focal and multifocal hard and bulging lesions, with grey to white or purple colors. In some samples, the involved areas were harder, white to grey and without production of lung fluid. In many other cases excessive production of lung fluid was observed.

In the samples of this study, cranioventral areas were mostly involved. However, in some cases, the infection was more severe and scattered in lung tissue. In other cases,

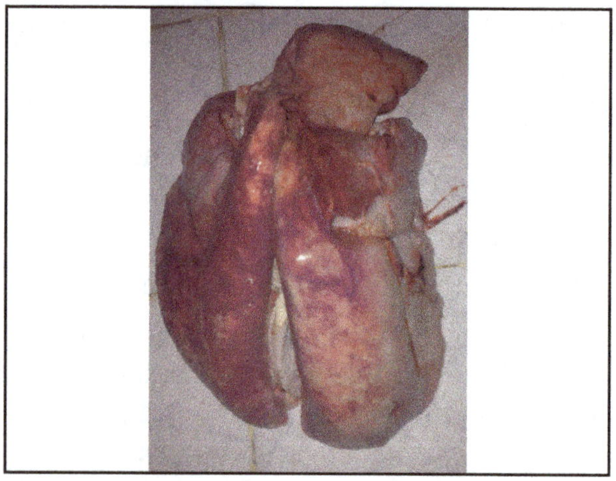

Figure 1. Pulmonary adenocarcinoma, dorsal and lateral view of ovine lung. Diffuse enlarged, grey to purple, edematous lesions.

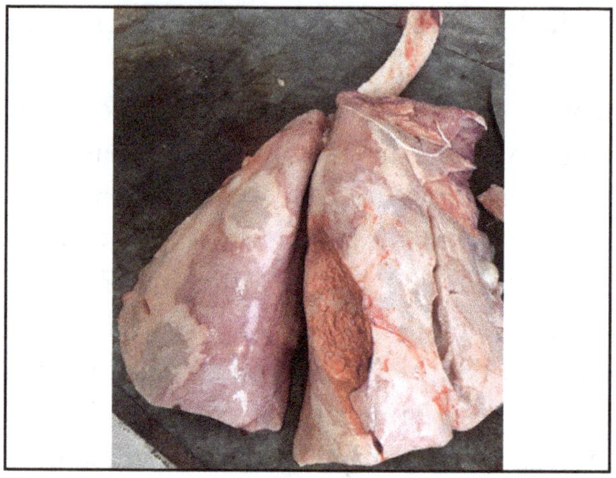

Figure 2. Demarcated white greyish nodules of various size in lung lobes.

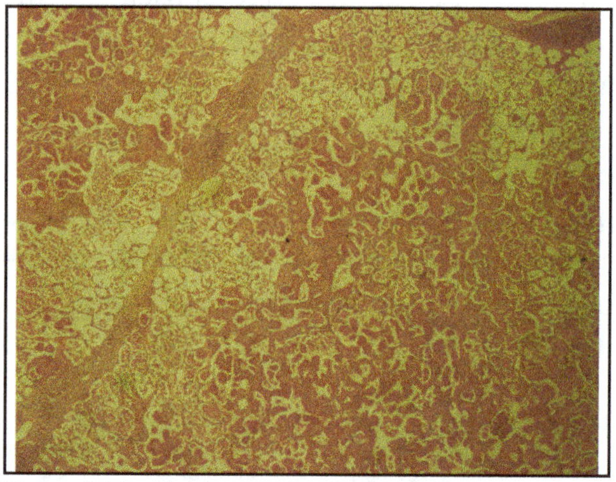

Figure 3. Neoplastic growth of epithelial cells in pulmonary alveoli and infiltration of alveolar macrophages in classical form of OPA, sheep lung. (H&E)(x40).

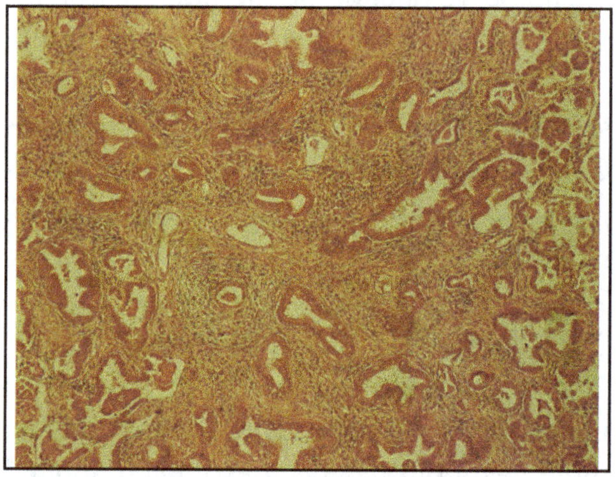

Figure 4. Neoplastic alveoli with proliferative connective tissue (fibrosis) and infiltration of mononuclear cells in atypical form of OPA, sheep lung. (H&E)(x100).

central necrosis and hemorrhage in tumoral areas were observed.

In 17 cases, heavy and large focal masses of white and grey color and some in purple, about 2 to 10 centimeters in diameter, surrounded by emphysematous parenchyma were observed. In some samples, several tumoral foci were joined together to form larger areas. Cross-cutting surfaces of these samples were moist with serous and foamy secretions on airways and parenchyma. These samples were categorized as classical OPA (Fig. 1).

In 8 samples single firm masses with few secretions in white to greyish about 3 to 7 centimeters in diameter were seen and were categorized as atypical OPA (Fig. 2).

Histopathological Findings: The samples were categorized into two forms of classical and atypical. The histopathological form of the classic adenocarcinoma presents small and large encapsulated neoplastic nodules with columnar to cuboidal cells in papillary to acinar growth. There was no sign of invasion. In most cases, large macrophages were seen in alveoli (Fig. 3). Histopathology of atypical adenocarcinoma is similar to classical forms except that

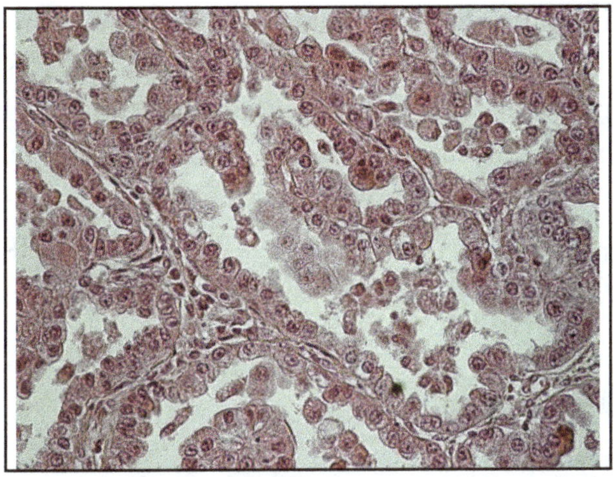

Figure 5. Acinar and papillar appearance of neoplastic alveoli with short cuboidal epithelial cells in classical non-mucinous form of OPA, sheep lung. (H&E)(x200).

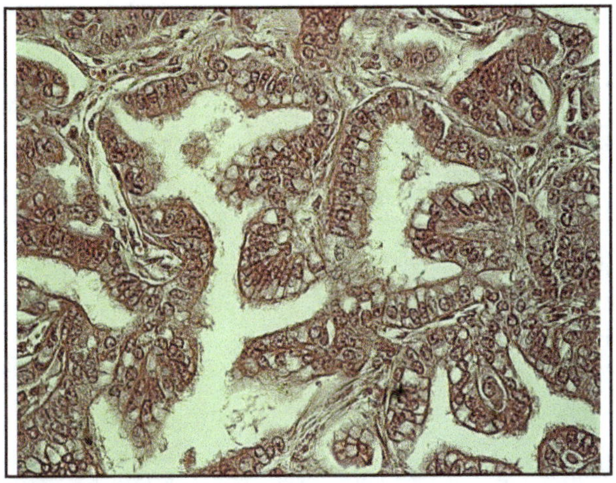

Figure 6. Neoplastic columnar cells with typical cytoplasmic mucin droplets lining alveoli, acinar to papillar growth related to classical mucinous form of OPA, sheep lung. (H&E)(x400).

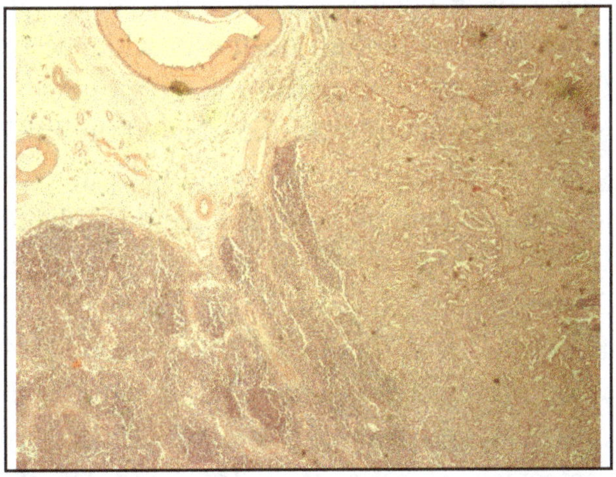

Figure 7. Mediastinal lymph node metastasis of OPA affected tissue, sheep mediastinal lymph node. (H&E)(x100).

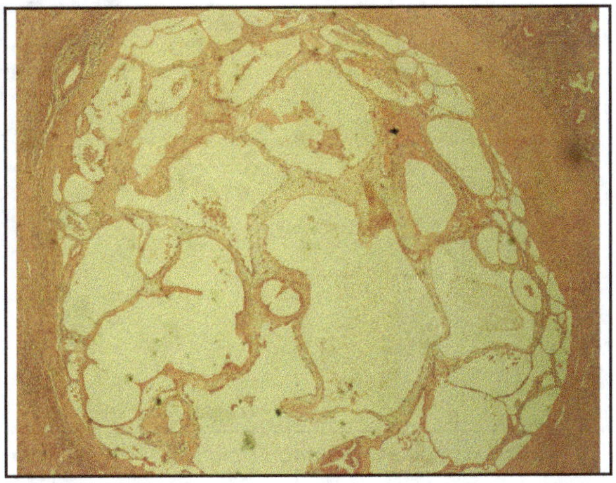

Figure 8. Cyctic growth of neoplastic epithelial cells and mucin secretion in OPA affected pulmonary tissue, sheep. (H&E)(x40).

neoplastic foci are often smaller and more limited in classic form. Severe infiltration of mononuclear cells and fibrosis can be seen in surrounding areas (Fig. 4). Macrophages and plasma cells are abundant in alveolar and interstitial spaces.

Another classification divides OPA into mucinous and non-mucinous forms. Non-mucinous adenocarcinomas are characterized by short columnar to cuboidal cells lining neoplastic alveolar walls (Fig. 5). Mucinous adenocarcinomas have long cylindrical cells with foamy cytoplasm filled with mucin secretions that push the nucleus to the cell border (Fig. 6). Invasion of tumoral cells from basal layers to lower layers were few in cases of the present study.

From 24 Adenocarcinomas of our study, just one Mediastinal lymph node metastasis was observed (Fig. 7). The neoplastic cells of this case were characterized by varying sizes, degrees of pleomorphism, big and bright nuclear and clear nucleoli. Mitotic figures were more significant.

Small and big cysts were observed in 4 lung tissues. Cyst walls were covered by columnar to cuboidal neoplastic cells. Mu-

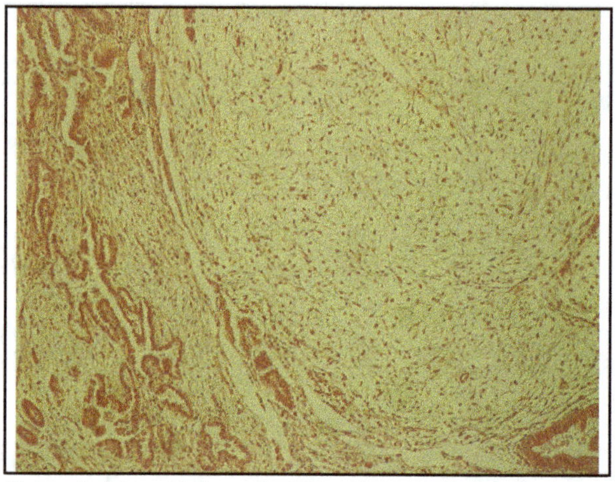

Figure 9. Myxoid tissue in OPA affected pulmonary tissue, sheep. (H&E)(x400).

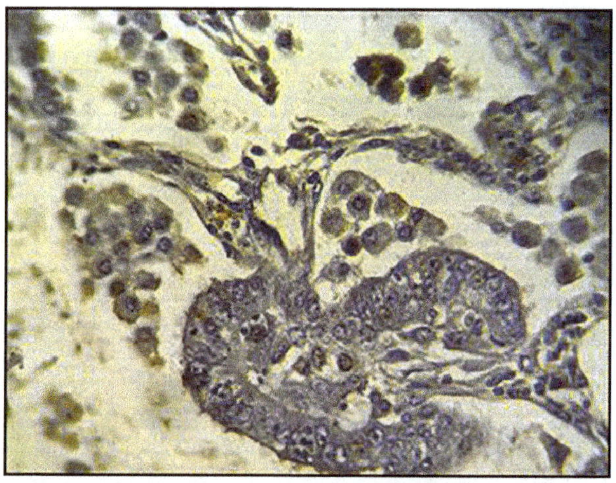

Figure 10. Immunohistochemical finding of Thyroid Transcription Factor (TTF-1) marker expression in neoplastic nuclei showing nuclear immunoreactivity. (x400).

cin secretions were also observed inside the cysts (Fig. 8). Three cases had shown some myxoid tissue in interstitial space of neoplastic alveoli (Fig. 9).

Big foamy macrophages were abundant in alveoli, which are more obvious in classic forms. Plasma cells and other mononuclear cells could be seen in tumoral and even non-tumoral interstitial space, while they were more frequent in atypical forms. Necrosis and severe infiltration of neutrophils were observed at some part of tumoral parenchyma.

Severe infiltration of mononuclear lymphocytes into the alveolar walls was seen in some tissue samples and even their mitosis division can be signs of simultaneous occurrence of pulmonary adenomatous and Maedi disease.

6 out of 8 examined cases for TTF1 marker staining were positive and 2 cases were negative for immunohistochemical test (Fig. 10).

Discussion

Ovine pulmonary adenocarcinoma is one of the many reasons of respiratory failure and pneumonia in sheep and less in goats. There have been some previous studies in other regions of Iran on the prevalence of this disease. In a period of six months in Khuzestan, a study was conducted on 3985 goats in which four goats showed macroscopic and histopathological lesions related to classic OPA (Sayyari and Mohamadian, 2012). In one study that was conducted in Fars province on lungs of 9400 sheep, 21% were diagnosed as OPA and showed both classical and atypical forms without any metastasis (Khodakaram-Tafti and Hematian, 2011). According to another study on lung tissues with OPA in Fars province, JSRV was detected by RT-PCR in all cases of suspected lungs (Khodakaram-Tafti et al., 2009). Another study in the northwest of Iran on the outbreak of pulmonary adenocarcinoma, and among 167 samples, 30 samples were positive. Finally, it was shown that this infection is highly prevalent in this part region of the country (Rezazadeh et al., 2012).

In the present study, from 7952 ovine lung tissues in a slaughterhouse during one year, 25 cases were positive histopathologically, indicating that the outbreak in that area was about 0.3 %.

According to available reports, there are two forms of OPA, including classical and atypical adenocarcinoma that could be identified clinically and histopathologically. Classical forms are often progressive to death while atypical forms remain subclinical. Histology of two forms is also similar, with the difference being that in the atypical form, infiltration of mononuclear cells, particular lymphocytes and plasma cells, and connective fibers to stromal are more (Martineau and Cousens Griffiths, 2010 - Summersa et al., 2012).

Some samples had different histological characteristics that indicate the intermediate state of classical and atypical forms or they are progressing neoplasms. Two cases of classic OPA explained small and large cysts with neoplastic cells. In mucinous form, long columnar cells were lining the alveoli walls with abundant cytoplasmic mucin and basal nuclei. In Non-mucinous forms, Clara cells and pneumocytes grow on alveolar wall and there was no stromal invasion (Palmarini and Fan 2001). In this study, mucinous forms were long cells with light and foamy cytoplasm, mucin secretion, acinar and papillary growth. In some parts of tissues, there were frequent large neoplastic cells and they filled alveoli. In non-mucinous forms short cells with pink cytoplasm were usually arranged in the walls of the alveoli. In some of the lesions both mucinous and non-mucinous forms existed. Furthermore, in two cases of lung lesions, some myxomatous nodules were observed.

One of 25 tumoral cases (4%), metastasized to mediastinal lymph node. This tumor was highly malignant with severe polymorphism, large nuclei, clear nucleoli with frequent mitotic figures. Usual organs for metastasis of OPA cells are intrathoracic metastases in the diaphragm, chest wall, heart and lymph node and metastases outside the chest area in the liver, kidney, adrenal glands, skeletal muscle, skin, digestive tract and spleen (Minguij_on, 2013).

TTF-1 (Thyroid transcription factor-1) expression is useful in distinguishing pulmonary from nonpulmonary tumors (Agoff, N.S., et al.). TTF-1, a nuclear protein, plays a role in transcriptional activation during embryogenesis in the thyroid, diencephalon, and respiratory epithelium (Bohinski RJ.,et al 1993 - Lazzaro D, et al,. 1991). In 6 out of 8 cases of our study, TTF 1 positive staining revealed pulmonary origin of these neoplasms.

Histological similarities between OPA and human lung tumors have been recognized for many years (Bonné, 1939), and OPA is regarded as a natural animal model for human lung adenocarcinomas of mixed subtypes (De las Heras et al., 2003 - Mornex et al., 2003 - Palmarini and Fan, 2001). A retroviral etiology for these human tumors has been suggested, and some cases have been shown to express an antigen related to betaretroviral Gag proteins (De las Heras et al 2000 - De las Heras, M., et al. 2007 - Hopwood et al., 2010). However, additional markers of retroviral infection in these patients have not been found (Hopwood et al., 2010). Antigen expression of virus Gap that causes lung adenocarcinoma is verified in some human tumors, but other evidence of beta-retroviral infections have not been observed. It is also shown that although the virus is present in human lung tumors, these viruses are not associated with beta-retrovirus. Other immunohistochemical studies suggest that some human lung carcinoma including bronchial alveolar carcinoma can be associated with JSRV retrovirus but no molecular study has been done to stabilize the expression (Hopwood et al., 2010).

Acknowledgments

The authors wish to thank laboratory of pathology department and Mr Samani for support and assistance. Dr Mohammad nejhad and Dr Jahaanzaad for science support. Meisam industrial slaughtered for tumor and normal lung sample collection.

References

Agoffs, N., Lamps, L.W., Philip, T., Amin, M.B. Schmidt, R.A., True, L.D., Folpe, A. (2000) Thyroid transcription factor-1 Is expressed in extrapulmonary small cell carcinomas but not in other extrapulmonary neuroendocrine tumors. Mod Pathol. 13: 238- 242.

Ahn, H.K., Jung, M., Ha, S.Y., Lee, J.I., Park, I., Kim, Y.S., Hong, J., Sym, S.J, Park, J., Shin, DB., Lee, J.H., Cho, E.K. (2014) Clinical significance of Ki-67 and p53 expression in curatively resected non-small cell lung cancer. Tumor Biol. 35: 5735-5740.

Amini, F., Mostafa-Tehrani, A. (2013) A Five-Year survey (2002-2007) on ovine pulmonary adenomatosis in a mixed-breed sheep flock. Bulg J Vet Med. 16: 139–142.

Azizi, S., Tajbakhsh, E., Fathi, F. (2014) Ovine pulmonary adenocarcinoma in slaughtered sheep: A pathological and polymerase chain reaction study. J S Afr Vet Assoc. 85: 4 Pages.

Bahari, A., Sabouri Ghannad, M., Dezfoulian, O., Rezazadeh, F., Sadeghi-Nasab, A. (2016) Detection of jaagsiekte sheep retrovirus in apparently healthy sheep by real-time TaqMan PCR in comparison with histopathological findings. J Vet Res. 60: 7-12.

Bejarano, P.A., Baughman, R.P., Biddinger, P.W., Miller, M.A., Fenoglio-Preiser, C., al-Kafaji, B., Di Lauro, R., Whitsett, J.A. (1996) Surfactant proteins and thyroid transcription factor-1 in pulmonary and breast carcinomas. Mod Pathol. 9: 445-52.

Beytut, E., So¨zmen, M., Ergı´nsoy, S. (2009) Immunohistochemical detection of pulmonary surfactant proteins and retroviral antigens in the lungs of sheep with pulmonary adenomatosis. J Comp Pathol. 140: 43e53.

Bohinski, R.J., Huffman, J.A., Whitsett, J.A., Lattier, D.L. (1993) Cis-active elements controlling lung cell-specific expression of human pulmonary surfactant protein B Gene. J Biol Chem. 268: 11160-6.

Bonné, C. (1939) Morphological resemblance of pulmonary adenomatosis (Jaagsiekte) in sheep and certain cases of cancer of the lung in man. Am J Cancer. 34: 491-501.

Cousens, C., Alleaume, C., Bijsmans, E., Martineau, M., Finlayson, J., Dagleish, M., Griffith, D. (2015) Jaagsiekte sheep retrovirus infection of lung slice cultures. Retrovirology. 12: 31.

De las Heras, M., Barsky, S.H., Hasleton, P., Wagner, M., Larson, E., Egan, J., Ortin, A., Gimenez-Mas, J.A., Palmarini, M., Sharp, J.M. (2000) Evidence for a protein related immunologically to the jaagsiekte sheep retrovirus in some human lung tumours. Eur Respir J. 16: 330-332.

De las Heras, M., Gonzalez, L., Sharp, J.M. (2003) Pathology of ovine pulmonary adenocarcinoma. Curr Top Microbiol Immunol. 275: 25-54.

De las Heras, M., Murcia, P., Ortín, A., Azúa, J., Borderías, L., Alvarez, R., Jiménez-Más, J.A., Marchetti, A., Palmarini, M. (2007). Jaagsiekte sheep retrovirus is not detected in human lung adenocarcinomas expressing antigens related to the gag polyprotein of betaretroviruses. Cancer Lett. 258: 22-30.

Griffiths, D.J., Martineau, H.M, Cousens, C.

(2010) Pathology and pathogenesis of ovine pulmonary adenocarcinoma. J Comp Pathol. 142: 260-83.

Holzinger, A., Dingle, S., Bejarano, P.A., Miller, M.A., Weaver, T.E., DiLauro, R., Whitsett, J.A. (1996) Monoclonal antibody to thyroid transcription factor-1: production, characterization, and usefulness in tumor diagnosis. Hybridoma. 15: 49-53.

Hopwood, P., Wallace, W.A., Cousens, C., Dewar, P., Muldoon, M., Norval, M., Griffiths, D.J. (2010) Absence of markers of betaretrovirus infection in human pulmonary adenocarcinoma. Hum Pathol. 41: 1631-1640.

Hopwood, P., William, A. H., Wallace, M., Cousens, C., Dewar, P., Muldoon, M., Norval, M., , David, J., Griffiths. (2010) Absence of markers of betaretrovirus infection in human pulmonary adenocarcinoma. Hum Pathol. 41: 1631-1640.

Jubb, Kennedy and pulmer's. (2007) Pahology of Domestic animals. (5th ed.). Elsevier saunders., USA.

Khodakaram-Tafti, A., Hematian, A. (2011) Ultrastructural Study of Naturally Occuring Ovine Pulmonary Adenocarcinoma In Fars Province, Iran. IJVR 2011 (Issue 4).

Khodakaram-Tafti, A., Mohammadi, A., Mansourian, M. (2009) Detection of the jaagsiekte sheep retrovirus by RT-PCR in naturally ovine pulmonary adenocarcinoma affected sheep and in apparently healthy in contact-sheep. Revue Méd Vét. 160: 319-323

Kojouri, G.H.A., Karimi, I. (2002) Sheep pulmonary adenomatosis: A study on prevalence and pathological findings. Pajouhesh-va-Sazandegi. (In Persian) 53: 64-67.

Lazzaro, D., Price, M., de Felice, M., Di Lauro, R. (1991) The transcription factor TTF-1 is expressed at the onset of thyroid and lung morphogenesis and in restricted regions of the foetal brain. Development. 113: 1093-104.

Linnerth-Petrik, N.M., Walsh, S.R., Bogner, P.N., Morrison, C., Wootton, S.K. (2014) Jaagsiekte sheep retrovirus detected in human lung cancer tissue arrays. BMC Res Notes. 7: 160.

Palmarini, M., Fan, H. (2001) Retrovirus-induced ovine pulmonary adenocarcinoma, an animal model for lung cancer. J Nat Cancer Inst. 93: 1603-1614.

Meuten, D.J. (2017) Tumor in Domestic Animals. (5th ed.). wiley-blackwell., USA.

Minguij_on, E., Gonz_alez, L., De las Heras, M., G_omez, N., Garc_ıa-Goti, M. ,Juste, R.A., Moreno, B. (2013) Pathological and aetiological studies in sheep exhibiting extrathoracic metastasis of ovine pulmonary adenocarcinoma (Jaagsiekte). J Comp Pathol. 148: 139-147.

Mornex, J.F., Thivolet, F., De las Heras, M., Leroux, C. (2003) Pathology of human bronchioloalveolar carcinoma and its relationship to the ovine disease. Curr Top Microbiol Immunol. 275: 225-248.

Palmarini, M., Fan, H. (2001) Retrovirus-induced ovine pulmonary adenocarcinoma, an animal model for lung cancer. J Natl Cancer Inst. 93: 1603-1614.

Rezazadeh, F., Zarrini, G.H., Cousens, C.H., Attarilar, N. (2012) Prevalence of jaagsiekte sheep retrovirus infection in north-west Iran. Glob Vet. 9: 535-540.

Sayyari, M., Mohamadian, B. (2012) Histopathological study of naturally occurring ovine pulmonary adenocarcinoma in native goat in Khuzestan, Iran. Iranian Journal of Veterinary Research, Shiraz University. Vol. 13, No. 4.

Summersa, C., Benitoa, A., Ortina, A., Garciade Jalona, J.A., Gonzalez, B.L., Norvalc, M., Sharpb, J.M., De las Heras, M. (2012) The dstribution of immune cells in the lungs of classical and atypical ovine pulmonary adenocarcinoma. Vet Immunol Immunopathol. 146: 1-7.

Tabata, K., Tanaka, T., Hayashi, T., Hori, T., Nunomura, S., Yonezawa, S., Fukuoka, J. (2014) Ki-67 is a strong prognostic marker of non-small cell lung cancer when tissue heterogeneity isconsidered. BMC Clin Pathol. 14: 23.

Zachary, J.F., McGavin, M.D. (2017) Pathologic Basis of Veterinary Disease. (5th ed). Penny Rudolph. Mosby, USA.

Monitoring the prevalence of the tetracycline efflux genes among *E. coli* isolated from chicken colibacillosis

Nouri Gharajalar, S.*, **Zare, P.**

Department of Pathobiology, Faculty of Veterinary Medicine, Tabriz University, Tabriz, Iran

Key words:
antibiotic resistance, colibacillosis, efflux genes, *E. coli*, tetracycline

Correspondence
Nouri Gharajalar, S.
Department of Pathobiology, Faculty of Veterinary Medicine, Tabriz University, Tabriz, Iran

Email: saharnouri@yahoo.com

Abstract:

BACKGROUND: Avian colibacillosis can lead to important economic losses in the poultry industry. *Escherichia coli*, the causative agent of this disease has acquired resistance to different antibiotics, including tetracycline. **OBJECTIVES:** This study was carried out to detect the distribution of tetracycline Group I efflux genes among *E.coli* isolates from from avian colibacillosis in Iran by PCR assay. **METHODS:** A total of 50 *E. coli* isolates from chicken colibacillosis were characterized by cultural, biochemical and PCR methods. Kirby-Bauer disk diffusion method was used to define the resistance of isolates to tetracycline, then the Frequencies of tetracycline resistance genes (*tetA*, *tetB*, *tetC*, *tetG*, *tetH*, *tetZ* and *tetE*) were also determined using PCR method. **RESULTS:** According to biochemical and molecular experiments, 50 isolates from 237 chicken samples were recognized as *E. coli*. Seventy-six (76%) of the isolates, however, were resistant to tetracycline. The distribution of tetracycline-resistance genes among *E. coli* isolates included *tetB* (34%), *tetA* (26%), *tetE* (16%), *tetC* (15%), *tetH* (12%), *tetG* (12%) and *tetZ* (6%). **CONCLUSIONS:** The present study highlights the prevalence of tetracycline resistant *E. coli* among chickens which is due to extensive use of this antibiotic for growth promotion in poultry industry.

Introduction

Widespread use of antibiotic agents is the most important factor causing emergence and dissemination of antimicrobial resistant bacteria (Van den Bogaard et al., 2001).

Antimicrobial drugs use in poultry production industries as a growth promotion factor, lead to the high resistance to antibiotic agents among avian infectious microorganisms (Romanus et al., 2012). Tetracycline is a broad - spectrum antibiotic that inhibits protein synthesis by binding to the bacterial ribosomes (Chopra and Roberts, 2001). There are four tetracycline resistance mechanisms in microorganisms including: efflux pumps, alteration in target receptors, ribosomal protection and enzymatic inactivation (Tuckman et al., 2007). Efflux pumps are transport proteins which could export antibiotics such as tetracycline from the cells to the outside (Webber and Piddock, 2003). Tetracycline efflux pumps belong to the six groups based on their amino acid sequences. Group 1 includes: *TetA*, *TetB*, *TetC*, *TetE*, TetD, *TetG*, *TetH*, *TetZ*, *TetJ* and *TetI* which are found exclusively in gram negative bacteria (Chopra and Roberts, 2001).

E. coli is an important microorganism among gram - negative bacteria (Sharma et al., 2013). Antibiotic resistance in *E. coli* strains isolated from human, animals and environment, has developed due to widespread use of antimicrobial agents for treatment of *E. coli* caused infections. (Wose Kinge et al., 2010). Among tetracycline resistance mechanisms, efflux proteins are the most important mechanism of resistance in *E. coli* (Tuckman et al. 2007).

Consequently, the increasing rate of antibiotic resistance among *E. coli* isolates complicates treatment of infections (Kibert and Abera, 2011).

Although in some studies the frequency of tetracycline resistance genes (*tetA*, *tetB*) in *E. coli* isolates recovered from commercial broiler chicken in east Azerbaijan were evaluated, there is not any complete study about the prevalence of other tetracycline efflux genes. So this work is the first study that evaluates the frequency of other efflux genes involved in tetracycline resistance in this area. The objective of the present study was to evaluate the occurrence of group I of tetracycline efflux genes in *E. coli* strains obtained from avian colibacillosis in east and west Azerbaijan in Iran.

Materials and Methods

Sample collection: During 2013-2015, a total number of 237 samples from chicken carcasses suspected of colibacillosis were collected from 11 poultry farms located in the provinces of east and west Azerbaijan. All chickens showed clinical signs including watery diarrhea, weakness, anorexia and weight loss before death. A thorough post-mortem examination of all dead birds was carried out. Liver and spleen samples were collected separately in sterile test tubes, then were used for bacteriological studies.

Isolation of *E. coli*: All samples were cultured on Mac Conkey (Sigma Aldrich, USA) and EMB agar (Sigma Aldrich, USA) then incubated for 24h at 37 °C. *E. coli* colonies were examined by biochemical tests like growth on triple sugar iron agar (TSI) or citrate utilization, fermentation of indol, methyl red test, motility and urease test and the *E. coli* isolates were confirmed (Sharma et al. 2013). All isolated bacteria were frozen in trypticase soy broth with 30% glycerol (Sigma Aldrich, USA) at -70 °C (Tadesse et al., 2012).

Molecular confirmation of *E. coli*: DNA extraction. All *E. coli* isolates were cultured overnight in Nutrient broth media (Sigma Aldrich, USA) and their chromosomal DNA was extracted using bacterial genomic DNA purification kit (INTRON, Korea).

Primers and PCR. *E. coli* 16s rRNA gene was detected through PCR method using universal Primer Sequences used for PCR identification of *E. coli* 16s rRNA gene were 5′- GTA TAG ATA CCC TGG TAG TCCA-3′ as forward and 5′- CCC GGG AAC GTA TTC ACC G-3′ as reverse primers.

The PCR assay was done in a total volume of 25 µl by using INTRON premix. The PCR conditions using DNA thermo cycler (MWG AG BIOTECHTHERMAL CYCLER, USA) were as follow: Three min at 95 °C followed by 26 cycles of 94 °C for 1 min, 55 °C for 1min and 72 °C for 10 min (Sharma et al., 2013). The PCR products were analyzed by electrophoresis in 1% agarose gel.

Antimicrobial susceptibility testing: After identification of *E. coli* isolates by

Table 1. Primer Sequences used for PCR identification of *tetB*, *tetA*, *tetE*, *tetC*, tetD, *tetG*, *tetH* and *tetZ*.

Primer	gene	Sequences
Forward	*tetA*	5′-GCGCGATCTGGTTCACTCG-3′
Reverse	*tetA*	5′-AGTCGACAGYRGCGCCGGC-3′
Forward	*tetB*	5′-TACGTGAATTTATTGCTTCGG-3′
Reverse	*tetB*	5′-ATACAGCATCCAAAGCGCAC-3′
Forward	*tetC*	5′-GCGGGATATCGTCCATTCCG-3′
Reverse	*tetC*	5′-GCGTAGAGGATCCACAGGACG-3′
Forward	*tetE*	5′-GTTATTACGGGAGTTTGTTGG-3′
Reverse	*tetE*	5′-AATACAACACCCACACTACGC-3′
Forward	*tetG*	5′-GCAGAGCAGGTCGCTGG-3′
Reverse	*tetG*	5′-CCYGCAAGAGAAGCAGAAG-3′
Forward	*tetH*	5′-CAGTGAAAATTCACTGGCAAC-3′
Reverse	*tetH*	5′-ATCCAAAGTGTGGTTGAGAAT-3′
Forward	*tetJ*	5′-CGAAAACAGACTCGCCAATC-3′
Reverse	*tetJ*	5′-TCCATAATGAGGTGGGGC-3′
Forward	*tetZ*	5′-CCTTCTCGACCAGGTCGG-3′
Reverse	*tetZ*	5′-ACCCACAGCGTGTCCGTC-3′

biochemical and molecular methods, the standard Kirby-Bauer disk diffusion method was used to determine the tetracycline resistance pattern among *E. coli* strains (Sayah et al., 2005).

Distribution of tetracycline resistance genes: All isolates which were resistant to tetracycline were examined further by the use of five PCR assays for the presence of *tetA*, *tetB*, *tetE*, *tetC*, *tetH*, *tetZ* and *tetG* genes. The primer sets used for amplification of these genes were shown in Table 2 (Aminov et al., 2002).

The first PCR assay used for amplification of *tetE*, consisted of initial denaturation at 94 °C for 1 min followed by 25 cycles at 94 °C for 1min, 1min of annealing at 50 °C and 72 °C for 10 min. The second PCR was performed for amplification of *tetB* as described above with the use of specific primers. The third assay was performed for amplification of *tetA* and *tetC* with annealing temperature of 48 °C.

The fourth assay was used to identify *tetG* as described above but the annealing temperature was 46 °C and finally the last amplification was carried out to identify *tetH* and *tetZ* genes using 46 °C as annealing temperature The PCR products were analyzed by agarose gel electrophoresis and the frequency of each tetracycline resistance determinants was determined.

Results

Out of 237 poultry carcasses samples suspected of colibacillosis, 21/09% (n=50) *E. coli* were isolated using culture and biochemical tests. Furthermore, molecular detection of *E. coli* isolates was carried out. 16s rRNA gene of *E. coli* was identified by PCR assay of extracted DNA using 16srRNA universal primers. Figure 1 shows the 16s rRNA gene of *E. coli* strains found at 612bp on 100bp DNA ladder.

As the antimicrobial susceptibility test shows 76% of *E. coli* isolates were resistant to tetracycline. The percentage of isolates susceptible to tetracycline was 24%, none of the isolates showed intermediate suscep-

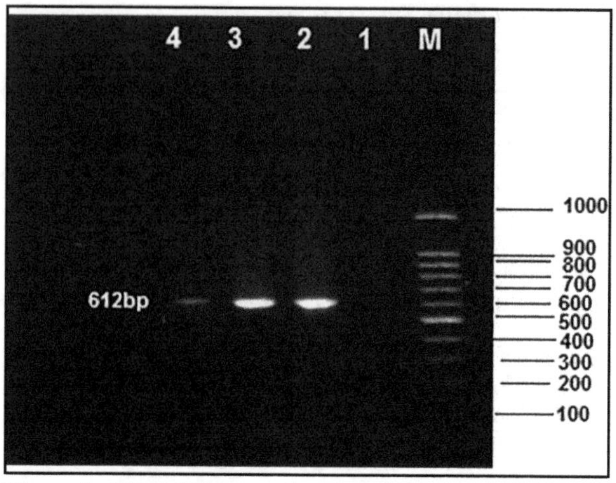

Figure 1. 16s rRNA gene found at 612bp on 1% agarose gel after PCR amplification. Lane M- 100bp ladder marker Lane 1- Negative control. Lane2- Positive control. Lane 3- *E. coli* 16s rRNA gene found at 612bp.

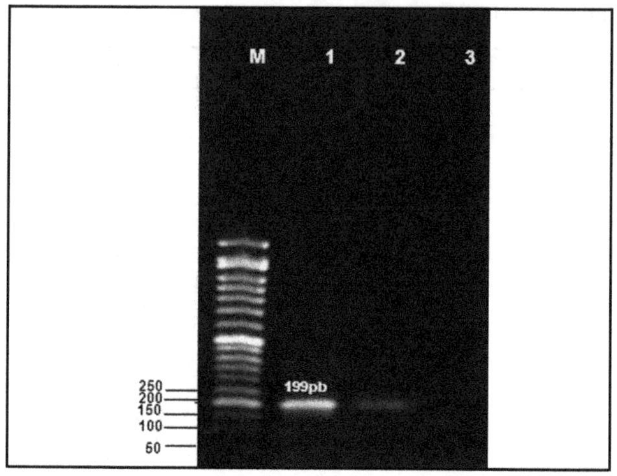

Figure 2. Representing agarose gel of PCR product from *E. coli* isolates, using primers for *tetE*. Lane M- 50bp Ladder marker. Lane 1- *tetE* gene found at 199bp. Lane 2- positive control. Lane 3- negative control.

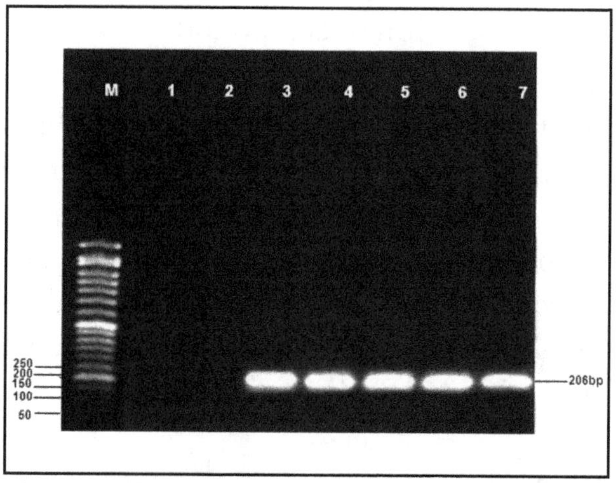

Figure 3. Gel electrophoresis of the PCR products of *tetB* gene. Lane M- 50bp Ladder marker. Lane 1- negative control. Lane 3- positive control. Lane 4, 7- *tetB* gene found at 206bp.

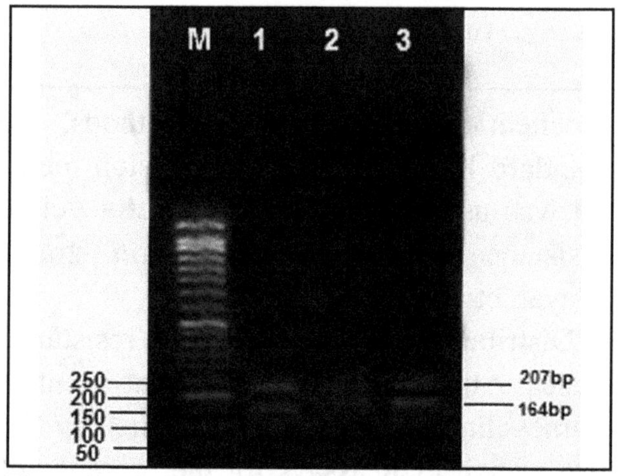

Figure 4. Gel electrophoresis of the PCR products of *tetA* and *tetC* determinants. Lane M- 50bp Ladder marker. Lane 1 to 3- *tetA* (164bp) and *tetC* (207bp).

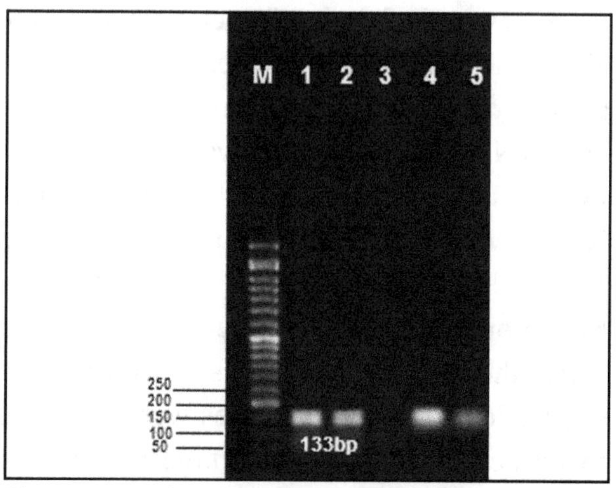

Figure 5. PCR detection of *tetG* marker in *E. coli* isolates Lane M- 50bp Ladder marker. Lane 1- positive control. Lane 3- negative control. Lane 4, 5- *tetG* (133bp).

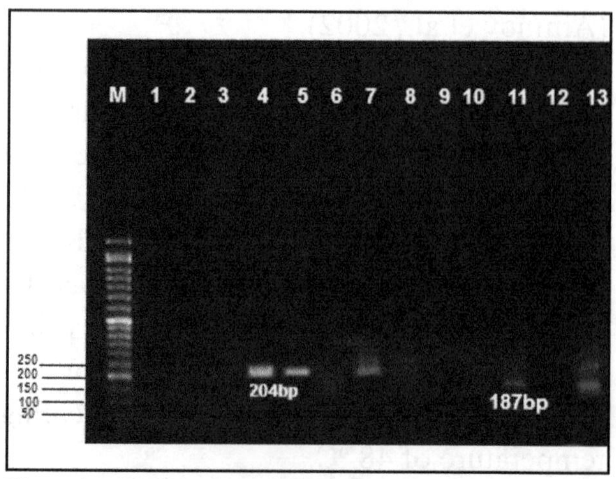

Figure6. PCR detection of tetH and tetZ markers in *E. coli* isolates.

tibility to the drug.

For detection of the tetracycline efflux genes frequency, among isolates, five PCR assays were used and results were shown in Fig. 2 to Fig. 6.

The most common determinants were *tetB* (34%) followed by *tetA* (26%). However, *tetH* (12%), *tetG* (12%), *tetC* (15%) and *tetE* (16%) were also found with different frequencies. The lowest Frequency among studied genes belonged to *tetZ* (6%).

Discussion

Among fifty *E. coli* isolates from chicken colibacillosis, 38 isolates were resistant to tetracycline. Study of the occurrence of tetracycline efflux genes showed that the *tetB* gene had the highest frequency among studied genes.

Antibiotics are usually used for treatment of bacterial infections in humans and animals. They are also used in commercial livestock and poultry food for promotion of growth. As a result, antimicrobial resistance among bacteria will be increased (Sayah et al., 2005).

Tetracyclines are broad spectrum antibacterials that have been used for a long period of time in humans and animals. But nowadays a widespread range of bacteria are showing resistance to tetracycline which encodes by several resistance genes (Trzcinski et al., 2000). Pathogenic strains of *E. coli* are common infectious microorganisms among gram negative bacteria, causing intestinal and extra intestinal infections. Many times, antibiotic therapy is needed for treatment of *E. coli* infections both in humans and veterinary medicine (Sharma et al., 2013). A great deal of evidence indicates that antimicrobial resistance in *E. coli* is the highest among other bacteria and tetracycline resistance is a very common resistance pattern in animal's coliforms (Taddesse et al., 2012).

Advances in molecular bacteriology lead to detection and use of new techniques for describing the genetic determinants responsible for antibiotic resistance in bacteria. Also, designing of specific primers have provided accurate and rapid detection of antibiotic resistance genes (Blake et al., 2003). According to prior studies, tetracycline efflux pumps are important resistance mechanisms in *E. coli* and among these determinants *tetB* gene was the most prevalent, responsible for tetracycline resistance (Tuckman et al., 2007). Our results also confirm the prevalence of tetracycline resistance and the predominant role of *tetB* resistance gene among *E. coli* isolated from animals.

In 2004 distribution of tetracycline resistance genes in *E. coli* strains from diverse human and animal sources was examined by Brayan et al. The most common genes found in their isolates were *tetB* and *tetA*. *tetC* and tetD were also found with lower frequencies. Also, Tuckman et al in 2007 monitored the prevalence of tetracycline resistance genes in *E. coli* strains by PCR assay. They revealed that *tetB* and *tetA* markers had the highest frequency among studied determinants. Our results are in accordance with their findings.

Momtaz et al in 2012 evaluated the distribution of antibiotic-resistant genes in *Escherichia coli* isolates from slaughtered commercial chickens in Iran by PCR. The distribution of *tetA* and *tetB* genes in the *E. coli* isolates were 52.63%. Also, Wang et al in 2013 investigated the prevalence of antimicrobial-resistant chicken *Escherichia coli* strains and the resistance genes in *E.*

coli. The detection rates of *tetA*, *tetB* genes were 95/3% and 97/4%. Here, we also used molecular PCR technique to determine the occurrence of tetracycline resistance genes in *E. coli* bacteria. Our results also indicate that *tetB* and *tetA* genes were the most frequent determinants for tetracycline resistance. Relative to the results obtained in the detection of antimicrobial resistance genes, in a study of *E. coli* isolated strains from broiler chickens in Brazil, Santos et al. (2014) observed the concomitant presence of *tetA* and *tetB* and genes. This is consistent with the detection of two resistance genes in the strains of *E. coli* in the present study.

The high percentage of phenotypes of *E. coli* isolates that were resistant to tetracycline, suggested that the widespread use of tetracycline in poultry creates the reservoir of resistant bacteria and resistance genes and may shorten the time that this antimicrobial agent will be available for effective treatment of infections in poultry.

Examining the frequency of tetracycline resistance genes among *E. coli* isolated from chicken colibacillosis, confirmed the presence of tetracycline resistance genes in most of the *E. coli* isolates and pictured the distribution pattern of these determinants which is very similar to the prior findings about these determinants.

Acknowledgments

This work was supported by Tabriz University, Tabriz, Iran.

References

Aminov, R.I., Chee-Sanford, J.C., Garrigues, N., Teferedegne, B., Krapac, I.J., White, B.A., Mackie, R.I. (2002) Development, validation and application of PCR primers for detection of Tetracycline Efflux genes of gram negative bacteria. Appl Environ Microbiol. 68: 1786-1793. DOI: 10.1128/aem.68.4.1786-1793.

Blake, D.P., Humphry, R.W., Scott, K.P., Hillman, K., Fenlon, D.R., Low, J.C. (2003) Influence of tetracycline exposure on tetracycline resistance and carriage of tetracycline resistance genes within commensal *Escherichia coli* populations. J Appl Microbiol. 94: 1087-1097. DOI: 10.1046/j.1365-2672.2003.01937.x.

Bryan, A., Shapir, N., Sadowsky, M.J. (2004) Frequency and distribution of tetracycline resistance genes in genetically diverse, none selected and nonclinical *Escherichia coli* strains isolated from diverse human and animal sources. Appl Environ Microbiol. 70: 2503-7. DOI:10.1128/aem.70.4.2503-2507.

Chopra, I., Roberts, M. (2001) Tetracycline antibiotics: mode of action, applications, molecular biology and epidemiology of bacterial resistance. Microbiol Mol Biol. 65: 232-60. DOI: 10.1128/mmbr.65.2.232-260.

Kibert, M., Abera, B. (2011) Antimicrobial susceptibility patterns of *E. coli* from clinical sources in northeast Ethiopia. Afr Health Sci. 11: 40-44. DOI:10.4314/ahs.v11i3.70069.

Momtaz, H., Rahimi, E., Moshkelani, S. (2012) Molecular detection of antimicrobial resistance genes in *E. coli* isolated from slaughtered commercial chickens in Iran. Vet Med. 57, 2 (4): 193-197. https://www.researchgate.net/publication/237047427.

Romanus, I., Chinyere, O.E., Amobi, N.E., Anthonia, O.E., Ngozi, A.F., Chidiebube, N.A., Eze, A.T. (2012) Antimicrobial resistance of *Escherichia coli* isolated from animal and human clinical sample. Global Res J Microbiol. 2: 85-89.

Santos, M.M., Alcantara, A.C.M., Perecmanis, S.I., Campos, A., Santana, A.P. (2014) Antimicrobial resistance of bacterial strains isolated from avian cellulitis. Braz J Poult Sci. 16: 13-18.DOI: 10.1590/s1516-635x2014000100002.

Sayah, R.S., Kaneene, J.B., Johnson, Y., Miller, R. (2005) Patterns of antimicrobial resistance observed in *Escherichia coli* isolates obtained from domestic and wild animal fecal samples, human septage, and surface water. Appl Environ Microbiol. 71: 1394- 1404.DOI: 10.1128/aem.71.3.1394-1404.

Sharma, S., Mahajan, B., Patidar, R.K., Sahare, K.N., Khare, M. (2013) Molecular detection of antimicrobial resistance genes in biofilm forming *Escherichia Coli*. Am J Pharm Health Res. 1: 2321-3647.

Tadesse, D.A., Zhoa, SH., Tong, E. Ayers, SH., Singh, A., Bartholomew, M.J., Mc Dermott, P.F. (2012) Antimicrobial drug resistance in *Escherichia coli* from humans and food animals, United States 1950-2002, Emerg Infect Dis. 18: 741-749. DOI:10.3201/eid1805.111153.

Trzysztof, K., Cooper, B.S., Hryniewicz, W., Dowson, C.G. (2000) Expression of resistance to tetracyclines in strains of methicillin-resistant Staphylococcus. J Antimicrob Chemother 2000; 45(6): 763-770. DOI: 10.1093/jac/45.6.763.

Tuckman, M., Petersen, P.J., Howe, A.Y.M., Orlowski, M., Mullen, S, Chan, K., Bradford, P.A. (2007) Hal Jones CH. Occurrence of tetracycline resistance genes among *Escherichia coli* isolated from the phase 3 clinical trials for tetracycline. Antimicrob Agents Chemother. 51: 3205-11. DOI: 10.1128/aac.00625-07.

Van den Bogaard, A.E., London, N., Driessen, C., Stobberingh, E.E. (2001) Antibiotic resistance of fecal *Escherichia Coli* in poultry, Poultry farmers and Poultry slaughteres. J Antimicrob Chemother. 47: 763-771.

Wang, J.Y., Tang, P., Cui, E.H., Wang, L.Q., Liu, W.H., Ren, J.J., Wu, N., Qiu, W.H., Liu, .HJ. (2013) Characterization of antimicrobial resistance and related resistance genes in *Escherichia coli* strains isolated from chickens in China during 2007-2012. Afr J Microbiol Res. 7: 5238-5247. DOI: 10.5897/AJMR2013.5860.

Webber, M.A., Piddock, L.J.V. (2003) The importance of efflux pumps in bacterial antibiotic resistance. J Antimicrob Chemother. 51: 9-11. DOI:10.1093/jac/dkg050.

Wose King, C.N., Njie Ateba, C., Tonderai Kawadza, D. (2010) Antibiotic resistance profiles of *Escherichia coli* isolated from different water sources in the mmabatho locality, north- West province. South Afr J Sci; 106 (1/2): 44- 49. DOI: 10.4102/sajs.v106i1/2.14.

18

Comparison of serum triiodothyronine, tetraiodothyronine and thyroid stimulating hormone concentrations in pregnant and lactating Beetal-cross and native goats in Garmsar township

Raoofi, A.[1*]**, Yourdkhani, S.**[2]**, Bokaie, S.**[3]

[1]Department of Internal Medicine, Faculty of Veterinary Medicine, University of Tehran, Tehran, Iran

[2]Department of Clinical Sciences, Faculty of Veterinary Medicine, Garmsar Branch, Islamic Azad University, Garmsar, Iran

[3]Division of Epidemiology and Zoonoses, Department of Food Hygiene and Quality Control, Faculty of Veterinary Medicine, University of Tehran, Tehran, Iran

Key words:

breed, goat, T3, T4, TSH

Correspondence

Raoofi, A.

Department of Internal Medicine, Faculty of Veterinary Medicine, University of Tehran, Tehran, Iran

Email: raoofi@ut.ac.ir

Abstract:

BACKGROUND: The preliminary survey made about congenital goiter in goats in Garmsar township indicated that the disease occurs much more in Beetal-cross than native goats raised in the same area. **OBJECTIVES:** The aim of the present study was to compare serum triiodothyronine (T3), tetraiodothyronine (T4) and thyroid stimulating hormone concentrations in pregnant and lactating Beetal-cross and native goats in Garmsar township. **METHODS:** One hundred Beetal-cross (n=50) and native (n=50) does in 4 groups (25 pregnant Beetal-cross, 25 lactating Beetal-cross, 25 pregnant native and 25 lactating native) were used in this study. Blood samples were obtained via jugular venipuncture and analyzed for serum T3, T4 and TSH concentrations. **RESULTS:** Breed had a significant ($p<0.05$) effect on T4 concentration and pregnancy had a significant ($p<0.05$) effect on T3 and TSH concentrations. No significant differences were seen for serum T3, T4 and TSH concentrations between pregnant and lactating native does. However, in the pregnant Beetal-cross, serum T3 and T4 concentrations were lower ($p<0.05$) and TSH concentration was higher ($p<0.05$) than lactating Beetal-cross does. **CONCLUSIONS:** The results of the present study highlight the relationships between thyroid activity and breed in the goat species that may play a role in more occurrence of congenital goiter in Beetal-cross in Garmsar township.

Introduction

The thyroid gland is unique in that it is the only tissue of the body which is able to accumulate iodine in large quantities and incorporate it into hormones. The thyroid hormones, triiodothyronine (T3) and tetraiodothyronine (T4) act on different target tissues, stimulating oxygen utilization and heat production in all types of body cells. The overall effects of these hormones are to increase the basal metabolic rate, to make more glucose available to cells, to stimulate protein synthesis, increase lipid metabolism and to stimulate cardiac and neural functions. Only the thyrotrophin (thyroid stimulating hormone, TSH) and the availability of iodine affect the rate of formation of the thyroid hormones (Capen and Martin, 1989). Metabolic differences during gestation and lactation are important when studying thyroid activity and making breed comparisons (Williams et al., 2004).

Goiter is an enlargement of the thyroid gland. In ruminants, goiter usually suggests attempted compensation for a hypothyroid state. Normally, low T4 and T3 output stimulates increased TSH output, which leads to increased iodine uptake from the blood and hyperplasia of the gland (Smith and Sherman, 2009). Congenital goiter is a non-inflammatory and non-neoplastic enlargement of thyroid gland in the fetus and is regarded as a common anomaly in goats (Al-Ani et al., 1998). The preliminary survey made about congenital goiter in goats in Garmsar township (center of Iran) indicated that the disease occurs much more in Beetal-cross than native goats and sheep raised in the same vicinity (Shakeri, 2004). The aim of the present study was to evaluate whether breed can affect serum T3, T4 and TSH concentrations in pregnant and lactating does. To our knowledge, there are no published data about the relationships between thyroid activity and breed in the goat species.

Material and Methods

The present study was carried out in Garmsar township located in the center of Iran. From 4 flocks at this area, 100 healthy Beetal-cross (n=50) and native (n=50) does in 4 groups (25 pregnant Beetal-cross, 25 lactating Beetal-cross, 25 pregnant native and 25 lactating native) aged between 3 and 6 years and with an average weight of 45 kg were used in this study. The goats were kept indoors and the diet used consisted of alfalfa hay, wheat straw and barley.

Blood samples were collected from the jugular vein in test tubes, and the blood was allowed to coagulate. Serum was then harvested following centrifugation, frozen and stored at -70 °C, until analyzed.

The serum total T3, T4 and TSH concentrations were measured by Enzyme-Linked Immunosorbent Assay (ELISA) kit (Diaplus Inc, USA). The mean intra-assay coefficients of variation (CV) were 4.0, 4.1 and 4.9%, the mean inter-assay CV were 4.2, 5.9 and 4.9% for serum T3, T4 and TSH, respectively.

Statistical analyses were performed using the SPSS version 16 statistical software package. Normality and homogeneity of variance assumptions for variables were satisfied and using two-way analysis of variance (ANOVA). Multiple comparisons were made by using post-hoc tests (LSD method) to find which groups were significantly different from each other, and $p<0.05$ was considered to be significant.

Results

The serum T3, T4 and TSH concentrations in the pregnant and lactating, native and Beetal-cross does are set out in Table 1. Breed had a significant ($p<0.05$) effect on T4 concentration and pregnancy had a significant ($p<0.05$) effect on T3 and TSH concentrations. No significant differences were seen for serum T3, T4 and TSH concentrations between pregnant and lactating native does. However, in the pregnant Beetal-cross, serum T3 and T4 concentrations were lower ($p<0.05$) and TSH concentration was higher ($p<0.05$) than lactating Beetal-cross does.

Two of the 25 pregnant Beetal-cross gave birth to 3 kids (1 single and 1 twin) with congenital goiter.

Discussion

Changes of blood thyroid hormone concentrations are an indirect measure of the changes in thyroid gland and extrathyreoidal deiodination activity (Todini, 2007). Variations in hormone concentration allow the animals to adapt their metabolic balance to different environmental conditions, variation in nutrient requirements and availability, and to homeorhetic changes during different physiological stages. Endogenous factors (breed, age, gender, body weight, physiological state), environmental factors (climate, season, photoperiod) and nutrition are able to affect thyroid activity and hormone concentrations in blood (Anderson and Harness, 1975; Riis and Madsen, 1985; Blaszczyk et al., 2004; Todini et al., 2006; Todini et al., 2007).

The present study indicated the significant effect of breed on T4 concentration in Beetal-cross and native Iranian goats. This may be related to differences in body size, length and amount of hair coat and body fat. Larger frame cattle and sheep have been shown to have higher circulating levels of T4 (Verde and Trenkle, 1987; Forbes et al., 1998).

Suffolk ewes had higher plasma T4 levels than Gulf Coast native ewes in the United States, which was positively associated with larger body size and enhanced growth rate potential (Forbes et al., 1998; Williams et al., 2004). Verde and Trenkle (1987) evaluated differences in metabolic hormone levels between large-frame Simmental crossbred steers and small-frame Angus crossbred steers, and found large-frame steers had higher plasma levels of T4.

The effect of breed on T4 concentration may be partly attributable to the lower length and amount of hairs, and lower body fat in Beetal-cross goats. These may be associated with means of thermoregulation. Higher plasma T4 concentrations in Assaf ewes than Merino and Rasa Aragonesa ewes have been related to differences in wool growth rate (Abecia et al., 2005).

Newborn Blackface lambs had greater plasma T3 and T4 concentrations than Suffolk lambs and this was associated with higher body temperature and better thermoregulatory ability (Dwyer and Morgan, 2006). Lambs breeds that are reared in hill regions (extensive conditions) have an improved thermoregulation than those reared in lowland (intensive conditions) and this is associated with birth coat characteristics and higher plasma T3 and T4 levels (Dwyer and Lawrence, 2005).

In sheep, the effects of breed on thyroid activity and thyroid hormones plasma concentrations have been described. The decrease in plasma T4 concentrations induced by feed restriction was greater in crossbreed ewes compared to native Indian sheep (Naqvi and Rai, 1991). Higher plasma concentrations of T3 and T4 in ram lambs have been related to higher prolificacy of the Outaouais breed than the Suffolk breed (Fallah-Rad and Connor, 1999). Cold stress in newborn Merino lambs have been associated with a higher increase of plasma T3 and T4 concentrations than Romney-Marsh lambs (Doubek et al., 2003).

There were no significant differences in serum T3, T4 and TSH concentrations between pregnant and lactating native does. However, these differences were signifi-

Table 1. T3, T4 and TSH concentrations in pregnant and lactating, native and Beetal-cross does. Values were expressed as mean ± SE. B= Breed, P= Pregnancy. ab Values with different symbol in each row are significantly different ($p<0.05$).

	Breed						
	Native		Beetal-Cross		Pvalue		
Parameters	Pregnant (n=25)	Lactating (n=25)	Pregnant (n=25)	Lactating (n=25)	B	P	B×P
T3 (ng/ml)	1.38±0.05^{ab}	1.27±0.03^{ab}	1.25± 0.07^{a}	1.40±0.05^{b}	0.975	0.684	0.014
T4 (ng/ml)	78.40±6.46^{ab}	93.08±7.38^{a}	60.96±5.82^{b}	80.36±6.39^{a}	0.023	0.011	0.719
TSH (μIU/ml)	0.92±0.23^{a}	0.87±0.24^{a}	1.07±0.21^{a}	0.26±0.04^{b}	0.254	0.032	0.058

cant in Beetal-cross. This may be associated with a higher average number and body size of fetuses in the pregnant Beetal-cross does. Plasma levels of thyroid hormones in goats at mid-pregnancy rose compared with the low levels observed just before estrus and mating. Then, during the second half of pregnancy, maternal hormone levels progressively decrease, probably because of the negative energy balance (Todini et al., 2007).

The iodine required for thyroid hormones synthesis in the fetal thyroid glands were taken up from the maternal circulation. Extraction of iodine from the maternal circulation, which would increase with the higher fetal number, would decrease iodine availability for the maternal thyroid glands that ultimately reduced maternal thyroid hormones synthesis and their total circulating concentrations (Manalu et al., 1997).

Plasma T4 concentrations in the twin-bearing does, which are often characterized by negative energy balance, had a greater reduction as compared to those in single-bearing does with less negative energy balance (Manalu et al., 1997). Different energy intakes significantly affect total plasma T4 concentrations, but not total plasma T3 levels. These findings suggest that the effects of energy intake on thyroid secretion of T4 are not always coupled to the corresponding changes in peripheral monodeiodinase activity (Todini et al., 2007).

The significant differences in serum T3, T4 and TSH concentrations between pregnant and lactating Beetal-cross does may be related to higher milk yield in the Beetal-cross does. An inverse relationship between blood thyroid hormone concentrations and milk yield has been observed in goats (Riis and Madsen, 1985). Blum et al (1983) evaluated thyroid hormones in relationship to milk yield in dairy cows and reported negative correlation between thyroid hormones and milk yield during several periods of lactation.

The drop in T4 secretion rate at the onset of lactation appears to be a homeostatic adaptation to a decreased fuel supply, similar to the situation with fasting or energy malnutrition (Riis and Madsen, 1985). These findings may support the meaning of blood thyroid hormone levels as indicators of the energy balance, and in lactating animals as well (Todini, 2007).

Under similar conditions, congenital goiter occurs much more in Beetal-cross than Iranian native goats (Shakeri, 2004). This may be related to significant lower serum concentrations of T3 and T4 in pregnant than lactating Beetal-cross does. This breed may be more susceptible to iodine deficiency compared to Iranian native goats. Iodine deficiency and feeding of goitrogens substances are two major mechanisms by which diet can cause development of goiters in goats.

Breeds of goats vary in sensitivity to iodine deficiency (Smith and Sherman, 2009). The Boer goat, a rapidly growing meat breed from South Africa, seems to be especially susceptible. It is possible that selection for resistance to iodine deficiency would be selection for slow growth rate (Van Jaarsveld et al., 1971). The Angora goat is apparently very susceptible to iodine deficiency (Smith and Sherman, 2009). In the Himalayas, where caprine goiter was extensively studied, indigenous strains were apparently more resistant to iodine deficiency than were goats (Barbari or Alpine) purchased from outside regions (Rajkumar, 1970).

Congenital goiters in Beetal-cross goats may have hereditary etiology. Inherited congenital goiter has been described in an inbred strain of Dutch goats (mixed Saanen and dwarf goats). The condition was inherited as an autosomal recessive trait (Kok, 1987).

Thyroglobulin, the normal precursor of the thyroid hormones T3 and T4, was not produced in the goat that was homozygous for this trait. As a consequence, the normal feedback mechanisms were impaired and continuous thyrotropin secretion led to development of a goiter (Smith and Sherman, 2009). The responsible mutation in the thyroglobulin gene has been characterized (Rivolta and Targovnik, 2006). Congenital goiters have also been suspected to be hereditary in Boer goats (Van Jaarsveld et al., 1971) and Shami dairy goats (Al-Ani et al., 1998).

The results of present study indicate breed and physiological state of the animal may influence the thyroid activity in Beetal-cross goats. The significant lower concentrations of serum T3 and T4 and higher concentration of TSH seen in pregnant Beetal-cross goats (compared to lactating does of this breed) suggests that the thyroid gland may be less active than in Iranian native goats. More research is needed to further characterize the etiology of congenital goiter and susceptibility to iodine deficiency in Beetal-cross breed.

Acknowledgments

Authors wish to thank Mr. Ali Motevalli for his contribution in the laboratory studies of this project.

References

Abecia, J.A., Valares, J.A., Forcada, F. (2005) The effect of melatonin treatment on wool growth and thyroxine secretion in sheep. Small Rumin Res. 56: 265-270.

Al-Ani, F.K., Khamas, W.A., Al-Qudah, K.M., Al-Rawashdeh, O. (1998) Occurrence of congenital anomalies in Shami breed of goats: 211 cases investigated in 19 herds. Small Rumin Res. 28: 225-232.

Anderson, R.R., Harness, J.R. (1975) Thyroid hormone secretion rates in growing and mature goats. J Anim Sci. 40: 1130-1135.

Blaszczyk, B., Udala, J., Gaczrzewicz, D. (2004) Changes in estradiol, progesterone, melatonin, prolactin and thyroxine concentrations in blood plasma of goats following induced estrus in and outside the natural breeding season. Small Rumin Res. 51: 209-219.

Blum, J.W., Kunz, P., Leuenberger, H., Gautschi, K., Keller, M. (1983) Thyroid hormones, blood plasma metabolites and haematological parameters in relationship to milk yield in dairy cows. Anim Sci. 36: 93-104.

Capen, C.C., Martin, S.L. (1989) The thyroid gland. In: Veterinary Endocrinology and Reproduction, fourth ed. McDonald, L.E., Pineda, M.H. (eds.). Lea and Febiger, Philadelphia, PA. p. 58-91.

Doubek, J., Slosarkova, S., Fleischer, P., Mala`,

G., Skrivanek, M. (2003) Metabolic and hormonal profiles of potentiated cold stress in lambs during early postnatal period. Czech J Anim Sci. 48: 403-411.

Dwyer, C.M., Lawrence, A.B. (2005) A review of the behavioural and physiological adaptations of hill and lowland breeds of sheep that favour lamb survival. Appl Anim Behav Sci. 92: 235-260.

Dwyer, C.M., Morgan, A. (2006) Maintenance of body temperature in the neonatal lamb: Effects of breed, birth weight, and litter size. J Anim Sci. 84: 1093-1101.

Fallah-Rad, A.H., Connor, M.L. (1999) Relationships of thyroid hormones, IGF-I and testosterone in breeds of ram lambs with low and high prolificacies. Can J Anim Sci. 79: 441-448.

Forbes, C.D., Fernandez, J.M., Bunting, L.D., Southern, L.L., Thompson Jr. D.L., Gentry, L.R., Chapa, A.M. (1998) Growth and metabolic characteristics of Suffolk and Gulf Coast Native yearling ewes supplemented with chromium tripicolinate. Small Rumin Res. 28: 149-160.

Kok, K., Van Dijk, J. E., Sterk, A., Baas, F., Van Ommen, G. J., De Vijlder, J. J. M. (1987) Autosomal recessive inheritance of goiter in Dutch goats. J Hered. 78: 298-300.

Manalu, W., Sumaryadi, M. Y., Kusumorini, N. (1997) Maternal serum concentrations of total triiodothyronine, tetraiodothyronine and cortisol in different status of pregnancy during late pregnancy in Ettawah-cross does. Asian-Australas J Anim Sci. 10: 385-390.

Naqvi, S. M. K., Rai, A. K. (1991) Influence of dietary energy-level on sheep for mutton during winter. 2. Effect on cardiorespiratory responses, rectal temperature, some blood metabolites, enzymes and thyroidal hormones. Indian J Anim Sci. 61: 1126-1131.

Rajkumar, S.S. (1970) Incidence of goiter in goats. Indian Vet J. 47: 185-187.

Riis, P.M., Madsen, A. (1985) Thyroxine concentration and secretion rates in relation to pregnancy, lactation and energy balance in goats. J Endocr. 107: 421-427.

Rivolta, C.M., Targovnik, H.M. (2006) Molecular advances in thyroglobulin disorders. Clin Chim Acta. 374: 8-24.

Shakeri, M. (2004) An abattoir survey on the frequency of goiter in small ruminants in Garmsar township, DVM Thesis, Faculty of Veterinary Medicine, Garmsar Branch, Islamic Azad University.

Smith, M.C., Sherman, D.M. (2009) Goat Medicine. (2nd ed.) Wiley-Blackwell, Ames, USA.

Todini, L., Delgadillo, J. A., Debenedetti, A., Chemineau, P. (2006) Plasma total T3 and T4 concentrations in bucks as affected by photoperiod. Small Rumin Res. 65: 8-13.

Todini, L. (2007) Thyroid hormones in small ruminants: effects of endogenous, environmental and nutritional factors. Animal. 1: 997-1008.

Todini, L., Malfatti, A., Valbonesi, A., Trabalza-Marinucci, M. Debenedetti, A. (2007) Plasma total T3 and T4 concentrations in goats at different physiological stages, as affected by the energy intake. Small Rumin Res. 68: 285-290.

Van Jaarsveld, P., Theron, C., Van Der Walt, B., Van Zyl, A. (1971) Congenital goitre in South African Boer goats. J S Afr Vet Med Assoc. 42: 295-303.

Verde, L.S., Trenkle, A. (1987) Concentrations of hormones in plasma from cattle with different growth potentials. J Anim Sci. 64: 426-432.

Williams, C.C., Calmes, K.J., Fernandez, J.M., Stanley, C.C., Lovejoy, J.C., Bateman, H.G., Gentry, L.R., Gantt, D.T., Harding, G.D. (2004) Glucose metabolism and insulin sensitivity in Gulf Coast native and Suffolk ewes during late gestation and early lactation. Small Rumin Res. 54: 167-171.

Effects of *Matricaria chamomille* and *Cichorium intybus* powder on performance, Rumen microbial population and some blood parameters of Dallagh sheep

Ghasemifard, M., Rahchamani, R.*, Ghanbari, F., Mostafalo, Y.

Department of Animal Sciences, College of Agriculture and Natural Resources, University of Gonbad Kavous, Gonbad Kavous, Iran

Key words:
blood metabolite, *Cichorium intybus* powder, microbial population, *Matricaria chamomille* powder, sheep

Correspondence
Rahchamani, R.
Department of Animal Sciences, College of Agriculture and Natural Resources, University of Gonbad Kavous, Gonbad Kavous, Iran

Email: r_rahchamani@yahoo.com

Abstract:

BACKGROUND: Manipulation of rumen microbial population for improving animal performance is done by several methods including medicinal plants. *Matricaria chamomille* (chamomile) and *Cichorium intybus* (chicory) are two medicinal plants with antibacterial effect, however, little information exists about the effects of them on rumen microflora. **OBJECTIVES:** The present study was carried out to evaluate the effects of chamomile and chicory powder on performance, ruminal microbial population and some blood parameters of sheep. **METHODS:** 9 Dallagh sheep were used in a change over design experiment at three 21-d periods (14 days as adaptation and 7 days for sample collection). Treatments were: 1) control (without additive), 2) chamomile (contained 10% chamomile powder) and 3) chicory (contained %10 chicory powder). Rumen fluid was collected before, 4 h and 8 h after morning feeding and a blood sample was obtained 3 h after morning feeding at the last day of each period. **RESULTS:** Weight gain, dry matter intake, feed conversion ratio, total count of bacteria, acid lactic bacteria, rumen pH, blood glucose and total protein were not affected by treatments. Diet containing 100g chicory significantly decreased plasma triglyceride versus chamomile but the difference was not significant compared with control. Coliforms in rumen fluid at 4 h after morning feeding were lower in chamomile treatment than control ($p<0.05$). Lambs that received chamomile and chicory powder had significantly higher rumen protozoa number before morning feeding. **CONCLUSIONS:** Although *Matricaria chamomille* and *Cichorium intybus* dry powder had some significant effects on rumen microbial population it had no effect on performance, growth and blood metabolites.

Introduction

Manipulation of rumen microbial ecosystem for enhancing fibrous feed digestibility, reducing methane emission and nitrogen excretion by ruminants to improve their performance are some of the most important goals for animal nutritionists (Patra et al., 2006). Medicinal herbs or Plant extracts with high concentration of secondary metabolites are good candidates for achieving one or more of these objectives (Wanapat et al., 2008).

Chamomile is a widely available herb with diverse therapeutic uses that has been used for centuries as a medicinal plant. The components of the essential oil extracted from chamomile flowers possess anti-inflammatory, anti-allergic, anti-spasmodic, anti-bacterial, anti-pyretic, ulcer-protective, anti-fungal, sedative, analgesic and anti-oxidant properties (Andishe et al., 2015). Several flavonoids and other phenolic compounds have been identified in various parts of the chamomile flower head. Apigenin (16.8%), quercetin (9.9%), patuletin (6.5%), luteolin (1.9%) and their glucosides are the major flavonoids present in the total flower (McKay and Blumberg, 2006). *Matricaria chamomille* extraction 5 ml Kg- body weight that were orally given to experimental infected lambs with *Ostertagia ostertagi* parasite showed favorable results in terms of antihelminthic in lambs (Bahrami et al., 2010).

Cichorium intybus commonly known as chicory, is an erect fairly woody perennial herb, around 1 m in height with a fleshy taproot of up to 75 cm in length and large basal leaves. Chicory is cultivated for numerous applications and can be divided into four main varieties or cultigroups according to their use: (1) "industrial" or "root" chicory produces the taproot as a coffee substitute or for inulin extraction; (2) "Brussels" or "witloof "chicory as industrial chicory for etiolated buds (chicons) by forcing; (3) "leaf "chicory is used as fresh or cooked vegetables; and (4) "forage"chicory, to intensify herbage obtainability in perennial pastures for livestock. Chicory is a medicinally important plant in Eurasia and in parts of Africa. The flowers of chicory contain saccharides, methoxy-coumarin cichorine, flavonoids, essential oils, and anthocyanins contributing to the blue color of the perianth. Chicory possess anti-inflammatory, anti-helminthic, anti-spasmodic, anti-bacterial, anti-oxidant, anti-diabetic, hepatoprotective and gastro protective properties (Street et al., 2013). In several studies the effect of chicory has been investigated on performance, carcass characteristics and gastrointestinal nematodes of lambs (Somasiri et al., 2015; Miller et al., 2011) and herbage intake and milk production of cows (Muir et al., 2015).

To the best of our knowledge, there is no study about the effect of chamomile and chicory as feed additive on rumen microflora and hematologic parameters in sheep. Thus the purpose of this study was to evaluate supplementation of these herbs on rumen microbial population, some hematologic parameters and performance of sheep.

Materials and Methods

Experimental design, diets and animals management: Nine adult male Dallagh sheep with an average initial BW of 35±3 kg were used in a change over design. The experiment consisted of three 21-day periods (14 days as adaptation and 7 days as sampling) and there were 3 treatments, each consisting of 9 replicates. At the start of the experiment sheep were weighted and randomly assigned to 1 of 3 treatments: 1) control (without additive), 2) chamomile (contained 10% chamomile powder) and 3) chicory (contained %10 chicory powder). Chamomile and chicory were collected from mountains around Minoodasht city, Golestan province, in the north of Iran.

These plants were shade-dried and ground through a 1 mm screen.

The basal diet was composed of 30% roughage and 70% concentrate, and the ingredients and nutrient composition of the basal diet (DM basis) is given in Table 1. Diets were fed as total mixed rations (TMR) and formulated according to NRC (1996) recommendations. The experimental diets were offered twice (08:00 and 18:00 h) daily for ad libitum intake (10% refusals) with one-half of the daily feed allotment offered at each feeding. Amounts of feed offered and refused were recorded daily for each animal throughout the trial. Body weight were measured at the beginning and the end of each period. The sheep were housed in individual stalls on mattresses bedded with straw in pens (2m× 1.5m) equipped with a water bowl. The pens were located in a covered barn. Each animal had free access to water at all times.

Measurements, sample collection and analysis: Average daily weight gain was calculated throughout the trial. Feed conversion ratio was calculated as the ratio between feed intake and weight gain.

Ruminal fluid was collected from animals at the last day of each period before morning feeding, and 4 h and 8 h after morning feeding via the esophagus using a 60 ml gavage syringe and a lubricated rubber tube. The first 20 ml of ruminal fluid content was discarded to ensure they were not polluted with saliva and then squeezed through four layers of cheesecloth. Rumen pH was measured immediately with a portable pH meter (Metrohm 691, Switzerland).

A 5-ml portion of the strained ruminal fluid was mixed with 5 ml of 0.2 N HCL. All samples were stored at -20 oC for subsequent analyses. The ruminal fluid concentration of NH3-N was determined using spectrophotometry by the phenol hypochlorite method of Broderick and Knag (1980). Serial 10-fold dilutions of strained ruminal fluid were prepared and used as inoculum on plate count agar (PCA), Modified Rogosa and Sharp Agar (MRSA) and Violent Red Bile Agar (VRBA) medium for total viable bacteria, acid lactic bacteria and coliforms count respectively (Ghoorchi et al., 2009).

Blood samples were collected at non-heparinized tube from the jugular vein at the end of each period (3 h after the morning feeding), samples were centrifuged (Denley BS400, England) at 10,000 rpm for 10 min and collected serum was frozen at -20°C until analysis. Serum concentration of glucose, total protein and triglyceride were determined using the commercial kits of Darmanfaraz Company (Isfahan, Iran) by spectrophotometry.

A 1-ml portion of the strained ruminal fluid was preserved using 9 ml of MFS (methyl green- formaldehyde- saline) solution for enumeration of protozoa. Protozoa samples were stored at room temperature in the dark until counting. Protozoa were enumerated microscopically in a Neubauer cytometer at ×40 magnification. Each sample was counted twice and if the average of the duplicates differed by more than 10%, the counts were repeated (Cedrola et al., 2015).

Statistical analysis: All data were statistically analyzed according to a change over design using the general linear model (GLM) procedure of SPSS software (version 18). Significant differences between means of treatments were assessed by the LSD test, and the differences among treatments were declared significant at $p<0.05$. Initial weight of sheep were used as covariate for weight gain data analysis.

Table1. Ingredient and nutrient composition of experimental diets (DM basis). [1] Contained: 21 g/kg Mg, 0.3 g/kg Zn, 2.2 g/kg Mn, 3 g/kg Fe, 0.3 g/kg Cu, 0.001 g/kg Se, 0.1 g/kg Co, 0.12 g/kg I, 195 g/Kg Ca, 80 g/Kg P, 600 IU/g of vitamin A, 200 IU/g of vitamin D, and 2.5 IU/g of vitamin E. *Treatments include: Control: without additive; Chamomile: contained 10% *Matricaria chamomile* powder; Chicory: contained 10% *Cichorium intybus* powder.

	Treatments*		
	Control	Chamomile	Chicory
Ingredient (%)			
Barley grain, ground	35	35	35
Alfa alfa	25	15	15
Chamomile dry power	-	10	-
Chicory dry powder	-	-	10
Wheat straw	18.5	18.5	18.5
Wheat bran	19	19	19
salt	0.5	0.5	0.5
Mineral-vitamin premix[1]	1	1	1
Pearl powder	1	1	1
Composition			
CP (%)	12	12.15	12.1
ME (Mcal/kg)	2.3	2.25	2.22
NDF (%)	42	43	43
Ash (%)	6.8	6.7	6.7
Ca (%)	0.80	0.83	0.82
P (%)	0.45	0.48	0.49

Table 2. Effect of *Matricaria chamomille* and *Cichorium intybus* powder on performance of sheep. *Treatments include: Control: without additive; Chamomile: contained 10% *Matricaria chamomile* powder; Chicory: contained 10% *Cichorium intybus* powder. *Standard error of means.

	Treatments*			
Item	Control	Chamomile	Chicory	SEM*
Initial weight (kg)	35.42	35.92	36.13	1.65
Final weight(kg)	38.62	38.05	38.37	1.74
Final weight gain (Kg)	3.18	2.13	2.24	0.50
Daily weight gain (g)	151.85	101.58	106.87	23.94
Daily dry matter intake (g)	857.53	830.95	825.42	93.71
Feed conversion ratio	6.58	7.46	9.24	2.08

Results

Dry matter intake and performance data are presented in Table 2. Initial and final BW did not differ among the experimental treatments and consequently, daily weight gain was not affected by treatments. Similarly, feed conversion ratio, expressed as feed: gain ratio (DMI to average daily gain ratio), was similar among treatments.

Mean of blood metabolites is shown in Table 3. Concentrations of serum glucose and total protein were not affected by additive treatments. Triglyceride level in chamomile treatment compared to chicory increased significantly but the differences were not significant compared with control.

Table 4 represents the effect of experimental treatments on rumen fluid pH, NH3-N and protozoa. Rumen fluid pH was not affected by treatments at before morning feeding, 4 h and 8 h after morning feeding. There was no significant difference in ruminal NH3-N concentration among treat-

Table 3. Effect of *Matricaria chamomille* and *Cichorium intybus* powder on some blood parameters of sheep. *Treatments include: Control: without additive; Chamomile: contained 10% *Matricaria chamomile* powder; Chicory: contained 10% *Cichorium intybus* powder. a-bMeans within the same row without common letters differ significantly (p<0.05). *Standard error of means.

	Treatments*				
Item	Control	Chamomile	Chicory	SEM*	p-value
Total protein (mg/dl)	5.58	5.27	5.18	0.48	0.83
Glucose (mg/dl)	70.60	67.65	87.90	7.47	0.14
Triglycerides (mg/dl)	21.27^{ab}	28.38^{a}	15.49^{b}	2.82	0.01

Table 4. Effect of experimental treatments on pH, NH3-N and protozoa of rumen fluid. *Treatments include: Control: without additive; Chamomile: contained 10% *Matricaria chamomile* powder; Chicory: contained 10% *Cichorium intybus* powder. * a-bMeans within the same row without common letters differ significantly (p<0.05). *Standard error of means.

Item	Time	Treatment*			SEM*	p-value
		Control	Chamomile	Chicory		
pH	Before feeding	6.91	6.79	6.82	0.07	0. 50
	4 hours after feeding	6.53	6.57	6.53	0.06	0.89
	8 hours after feeding	6.57	6.54	6.56	0.07	0.95
NH3-N	Before feeding	2.67	2.52	2.61	0.27	0.92
(mg dl^{-1})	4 hours after feeding	2.49	4.19	1.99	1.24	0.43
	8 hours after feeding	2.25	2.20	2.01	0.17	0.60
Protozoa	Before feeding	4.96^{a}	7.65^{b}	7.65^{b}	0.90	0.04
(×10^{5} ml^{-1})	4 hours after feeding	6.91	8.98	8.51	1.16	0.29
	8 hours after feeding	6.53	9.40	9.03	1.13	0.48

Table 5. Effect of *Matricaria chamomille* and *Cichorium intybus* powder on rumen bacteria (Log$^{cfu/ml}$) of sheep. * Treatments include: Control: without additive; Chamomile: contained 10% *Matricaria chamomile* powder; Chicory: contained 10% *Cichorium intybus* powder * a-bMeans within the same row without common letters differ significantly (p<0.05). * Standard error of means.

Item	Time	Treatments*			SEM*	p-value
		Control	Chamomile	Chicory		
	Before feed	9.91	10.08	10.16	0.13	0.64
Total bacteria	4 hours after feed	9.95	9.86	9.99	0.14	0.82
	8 hours after feed	10.02	9.82	9.93	0.12	0.55
	Before feed	3.58	3.33	3.59	0.09	0.10
Coliform bacteria	4 hours after feed	4.08^{a}	3.55^{b}	3.93^{ac}	0.11	0.01
	8 hours after feed	3.74	3.91	4.04	0.15	0.40
	Before feed	5.46	5.46	5.62	0.61	0.71
Lactic acid bacteria	4 hours after feed	5.22	5.21	5.51	0.12	0.15
	8 hours after feed	5.41	5.27	5.29	0.15	0.79

ments. The rumen protozoan was significantly lower in control compared to chamomile and chicory treatment before morning feeding but the differences was not significant among three treatments at 4 and 8 h after the morning feeding.

Table 5 summarize data obtained on the effects of experimental diets on rumen microbial population. Total viable bacterial count and Acid lactic bacteria had no significant difference before feeding, 4h and 8 h after feeding. Coliforms count was influenced by treatments. Coliforms count was significantly lower in chamomile treatment compared with control and chicory treatment 4 h after morning feeding. But Before morning feeding and at 8 h after feeding there was no significant difference among treatments.

Discussion

Feed intake and performance: There is little information on the effects of chamomile and Chicory 10% on DMI and performance in sheep so we must compare the results of this study with other medicinal plants and species. Somasiri et al. (2015) found that both Plantain mix and Chicory mix lambs had greater live weight gains and were heavier at slaughter and displayed greater carcass weights and dressing-out percentages compared to the Pasture mix lambs. In a study lambs grazing chicory had increased performance and average daily gain and reduced gastrointestinal infection compared to those grazing Cynodon dactylon (Miller et al., 2011). Torabi Goudarzi et al., (2010) reported that mixture of chicory and anise significantly increased rate of appetite, frequency and strength of ruminal contractions in cattle. Payvastegan et al. (2015) showed that 10 and 20 g/d *Satureja hortensis* dry powder had no significant effect on dry matter intake, average daily gain, and feed conversion of kids. The findings of present study for DMI were in line with previous researches in growing lambs (Chaves et al., 2008a), sheep (Distel et al., 2007; Nolte and Provenza, 1992) and cattle (Benchaar et al., 2007; Beauchemin and Mcginn, 2006) who found no effect of essential oil (EO) on DMI. In contrast with our results, Demir et al. (2003) reported that pennyroyal EO increased nutrient absorption, growing and weight gain. Ghahari et al. (2016) showed that inclusion of *Mentha spicata* and *Mentha pulegium* calves diet significantly decreased dry matter intake. Our result confirmed the report which showed that *Leucaena leucocephalaon* and *Salix babylonica* had no effect on weight gain in growing lamb (Salem et al., 2011). The effects of EO on DMI might vary with EO source, type of diet, diet interaction or adaptation of rumen microbial population to EO (Yang et al., 2010a; b; Geraci et al., 2012). Furthermore, it has been reported that it can be affected by a number of dietary or management factors such as body weight, animal growth stage, and specific physical and chemical characteristics of diet or rumen fermentation metabolites (Allen, 1997; Yang et al., 2010b).

Blood metabolites: Payvastegan et al. (2015) showed that 10 and 20 g/d *Satureja hortensis* dry powder had no significant effect on glucose, total protein, triglyceride, cholesterol and HDL in kids. Our results are in agreement with some studies that declared peppermint and dill oil feeding at 0.05% DM had no effect on blood glucose in Kordi breed growing lamb (Tohidi, 2014) and peppermint EO feeding did not affect blood metabolites significantly (Hosoda et al., 2006). In our study serum triglyceride was increased by chamomile compared to chicory supplementation which was in contrast to some researches (Tohidi, 2014; Hosoda et al., 2006). Ghahari et al. (2016) showed that supplementation of 20 g/d *Mentha spicata* and *Mentha pulegium* dry powder had no significant effect on plasma glucose, triglyceride and total protein in calves. The result of total serum protein in this study was in agreement with Ahmadi Naghadehi et al. (2014) who reported that 100 and 200 mg peppermint EO did not significantly change total serum protein of sheep. It has been reported that concentration of some blood metabolites such as triglyceride can be influenced by EO supplementation via changing of feed intake (Yang et al., 2010b) and no change in blood metabolites in present study may have contributed to lack of DMI alteration by dry powder.

Rumen pH, NH3-N and protozoa: Rumen pH is a resultant of produced volatile fatty acids (acetate, propionate and lactate), ammonia, rumen buffers and saliva (Vansoet, 1994) and an index for fermentation. Payvastegan et al. (2015) found that 20 g/d dry powder and 200 mg/d essential oil of *Satureja hortensis* decreased rumen pH. 100 and 200 mg peppermint EO feeding did not affect rumen pH in sheep (Ahmadi Naghdahi et al., 2014). In agreement with our result peppermint feeding at 5% DM (Hodosa et al., 2006) and peppermint EO feeding at 0.025% DM (Tohidi, 2014) had no effect on rumen pH in steers and sheep respectively. In contrast with our study, peppermint feeding (200 g/day) decreased rumen pH and protozoa count in steers (Ando et al., 2003). Variable effects of EO on rumen pH can result from different diets and levels of EO in studies as when EO was added to diets with higher roughage/concentrate ratio, rumen pH increased (Meyer et al., 2009).

Similarly, supplementation with 0.2g/kg (DM basis) of carvacrol and cinnamaldehyde did not alter ruminal ammonia in growing lamb (Chaves et al., 2008b). In contrast, in a study it was reported that free thymol and sustained release thymol decreased plasma urea concentration and rumen ammonia at 5, 7 h after feeding (Zamani et al., 2015). Taherinia et al., (2015) showed that supplementation of garlic powder at 2% DM had no effect on blood urea nitrogen and rumen ammonia. Hosoda et al. (2006) found that peppermint feeding at 5% of the diet (DM basis) significantly increased rumen ammonia in Holstein steers. Also, this is in disagreement with the in vitro results of Newbold et al. (2004), who observed a decrease in ruminal ammonia when rumen contents of cows or sheep supplemented with EO and acid hydrolyzed protein were incubated for 24-48 h in strained ruminal fluid (1 or 110 mg/d, respectively).

Wanapat et al. (2013) reported that lemongrass supplementation at 100g/d alone or plus peppermint powder at 10 g/d with or without garlic powder 40g/d decreased rumen protozoa. Busquet et al. (2005) showed in vivo that 200 g peppermint powder decreased rumen protozoa. In a study it was reported that peppermint decreased rumen protozoa and ammonia nitrogen (Bach et al., 2005). Our result was in agreement with some researchers (Newbold et al., 2004; Benchaar et al., 2007) who reported that EO feeding had no effect on rumen protozoa in sheep. Similarly, Djouvino et al. (1997) reported that 450 g/d peppermint did not influence protozoa count in sheep.

Rumen bacteria: Rumen microbiome plays a key role in rumen feed fermentation, methane production and, nitrogen utilization. Its activity directly affects ruminant performance, health, and welfare, but it is still poorly understood. Rumen microbial populations are highly dynamic and are able to adapt to a wide range of nutritional strategies or host physiological status so it is often difficult to understand the interactions between dietary components and rumen microbial populations (Cobellis et al., 2016). Considering the large number of different groups of chemical compounds present in essential oils, it is most likely that their antibacterial activity is not attributable to one specific mechanism but that there are several targets in the cell (Brenes and Roura, 2010). In one study a mixed EO did not change rumen microbial population (Benchaar et al., 2007). Also, it was reported that EO inhibited rumen bacteria (Mcintosh et al., 2003). Factors such as EO type, diet property, species, and geographical situation affect variability and bacterial count including lactic acid bacteria of rumen (Dehority et al., 2003). In our study chamomile decreased coliforms which was in disagreement with a study that showed clove and garlic EO did not affected rumen coliforms (Ghoorchi et al., 2009).

Conclusions: The results of this study showed that although chamomile 10% decreased coliform bacteria 4 h after feeding but chamomile and chicory 10% had no effect on performance, blood metabolites, rumen pH, NH3-N and protozoa count. More in vivo studies are required to investigate the effects of different supplementations levels on rumen microbial fermentation and blood metabolites to improve nutrient utilization and growth performance in sheep.

Acknowledgments

This work was financially supported by University of Gonbad Kavous, Iran which is gratefully acknowledged.

References

Ahmadi Naghadehi, A.A., Pirmohammadi, R., Sahrae Belverdi, M., Parsaemehr, K. (2014) Effect of peppermint (*Mentha piperita*) on digestibility and rumen fermentation of Makuei sheep. Iranian J Anim Sci. 106: 65-70. (In Persian)

Allen, M.S. (1997) Relationship between fermentation acid production in the rumen and the requirement for physically effective fiber. J Dairy Sci. 80: 1447-1462.

Andishe, A., Pourshahidi, S., Ebrahimi, H., Hajipour, Z., Reza, M., Shirazian, S. (2015) The effect of *Matricaria chamomilla* (chamomile) extract in Orabase on minor aphthous stomatitis, a randomized clinical trial. J Herb Med. 5: 71-76.

Ando, S., Nishida, T., Ishida, M., Hosoda, K., Bayaru, E. (2003) Effect of peppermint feeding on the digestibility, ruminal fermentation and protozoa. Livest Prod Sci. 82: 245-248.

Bach, A., Calsamiglia, S., Stern, M.D. (2005) Nitrogen metabolism in rumen. J Dairy Sci. 88: 9-21.

Bahrami, A.M., Doosti, A., Moosavi, A.B. (2010) Effect of *Matricaria chamomile* L. plant extraction on experimental infected lamb with *Ostertagia ostertagi* parasites. Int J Pharmacol. 6: 712-718.

Beauchemin, K.A., McGinn, S.M. (2006) Methane emissions from beef cattle: Effects of fumaric acid, essential oil, and canola oil. J Anim Sci. 84: 1489-1496.

Benchaar, C., Calsamiglia, S., Chaves, A.V., Fraser, G.R., Colombatto, D., McAllister, T.A., Beauchemin, K.A. (2007) A review of plant-derived essential oils in ruminant nutrition and production. Anim Feed Sci Technol. 145: 209-228.

Brenes, A., Roura, E. (2010) Essential oils in poultry nutrition: main effects and mod of actions. Anim Feed Sci Technol. 158: 1-14.

Broderick, G.A. and Kang, G.H. (1980) Automated simultaneous determination of ammonia and total amino acids in ruminal fluid and in vitro media. J Dairy Sci. 63: 64-75.

Busquet, M.S., Calsamiglia, A., Kamel, C. (2005) Screening for the effects of natural plant extracts and secondary plant metabolites on rumen microbial fermentation in continuous culture. Anim Feed Sci Technol. 123: 597-613.

Cedrola, F., Rossi, F., Dias, R.J.P., Martinele, M. Agosto, M. (2015) Methods for taxonomic study of rumen ciliates (Aleolata: Ciliofora): a brief review. Zool Sci. 32: 8-15.

Chaves, A.V., Stanford, K., Dugan, M.E.R., Gibson, L.L., McAllister, T.A., Van Herk, F., Benchaar, C. (2008a) Effects of cinnamaldehyde, garlic and juniper berry essential oils on rumen fermentation, blood metabolites, growth performance, and carcass characteristics of growing lambs. Livest Sci. 117: 215-224.

Chaves, A.V., Stanford, K., Gibson, A.A., Mcallister T.A., Benchaar, C. (2008b) Effects of caracole and cinnamldehyde on intake, rumen fermentation, growth performance, and carcass characteristic of growing lambs. Anim Feed Sci Technol. 145: 396-408.

Cobellis, G., Trabalza-Marinucci, M., Yu, Z. (2016) Science of the total environment critical evaluation of essential oils as rumen modifiers in ruminant nutrition: A review. Sci Total Environ. 545-546: 556-568.

Dehority, B.A. (2003) Rumen Microbiology. (1st ed.) Nottingham University Press. Nottingham, UK.

Demir, E., Sarica, S., Ozcan, M.A., Suimez, M. (2003) The use of natural feed additives as alternative for an antibiotic growth promoter in broiler diets. Br Poult Sci. 44: 44-45.

Distel, R.A., Iglesias, R.M.R., Arroquy, J., Merino, J. (2007) A note on increased intake in lambs through diversity in food flavor. Appl Anim Behav Sci. 130: 232-237.

Djouvinov, D., Palvov, D., Ilchev, A., Envev E. (1997) Peppermint (*Mentha piperita* Huds.) and basil (*Ocimum basilicum* L.) etheric oil by-products as roughage for sheep feeding. Anim Feed Sci Technol. 68: 287-294.

Geraci G.I., Garciarene A.C., Gagliostro, G.A., Beauchemin K.A., Colombato D. (2012) Plant extract containing cinnamaldehyde, eugenol and capsicum oleoresin added to feedlot cattle diet: ruminal environment, short term intake pattern and animal performance. Anim Feed Sci Technol. 176: 123-130.

Ghahari, N., Ghoorchi, T., Vakili, S.A. (2016) Effect of adding herbs (*Ziziphora clinopodioides, Menta spicata* and *Menthe pulegium*) in milk on performance, blood metabolites and fecal microbial population of Holestein calves. Iran J Anim Sci Res. 8: 57- 71. (In Persian)

Ghalamkari, G.R., Toghyani, M., Landy, N., Tavalaeian, E. (2012) Investigation the effects using different levels of *Mentha pulegium* L. (pennyroyal) in comparison with an antibiotic growth promoter on performance, carcass traits and immune responses in broiler chickens. Asian Pac J Trop Biomed. 2: S1396-S1399.

Ghoorchi, T., Ghanbari, F., Khamiri M., Ebrahimi, T. (2009) Survey on effects of clove and garlic essential oils on degradability of dry matter and rumen microbial population in sheep. Gorgan University of Agricultural Sciences and Natural Resources. Research report. 62 p. (In Persian)

Hosoda, K., Kuramoto, K., Eruden, B., Nishida, T., Shona, S. (2006) The effects of three herbs as feed supplements on blood metabolites, hormones, antioxidant activity, IgG concentration and ruminal fermentation in Holstein steers. J Anim Sci. 19: 35-41.

Mcintosh, F.M., Williams, P., Losa, R., Wallace, R.J., Beever, D.A., Newbold, C.J. (2003) Effect of essential oils on ruminal microorganisms and their protein metabolism. J Appl Environ Microbiol. 69: 5011-5014.

Mckay, D.L., Blumberg, J.B. (2006) A review of the bioactivity and potential health benefits of chamomile tea (*Matricaria recutita* L.). Phytother Res. 20: 519-530.

Meyer, N.F., Erickson, G.E., Klopfenstein, T.J., Greenquist, M.A., Luebbe, M.K., Williams, P., Engstrom, M.A. (2009) Effect of essential oils, tylosin, and monensin on finishing steer performance, carcass characteristics, liver abscesses, ruminal fermentation, and digestibility. J Anim Sci. 87: 2346-2354.

Miller, M.C., Duckett, S.K., Andrae, J.G. (2011) The effect of forage species on performance and gastrointestinal nematode infection in lambs. Small Rumin Res. 95: 188-192.

Muir, S.K., Ward, G.N., Jacobs, J.L. (2015) Herbage intake and milk production of late-lactation dairy cows offered a second-year chicory crop during summer. J Dairy Sci. 98: 1-11.

Newbold, C.J., McIntosh, F.M., Williams, P., Losa, R., Wallace, R.J. (2004) Effects of a specific blend of essential oil compounds on rumen fermentation. Anim Feed Sci Technol. 114: 105-112.

Nolte, D.L., Provenza, F.D. (1992) Food preferences in lambs after exposure to flavors in solid foods. Appl Anim Behav Sci. 32: 337-347.

Patra, A.K., Kamra, D.N., Agarwal, N. (2006) Effect of plant extracts on in vitro methanogenesis, enzyme activities and fermentation of feed in rumen liquor of buffalo. Anim Feed Sci Technol. 128: 276-291.

Payvastegan, S., Farhoomand, P., Talatapesh, A., Sahraei, M. (2015) The effects of different levels of summer savory (*Satureja hortensis* L.) dry powder and essential oil on performance, ruminal fermentation and blood metabolites of west Azerbayjan native kids. Anim Sci J. (Pajouhcsh & sazandegi) 105: 53-66. (In Persian)

Rafii, F., Shahverdi, A. (2007) Comparison of essential oils from three plants for enhancement of antimicrobial activity of nitrofurantoin against enterobacteria. Chemotherapy. 53: 21-25.

Salem, A., Olivares, M., Lopez, S., Gonzalez-Ronquillo, M., Rojo, R., Camacho, L., Cerrillo, S., Mejia, H. (2011) Effect of natural extracts of *Salix babylonica* and *Leucaena leucocephalaon* on nutrient digestibility and growth performance of lambs. Anim Feed Sci Technol. 170: 27-34.

Somasiri, S.C., Kenyon, P.R., Kemp, P.D., Morel, P.C.H., Morris, S.T. (2015) Growth performance and carcass characteristics of lambs grazing forage mixes inclusive of plantain (*Plantago lanceolata* L.) and chicory (*Cichorium intybus* L.). Small Ruminant Res. 127: 20-27.

Street, R.A., Sidana, J., Prinsloo, G. (2013) *Cichorium intybus*: Traditional Uses, Phytochemistry, Pharmacology, and Toxicology. Evid based complement alternat Med. 2013: 1-13.

Taherinia, M.H., Chaji, M., Mohamad Aabadi, T., Islami, M., Sari, M. (2015) Effect of garlic powder supplementation on digestibility, rumen fermentation and protozoa population. Iranian J Anim Res Sci. 6: 324-332 (In Persian).

Tohidi A. (2015) Effect of addition of *Mentha spicata* and *Anethum graveolens* (dill) essence on ruminal fermentation parameters, blood metabolites and performance of growing Kordi lambs. M.Sc. thesis of Gonbad Kavous University, Iran.

Torabi Goudarzi, M., Bahonar, A.R., Raoofi, A., Akbari, H., Haghi, G.H. (2010) Clinical evaluation of chicory (*Cichorium intybus* L.) and anise (*Pimpinella anisum* L.) on cattle appetite and comparison with common product. Iranian J Med Aro Plant. 26: 275-282. (In Persian).

VanSoest, P.J. (1994) Nutritional Ecology of the Ruminant. Cornel University Press. Ithaca,

New York, USA.

Wanapat, M., Kang, S., Khejornsart, P., Wanapat, S. (2013) Effects of plant herb combination supplementation on rumen fermentation and nutrient digestibility in beef cattle. Asian Austrlas J Anim Sci. 26: 1127-1136.

Wanapat, M., Cherdthong, A., Pakdee, P., Wanapat, S. (2008) Manipulation of rumen ecology by dietary lemongrass (*Cymbopogon citratus* Stapf.) powder supplementation. J Anim Sci. 86: 3497-3503.

Yang, W.Z., Ametaj, B.N., He, M.L., Benchaar, C., Beauchemin, K.A. (2010a) Cinnamaldehyde in feedlot cattle diet: intake, growth performance, carcass characteristics, and blood metabolites. J Anim Sci. 88: 1082-1092.

Yang, W.Z., Benchaar, C., Ametaj, B.N., Beauchemin, K.A. (2010b) Dose response to eugenol supplementation in growing beef cattle ruminal fermentation intestinal digestion. Anim Feed Sci Technol. 158: 57-64.

Zamani, Z., Alipour, D., Moghimi, H.R., Mortazavi, S.A., Zolhavarieh, S.M. (2015) Effect of free thymol and sustained release thymol on rumen fermentation and plasma metabolites in sheep. Anim Prod Res. 3: 75-88. (In Persian).

Alterations of the electrocardiographic parameters in relation to circulating electrolytes and cardiac enzymes during different productive states of high producing Holstein dairy cows

Chalmeh, A.*, Hajimohammadi, A., Asadollahpour, S., Mazrouei Sebdani, M.

Department of Clinical Sciences, School of Veterinary Medicine, Shiraz University, Shiraz, Iran

Key words:
cardiac enzymes, dairy cows, electrolytes, electrocardiography, physiological periods

Correspondence
Chalmeh, A.
Department of Clinical Sciences, School of Veterinary Medicine, Shiraz University, Shiraz, Iran

Email: achalmeh81@gmail.com

Abstract:

BACKGROUND: Dairy cows undergo physiological changes during pregnancy and lactation and cardiovascular system may alter during these periods. **OBJECTIVES:** Understanding the physiological effects of production periods of dairy cows on heart electrical activities can aid in better monitoring the cardiovascular system in these animals. **METHODS:** Five multiparous Holstein dairy cows were studied from early lactation to close-up dry periods. Electrocardiogram recordings and blood samplings were performed from each cow at their different productive states. Sera were separated and the concentrations of sodium, potassium, chloride, calcium, magnesium, phosphorus, aspartate aminotransferase, alanine transaminase and lactate dehydrogenase were evaluated in all specimens. **RESULTS:** There were no significant changing patterns in P, Q, S and T amplitude from early lactation to close-up dry periods ($p>0.05$); however, the R amplitude was significantly increased from early to late lactation and then decreased to close-up dry period, subsequently ($p<0.05$). P wave had the longest and Q wave had the shortest durations during different productive states. There were no significant changing patterns in PR, QT and ST intervals from early lactation to close-up dry periods ($p>0.05$) but RR interval in dry periods was significantly longer than lactating ones. Serum concentrations of calcium, phosphorus, sodium, chloride, potassium, aspartate aminotransferase, alanine transaminase and lactate dehydrogenase were decreased significantly from lactating cows to non-lactating ones ($p<0.05$). **CONCLUSIONS:** The heart electrical activities of dairy cows at each production period were different from another one. The differences among serum electrolyte levels may affect the electrocardiographic findings at each production period which may alter the production and conduction of cardiac electrical impulses. Furthermore, the cardiac activities in different production periods could have a significant impact on the levels of circulating cardiac enzymes.

Introduction

Dairy cows undergo physiological changes during pregnancy and lactation (Tanritanir et al., 2009). Each state has characteristics which are different from those of others.

Two to three weeks before parturition, a phase of catabolism starts to prepare the cow for parturition and the initiation of lactation. Immediately after the calving, they commence lactogenesis at the high levels which is associated with decreasing the body condition score (BCS), subsequently (Wathes et al., 2009). The last period of the production year is a phase of anabolism where the emphasis is put on increased weight gain as a long term preparation for the next lactation. Pregnancy and fetal growth at this period can also influence the physiological pathways of dairy cows (Piccione et al., 2012). Information regarding the physiological alterations in each productive period can lead to better manage the high producing dairy cows (Duffield, 2000).

Cardiovascular system has a key role in reproductive performance, pregnancy and lactogenesis. We hypothesized that this system may alter during physiological alteration of dairy cows from early lactation to close-up dry periods. Hence, we used the electrocardiography to evaluate the cardiac electrical activities of dairy cows at different productive states. The electrocardiogram (ECG) is a noninvasive and inexpensive diagnostic technique which measures and evaluates the heart electrical activities. Some of the cardiac problems can be detected by clinical evaluation such as auscultation but the executive details of cardiac electrical performance should be detected by using ECG (Radostits et al., 2007; Jafari Dehkordi et al., 2014a,b). The majority of conduction disturbances can be detected on clinical examination (Radostits et al., 2007) but several researchers recorded the cardiac abnormalities of the large animals which have not been detected by clinical investigations (Pourjafar et al., 2012; Chalmeh et al., 2014; Chalmeh, 2015; Trenk et al., 2015). Alterations of the heart electrical activities in large animals include physiological and pathological abnormalities (Radostits et al., 2007; Yoshida et al., 2015) in which physiological variations in normal animals may be detected electrocardiographically due to autonomic influence, primary myocardial disease and acid-base and electrolyte imbalances (Radostits et al., 2007); therefore, we also assessed the serum electrolytes and cardiac enzymes following the alterations of physiological states of dairy cows to better understand the heart electrical activities. Based on the author's knowledge, there are several studies on bovine ECGs alone without the interrelationships with electrolyte and cardiac enzymes (Deroth, 1980; Pourjafar et al., 2012; Chalmeh et al., 2014; Chalmeh, 2015). However, information regarding the electrocardiographic alterations during the different physiological periods of the same dairy cows is lacking. Therefore, the current research was designed to present the alterations of the electrocardiographic parameters in relation to circulating electrolytes and cardiac enzymes during different production states of high producing Holstein dairy cows.

Materials and Methods

Animals: The present experimental study was carried out in 2015 on 5 multiparous Holstein dairy cows from a high producing industrial dairy farm around Shiraz, in the southwest of Iran. The animals had 3 and/ or 4 times parturition. Cows were housed in open-shed barns with free access to water and shade. The total mixed rations were formulated and prepared for all animals at different productive states according to

National Research Council (NRC) requirements (Table 1). In this farm, a dry period of 60 days has been considered. Milk production was about 10,000 kg per year per head, an average of 3.6 of milk fat %, and 3.3 of milk protein %. All the animals were clinically healthy, had no history of debilitating disease and clinical signs of heart diseases (edema, jugular distension or pulsation and cardiac murmurs), coughing, exercise intolerance, and were free from internal and external parasites due to routine antiparasitic programs at this farm. BCS was estimated based on 0-5 system. We selected these 5 cows at their far-off dry period (281.9 ± 5.4 days after calving, 228.4 ± 8.6 days of pregnancy, with 3.5 ± 0.25 BCS) and studied them from this period to close-up dry periods (312.1 ± 8.3 days after calving, 255.6 ± 6.3 days of pregnancy, with 3.5 ± 0.25 BCS), early (30.2 ± 5.7 days after calving, with 3.25 ± 0.25 BCS), mid (108.1 ± 8.4 days after calving, with 3.25 ± 0.25 BCS) and late lactations (184.5 ± 5.7 days after calving, with 3.5 ± 0.25 BCS).

Electrocardiographic studies: The ECGs were recorded at 07:00 AM, 3 h after morning meal, on a bipolar base apex lead, using limb lead I (Fig. 1). Animals were kept standing without any sedation and minimum restraint. When animals became calm (decrease in panting behavior and muscle tremors), the ECGs were recorded, using alligator-type electrodes which were attached to skin after cleaning it with ethanol and applying electrocardiographic jelly to improve skin contact. The positive electrode (left arm) was placed over cardiac apex on the 5th left intercostal space at the level of the elbow, the negative electrode (right arm) was placed on the left jugular furrow at the top of heart base, and the neutral electrode was placed on the dorsal spine or another site away from the heart (Radostits et al., 2007). All ECGs were obtained in a single channel electrocardiographic machine (Kenz-line EKG 110, Suzuken Co., Ltd., Japan) with paper speed of 25 mm/sec and calibration of 10 mm/1 mV. The precision of duration was 0.02 s, the amplitude 0.05 mV.

Blood sampling and biochemical assays: Blood sampling was performed after ECG was recorded from each animal via middle coccygeal vein. Immediately after blood collections, sera were separated by centrifugation for 10 min at 3000g and stored at -22 °C until assayed. Serum chloride and phosphorus were analyzed using routine biochemical procedures (Burtis and Ashwood, 1994). The serum concentrations of sodium and potassium were measured by the flame photometry (Flame Photometer, FLM, Ontario, Canada). The samples were also analyzed for magnesium and calcium by atomic absorption spectroscopy (Shimadzo AA-670, Japan). Values of serum aspartate aminotransferase (AST), alanine transaminase (ALT) and lactate dehydrogenase (LDH) were measured with Integra 800 auto-analyzer (Roche-Cobes, Switzerland).

Statistical analyses: Data were expressed as mean ± standard deviation (SD). Statistical analyses were performed using one-way ANOVA with LSD post-hoc test to compare mean concentrations of different electrocardiographic parameters and serological factors among different groups. Repeated measures ANOVA was also used to study the changes in pattern of different electrocardiographic parameters and serum electrolytes and enzymes during the productive states of the cows, using SPSS

Table 1. The basic nutrient content of rations in different physiological states of studied high producing Holstein dairy cows. DMI: dry matter intake; NEL: net energy lactation; CP: crude protein; RDP: rumen degradable protein; RUP: rumen undegraded protein; MP: metabolizable protein; ME: metabolizable energy; NDF: neutral detergent fiber; ADF: acid detergent fiber; NFC: non-fiber carbohydrate. Trace mineral added to ration (expressed as ppm): cobalt: 0.11; copper 10-18; iodine: 0.3-0.4; iron: 13-130; manganese: 14-24; selenium: 0.30 and zinc: 22-70.

Nutrient	Early lactation	Mid lactation	Late lactation	Far-off dry	Close-up dry
DMI (kg/day)	30	24	20	14	10
NEL (Mcal/kg)	1.61	1.47	1.36	1.32	1.43
Fat (%)	7	6	4	3	4
CP (%)	16.7	15.2	14.1	9.9	12.4
RDP (%)	9.8	9.7	9.5	7.7	9.6
RUP (%)	6.9	5.5	4.6	2.2	2.8
MP (%)	11.6	10.2	9.2	6.0	8.0
NDF (%)	28	30	32	40	35
ADF (%)	19	21	24	30	25
NFC (%)	38	35	32	30	34
Calcium (%)	0.60	0.61	0.62	0.44	0.48
Phosphorous (%)	0.38	0.35	0.32	0.22	0.26
Magnesium (%)	0.21	0.19	0.18	0.11	0.40
Chlorine (%)	0.29	0.26	0.24	0.13	0.20
Sodium (%)	0.22	0.23	0.22	0.10	0.14
Potassium (%)	1.07	1.04	1.00	0.51	0.62
Sulfur (%)	0.20	0.20	0.20	0.20	0.20
Vitamin A (IU/day)	75,000	75,000	75,000	80,300	83,270
Vitamin D (IU/day)	21,000	21,000	21,000	21,900	22,700
Vitamin E (IU/day)	545	545	545	1,168	1,200

software (SPSS for Windows, version 11.5, SPSS Inc, Chicago, Illinois). The level of significance was set at $p<0.05$.

Results

Electrocardiographic parameters and circulating electrolytes and cardiac enzymes (mean±SD) of high producing Holstein dairy cows at their different productive states are presented in Table 2. Furthermore, the changing patterns of the electrocardiographic parameters and serum electrolytes and cardiac enzymes during different productive states of studied high producing Holstein dairy cows are drawn in Fig. 2 and 3.

Based on the findings, there were no significant changing patterns in P, Q, S and T amplitude from early lactation to close-up dry periods ($p>0.05$; Fig. 2); However, the R amplitude was significantly increased from early to late lactation and then decreased to close-up dry period, subsequently ($p<0.05$). R wave had the highest and S wave had the lowest amplitude at all studied productive states (Fig. 2). There were no significant changing patterns about electrocardiographic durations from early lactation to close-up dry periods ($p>0.05$; Fig. 2). P wave had the longest and Q wave had the shortest durations during different productive states. There were no significant changing patterns in PR, QT and ST intervals from early lactation to close-up dry periods ($p>0.05$; Fig. 2) but RR interval in dry periods was significantly longer than lactating ones. Serum concentrations of calcium and

Table 2. Electrocardiographic parameters and circulating electrolytes and cardiac enzymes (mean ± SD) of high producing Holstein dairy cows (n=5) at their different productive states. [a,b,c] Different letters indicate significant difference among groups at similar parameter (p<0.05).

Parameters	Early lactation	Mid lactation	Late lactation	Far-off dry	Close-up dry
P-amplitude (mV)	0.18±0.02	0.17±0.04	0.16±0.04	0.13±0.03	0.15±0.03
Q-amplitude (mV)	0.16±0.12	0.15±0.09	0.10±0.05	0.12±0.07	0.12±0.09
R-amplitude (mV)	0.87±0.16[a]	0.99±0.27[a]	1.07±0.13[a]	0.74±0.18[b]	0.70±0.10[b]
S-amplitude (mV)	0.02±0.03	0.05±0.04	0.00±0.01	0.02±0.02	0.03±0.04
T-amplitude (mV)	0.40±0.08[a]	0.40±0.17[a]	0.44±0.13[a]	0.28±0.09[b]	0.25±0.05[b]
P-duration (Sec)	0.09±0.01	0.10±0.01	0.10±0.01	0.10±0.01	0.09±0.01
Q-duration (Sec)	0.02±0.01	0.02±0.01	0.02±0.01	0.02±0.01	0.02±0.01
R-duration (Sec)	0.06±0.01	0.06±0.01	0.06±0.01	0.05±0.01	0.05±0.01
S-duration (Sec)	0.02±0.01	0.03±0.02	0.03±0.01	0.03±0.02	0.03±0.02
T-duration (Sec)	0.07±0.01	0.07±0.01	0.07±0.01	0.07±0.02	0.06±0.01
PR-interval (Sec)	0.24±0.02	0.22±0.01	0.20±0.02	0.22±0.01	0.22±0.01
RR-interval (Sec)	0.78±0.02[a]	0.72±0.06[a]	0.69±0.06[a]	1.16±0.16[b]	0.93±0.18[b]
QT-interval (Sec)	0.40±0.01	0.37±0.03	0.36±0.04	0.45±0.03	0.41±0.05
ST-interval (Sec)	0.31±0.03	0.25±0.03	0.29±0.04	0.33±0.05	0.30±0.03
Calcium (mg/dL)	9.60±0.65[a]	9.48±0.21[a]	9.25±0.48[a]	9.84±0.38[b]	4.72±1.47[b]
Magnesium (mg/dL)	2.64±0.25[a]	2.42±0.16[a]	2.34±0.22[a]	2.30±0.18[b]	1.20±0.48[b]
Phosphorous (mg/dL)	7.17±1.03[a]	5.87±0.37[a]	7.04±0.89[a]	5.37±1.13[a]	3.52±1.30[b]
Sodium (mmol/L)	143.85±7.69[a]	142.71±7.95[a]	149.28±9.92[a]	141.28±0.95[a]	58.42±30.28[b]
Chloride (mmol/L)	105.57±3.20[a]	103.14±1.77[a]	102.00±1.63[a]	106.57±1.39[a]	55.92±18.14[b]
Potassium (mmol/L)	4.70±0.25[a]	4.60±0.21[a]	4.74±0.88[a]	4.70±0.24[a]	2.12±1.09[b]
AST (U/L)	75.71±14.20[a]	73.57±9.34[a]	77.42±10.96[a]	64.00±17.45[b]	28.28±10.98[c]
ALT (U/L)	24.42±5.12[a]	29.28±3.49[a]	31.28±8.82[a]	18.71±4.02[b]	10.85±6.01[c]
LDH (U/L)	1751.42±121.85[a]	1800.00±178.79[a]	1894.28±273.12[a]	1460.00±215.48[b]	530.85±231.60[c]

phosphorus were decreased significantly from lactating cows to non-lactating ones (p<0.05; Fig. 3). The levels of these electrolytes in dry cows were significantly lower than lactating groups and their concentrations were detected at the lowest levels in close-up dry period, significantly (p<0.05; Table 2). The significant decreasing patterns of sodium, chloride and potassium were detected from early lactation to close-up dry period and their concentrations in close-up dry group were significantly lower than other groups (p<0.05; Fig. 3; Table 2). The circulating levels of AST, ALT and LDH in close-up dry period were significantly lower than other periods and there were significant decreasing patterns of them from early lactation to close-up dry cows (p<0.05; Fig. 3; Table 2).

Discussion

There were differences among electrocardiographic amplitudes, durations and intervals at several productive states of high producing Holstein dairy cows. The higher amplitudes can draw the following powerful cardiac contractions and thin thorax (Deroth, 1980). In this study, lactating cows had lower BCS in comparison with dry ones; furthermore, the demands of the mammary glands for more blood supply for lactogenesis may increase the cardiac contractility in lactating periods, hence, the amplitudes in early, mid and late lactations were significantly recorded higher than far-

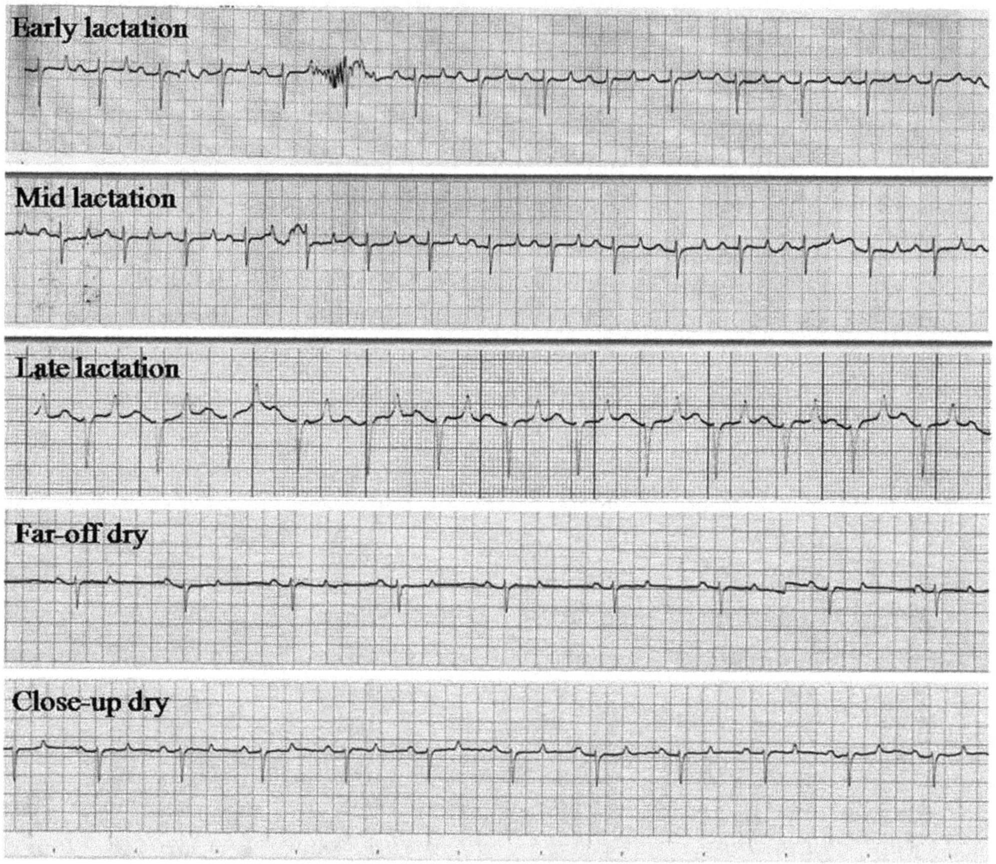

Figure 1. Normal electrocardiograms tracing from an adult multiparous high producing Holstein dairy cow at her different productive states from early lactation to close-up dry periods (base apex lead, paper speed 25 mm/sec, sensitivity 10 mm/mV).

off and close-up dry periods. Increasing the BCS and fattening the cows can act as the insulation and electrical impulses recorded with lower amplitudes (Too et al., 1966). The cardiac contractile activities in lactating cows are higher than non-lactating ones and these powerful contractions may cause the higher recorded amplitudes. P wave had the longest duration at all productive states. This wave was recorded along with the atrial depolarization and before atrial contraction commencement (Radostits et al., 2007).

Transferring the electrical impulses from sinoatrial to atriaoventricular node delay is due to the large atrium of dairy cattle, which records the long P wave in comparison with other waves (Rezakhani et al., 2004). P wave duration in mid lactating cows was longer than other groups, non-significantly. It may be suggested that this finding may be due to physiological alterations of cardiac musculature in order to compensate the lactating demands of dairy cows at mid lactation period. There were no significant changing patterns in PR, QT and ST intervals from early lactation to close-up dry periods; however, RR interval in lactating cows was significantly lower than non-lactating ones. RR interval reveals the distance between two heart rates and increasing this interval shows the low heart rate (Radostits et al., 2007). Transitioning the cows from lactating to non-lactating periods can cause the lower mammary gland demands to blood

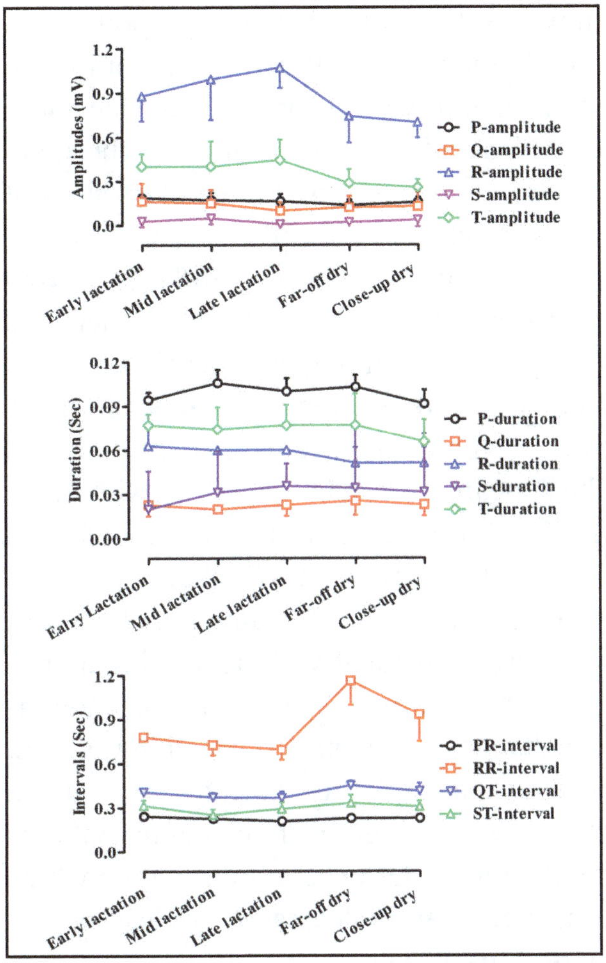

Figure 2. Changing pattern of electrocardiographic amplitudes, durations and intervals (mean ± SD) from early lactation to close-up dry periods of 5 adult multiparous high producing Holstein dairy cows.

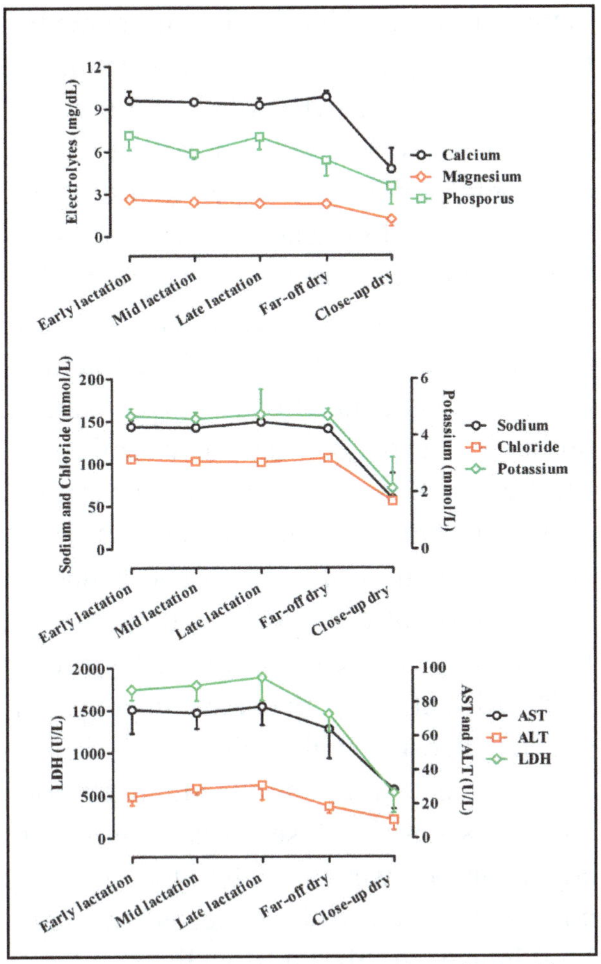

Figure 3. Changing pattern of serum electrolytes and cardiac enzymes (mean ± SD) from early lactation to close-up dry periods of 5 adult multiparous high producing Holstein dairy cows.

in order for lactogenesis; hence, the heart rate reduces in dry periods. RR interval was decreased at the close-up dry cows which may be due to the needs of gravid uterus and lactogenesis commencement. Decreasing the RR interval is equal to increasing the heart rate. Cardiac output follows from the heart rate and increasing the heart rate can cause the high cardiac output (Radostits et al., 2007).

Resolving the fetal growth and lactogenesis demands in close-up dry cows could be done due to increasing the cardiac output which followed from higher heart rate and lower RR interval in this group in comparison with far-off dry cows. Serum concentrations of calcium and phosphorus in non-lactating groups were lower than lactating cows and their levels at close-up dry period were significantly lower than others. Comparing the low calcium and phosphorus amount in the ration of non-lactating cows (Table 1), and the presence of sub-clinical hypocalcemia in these animals (Radostits et al., 2007), may explain the lower circulating levels of calcium and phosphorus in dry period.

Failure to secrete sufficient levels of parathyroid hormone was the primary defect in cows with hypocalcemia. While it is accepted that the calcium homeostatic mechanisms regulated by parathyroid hormone fail to maintain normal blood calcium concentrations resulting in severe hypocalcemia, the nature of this endocrine defect is not well understood. It was also once thought that calcitonin, a hormone which inhibits bone calcium resorption was a cause of milk fever but this has not been demonstrated in cows with clinical hypocalcemia. Systemic acidification induced by anionic supplementation affects the function of the parathyroid hormone. The major effect of systemic acidification is to cause an increased response to parathyroid hormone which results in increased retention of calcium and enhanced mobilization of calcium from bone. A total DCAD in the range of -100 to -200 mEq/kg feed DM is effective in controlling hypocalcemia (Radostits et al., 2007).

Serum concentrations of sodium, chloride and potassium in close-up dry cows were significantly lower than other groups. Dairy cows receive electrolytes needs from their food intake. In this study, sodium, chloride and potassium amounts in the balanced ration of dry cows were lower than lactating ones. Furthermore, based on the large size of gravid uterus, the capacity of gasterointestinal tract to food intake is reduced, which causes the reduction of received electrolytes to the cow at close-up dry period. Due to the distribution of the main intra and extracellular electrolytes such as sodium, potassium and chloride, the interior of the cardiac cells is more negative than the exterior. In myocardial cells, the interior is maintained more negative than the exterior by the extrusion of 3 sodium ions for every 2 potassium ions pumped in by the sodium/potassium ATPase pump. Movement of electrolytes across the impermeable cell membrane is through a number of channels (sodium and potassium channels, e.g.) that permit or prevent the movement of ions depending upon transmembrane voltage. Whereas calcium is the main electrolyte responsible for pacemaker cell depolarization, sodium is the main electrolyte responsible for depolarization of myocardial cells and cells dedicated to conduction of impulses (Fisch, 1984). The lower potassium concentrations were detected at dry periods. In humans, hypokalaemia is known to produce typical changes in the T wave, in particular decreased amplitude and the appearance of a U wave (Surawicz et al., 1957). Similar changes have been observed in hypokalaemic dogs (Felkai, 1985). In Hanton et al.'s (2007) study, hypokalaemia was also associated with decreasing amplitude of the T wave and with morphological changes in tracings recorded in CV5RL. The results of the present study showed that there were no significant changing patterns in all amplitudes except R amplitude which was significantly decreased at close-up dry period ($p<0.05$).

Potassium plays a key role in electrophysiological phenomena and, in particular, in the repolarization of the ventricular cells (Gadsby et al., 1995). Hypokalaemia increases the duration of cardiac action potential and, consequently, prolongs QT interval. The inhibition of cardiac repolarization associated with a decrease in extracellular potassium is assumed to be related to faster inactivation of potassium channels responsible for delayed potassium outflow and consequent inhibition of repolarization currents (Yang et al., 1997). The PR interval can be prolonged along with an increase in the amplitude of the P wave (Drighil et al., 2007). In the present research, the RR interval was increased significantly at dry periods when potassium levels in these periods were significantly lower than lactating ones

($p<0.05$). Akita et al. (1998) demonstrated that the ECG changes that are induced by hypokalemia in the rat, including suppression of conduction in most parts of the heart, prolong the QT interval, and decrease the amplitude of all waves except P waves. A prolonged QT interval is also a typical ECG manifestation of hypokalemia. A low extracellular potassium concentration produced a prolonged action potential and increased the time of diastolic depolarization (Gettes and Surawicz, 1968). In humans, the cardiac effect of hypokalaemia is well documented. Decreases in potassium plasma levels might occur in different pathological states and may be produced by a number of drugs (Cohen et al., 2002). Hypokalaemia could have a major effect on cardiac repolarization and ECG durations (Yelamanchi et al., 2001). Hyponatraemia would have a QT prolongation effect similar to that of hypokalaemia (Yelamanchi et al., 2001). However, sodium produces electrophysiogical abnormalities only at a concentration well outside the physiological range (Surawicz, 1980). Theoretically, reduction of the extra cellular concentration of sodium should slow cardiac pacemaker activity. In animal models, wide QRS complexes, either through hyperkalemia or quinidine administration have been documented (Surawicz, 1980). Hyponatremia plays as a role in the pathogenesis of the cardiac conduction defect. In the present study, sodium concentrations were decreased from lactating to non-lactating periods, significantly, which may be responsible for some electrocardiographic alterations at these periods.

Based on several researches, the solubility and absorption of Mg in acid solutions is higher than other ones. For instance, Ben-Ghedalia et al. (1975) observed that the solubility of Mg within the small intestine is maximal between the pylorus and 7 meters after the pylorus within the pH range from 2.6 to 7.02 and decreased according to the rise in pH. This also appears to be the case with caecal digesta and rumen contents in which a decrease in pH has been associated with an increase in Mg solubility, reflecting the greater solubility of Mg in acid solutions (Grace et al., 1977; Hom and Smith, 1978; Dalley et al., 1997). Acidification of the rumen contents occurs with fermentation and degradation of organic matter and this effect could enhance Mg solubility and therefore availability for absorption (Ben-Ghedalia et al., 1975; Hom and Smith, 1978). The major change in solubility observed in vitro occurs around pH 5.5-6.0 and pH 6.5-7.0 for ruminal and caecal samples, respectively (Dalley et al., 1997). It may explain the low level of serum Mg of close up cows, despite of 0.4% in their DMI.

The circulating levels of cardiac enzymes in dry cows were significantly lower than lactating ones and their concentrations in close-up were lower than far-off dry group, significantly. Based on the high myocardial activity of dairy cows at their lactating periods, the high serum levels of cardiac enzymes were detected in lactating groups. However, according to clinical healthiness of the studied cows at all production cycles, it may be suggested that the elevation of cardiac enzymes at lactating periods was physiologic and not related to myocardial injuries. LDH activity rises slowly after myocardial infarction (Ohman et al., 1982). Determinations of LDH activity have been used diagnostically to determine whether acute myocardial infarction occurred in the days before a patient was evaluated (Adams et al., 1993). In the diagnosis of acute myocardial infarction, the measurement of elevated levels of LDH is well known (Jaffe et al., 1984). Measurements of AST and ALT activities are common laboratory tests, usually requested as an aid for diagnosis and surveillance of cardiac problems and both AST and ALT activities rise after an acute myocardial infarction (Ohman et al., 1982). AST lacks organ specificity but is present in skeletal muscle, cardiac muscle and liver of large animals; the pathological changes in these organs elevate the activity of AST in the blood (Kaneko et al., 2008). AST is also an intracellular enzyme involved in amino acid and carbohydrate metabolism, and its elevated levels show the damage in the organ whose cells are rich in this enzyme such as the heart (Aziz and Mahboob, 2010). In contrast, elevation in ALT levels is widely viewed as a specific indicator of liver necrosis and cardiac injuries. Elevated ALT activity is associated with the high risk of chronic heart disease. Both AST and ALT activities rise after an acute myocardial infarction (Ohman et al., 1982).

In conclusion, it could be stated that the heart electrical activities of dairy cows at each production period were different from other ones which may be related to lactogenesis, pregnancy and fetal growth. The differences among serum electrolyte levels may affect the electrocardiographic findings at each production period which could alter the production and conduction of cardiac electrical impulses. Furthermore, the cardiac activities in different production periods could have a significant impact on the levels of circulating cardiac enzymes. However, based on the clinical healthiness of studied cows, all of the electrocardiographic, serum electrolytes and enzymes alterations may be considered as physiological events. Furthermore, these findings could be used as guidelines to evaluate the cardiac electrical activities of high producing Holstein dairy cows at different production states.

Conflict of interest: The authors declare that there is no conflict of interest.

Acknowledgments

The authors would like to appreciate Shiraz University for their financial support of this research.

References

Adams, J., Abendschein, D.R., Jaffe, A.S. (1993) Biochemical markers of myocardial injury. Is MB creatine kinase the choice for the 1990s? Circulation. 88: 750-763.

Akita, M., Kuwahara, M., Tsubone, M.H., Sugano, S. (1998) ECG changes during furosemide induced hypokalemia in the rat. J Electrocardiol. 31: 45-49.

Aziz, R., Mahboob, T. (2010) Relation between preeclampsia and cardiac enzymes. ARYA Atheroscler. 4: 29-32.

Ben-Ghedalia, D., Tagari, H., Zamwel, S., Bondi, A. (1975) Solubility and net exchange of calcium, magnesium and phosphorus in digesta flowing along the gut of the sheep. Br J Nutr. 33: 87-94.

Burtis, C.A., Ashwood, E.R. (1994) Tietz Textbook of Clinical Chemistry. (2nd ed.) W.B. Saunders Co, Philadelphia, USA.

Chalmeh, A. (2015) Changes of the electrocardiographic parameters during aging in clinically healthy Holstein cattle. Bulg J Vet Med. 18: 105-111.

Chalmeh, A., Pourjafar, M., Naghib, M. (2014) Comparison of ST-segment duration and morphology between clinically healthy and diarrheic Holstein dairy calves. J Fac Vet Med Istanbul Univ. 40: 162-167.

Cohen, J.D., Blumenthal, R., Horn, H.R., Weintraub, H., Weglicki, W. (2002) Torsades de pointes, a potential complication of diuretic-induced hypokalemia and hypomagnesemia in patients with congestive heart failure. Conference presentation of a generic patient. Current Curr Ther Res Clin Exp. 63: 803-809.

Dalley, D.E., Isherwood, P., Sykes, A.R., Robson, A.B. (1997) Effect of intraruminal infusion of potassium on the site of magnesium absorption within the digestive tract in sheep. J Agric Sci. 129: 99-105.

Deroth, L. (1980) Electrocardiographic parameters in the normal lactating Holstein cow. Can Vet J. 21: 271-277.

Drighil, A., Madias, J.E., El mosalami, H., El badaoui, N., Mouine, B., Fadili, W., Ramdani, B., Bennis, A. (2007) Impact of hemodialysis on P-wave amplitude, duration, and dispersion. Indian Pacing Electrophysiol J. 7: 85-96.

Duffield, T. (2000) Subclinical ketosis in lactating dairy cattle. Vet Clin North Am Food Anim Pract. 16: 231-53.

Felkai, F. (1985) Electrocardiographic signs in ventricular repolarization of experimentally induced hypokalaemia and appearance of the U-wave in dogs. Acta Vet Hung. 33: 221.

Fisch, C. (1984) Electrocardiography and vectorcardiography. In: Heart Disease: A Textbook of Cardiovascular Medicine. E.U. Braun-wald. (2nd ed.) W.B. Saunders, Philadelphia, USA. p. 195.

Gadsby, D.C., Karagueuzian, H.S., Wit, A.L. (1995) Normal and abnormal electrical activity in cardiac cells. In: Cardiac Arrhythmias. W. J. Mandel, Lippincott, Philadelphia, USA. p. 55.

Gettes, L., Surawicz, B. (1968) Effects of low and high concentrations of potassium on the simultaneously recorded Purkinje and ventricular action potentials of the perfused pig moderator band. Circ Res. 23: 717-729.

Grace, N.D., Davies, E., Momo, J. (1977) Association of Mg, Ca, P, and K with various fractions in the diet, digesta, and faeces of sheep fed fresh pasture. New Zeal J Agr Res. 20: 441-448.

Hanton, G., Yvon, A., Provost, J., Racaud, A., Doubovetzky, M., 2007. Quantitative relationship between plasma potassium levels and QT interval in beagle dogs. Lab Anim Res. 41: 204-217.

Hom, J.P., Smith, R.H. (1978) Absorption of magnesium by the young steer. Br J Nutr. 40: 473-484.

Jafari Dehkordi, A., Mohebi, A.N., Heidari Soreshjani, M. (2014a) Frequency of cardiac arrhythmias in high- and low- yielding dairy cows. Vet Res Forum 5: 1-5.

Jafari Dehkordi, A., Mohebbi, A.N., Balali Dehkordi, Sh. (2014b) Evaluation of dysrhythmias and myocardial biomarkers in high and low-yielding dairy cows. Iran J Vet Med (University of Tehran). 8: 101-109.

Jaffe, A.S., Garfinkel, B.T., Ritter, C.S., Sobel, B.E. (1984) Plasma MB creatine kinase after vigorous exercise in professional athletes. Am J Cardiol. 53: 856-858.

Kaneko, J.J., Harvey, J.W., Bruss, M.L. (2008) Clinical Biochemistry of Domestic Animals. Academic press. California, USA.

Ohman, E., Teo, K., Johnson, A., Collins, P., Dowsett, D., Ennis, J., Horgan, J. (1982) Abnormal cardiac enzyme responses after strenuous exercise: alternative diagnostic aids. Br Med J. 285: 1523-1526.

Piccione, G., Mesina, V., Marafioti, S., Casella, S., Giannetto, C., Fazio, F. (2012) Changes of some haematochemical parameters in dairy cows during late gestation, post partum, lactation and dry periods. Vet Med Zoot. 58: 59-64.

Pourjafar, M., Badie, K., Chalmeh, A. (2012) Evaluation of ST-segment duration and morphology of standard base apex lead electrocardiograms in different age groups of apparently healthy Holstein cattle. J Fac Vet Med Istanbul Univ. 38: 51-58.

Radostits, O.M., Gay, C.C., Hinchcliff, K.W., Constable, P.D. (2007) Diseases of the Cardiovascular System. In: Veterinary Medicine: A Text Book of the Diseases of Cattle, Horses, Sheep, Pigs and Goats. (10th ed.) Elsevier. Philadelphia, USA. p. 399-438, 543-574.

Rezakhani, A., Paphan, A.A., Shekarfroush, S. (2004) Analysis of base apex lead electrocardiograms of normal dairy cows. Vet Arhiv. 74: 351-358.

Surawicz, B. (1980) The interrelationship of electrolyte abnormalities and arrhythmias. Cardiac Arrhythmias: Their Mechanisms, Diagnosis, and Management. JB Lippincott Company, Philadelphia, USA. p. 83-106.

Surawicz, B., Braun, H.A., Crum, W.B., Kemp, R.L., Wagner, S., Bellet, S. (1957) Quantitative analysis of the electrocardiographic pattern of hypopotassemia. Circulation. 16: 750-763.

Tanritanir, P., Dede, S., Ceylan, E. (2009) Changes in some macro minerals and biochemical parameters in female healthy siirt hair goats before and after parturition. J Anim Vet Adv. 8: 530-533.

Too, K., Kanagawa, H., Kawata, K. (1966) Fetal electrocardiogram in dairy cattle: 3. Variations in fetal QRS pattern. Jpn J Vet Res. 14: 103-113.

Trenk, L., Kuhl, J., Aurich, J., Aurich, C., Nagel, C. (2015) Heart rate and heart rate variability in pregnant dairy cows and their fetuses determined by fetomaternal electrocardiography. Theriogenology 84: 1405-1410.

Wathes, D.C., Cheng, Z., Chowdhury, W., Fenwick, M.A., Fitzpatrick, R., Morris, D.G., Patton, J., Murphy, J.J. (2009) Negative energy balance alters global gene expression and immune responses in the uterus of postpartum dairy cows. Physiol Genomics. 39: 1-13.

Yang, T., Snyders, D.J., Roden, D.M. (1997) R apid inactivation determines the rectification and [K+]o dependence of the rapid component of the delayed rectifier K+ current in cardiac cells. Circ Res. 80: 782-789.

Yelamanchi, V.P., Molnar, J., Ranade, V., Somberg, J.C. (2001) Influence of electrolyte abnormalities on interlead variability of ventricular repolarization times in 12-lead electrocardiography. Am J Ther. 8: 117-122.

Yoshida, M., Onda, K., Wada, Y., Kuwahara, M. (2015) Influence of sickness condition on diurnal rhythms of heart rate and heart rate variability in cows. J Vet Med Sci. 77: 375-379.

The effect of enzymatic pre-treatment of corn or soybean meal on their phytate content under different *in vitro* conditions

Rahimi, Z.S., Modirsanei, M.*, Mansoori, B., Rezaeian, M., Farkhoy, M., Honarzad, J.

Department of Animal and Poultry Health and Nutrition, Faculty of Veterinary Medicine, University of Tehran, Tehran, Iran

Key words:
bio-phytase, phytate, pre-treatment, rovabio excel AP, rovabio max AP

Correspondence
Modirsanei, M.
Department of Animal and Poultry Health and Nutrition, Faculty of Veterinary Medicine, University of Tehran, Tehran, Iran

Email: msaneii@ut.ac.ir

Abstract:

BACKGROUND: Phosphorous is one of the expensive nutrients in poultry feed. Therefore, improving the bioavailability of this nutrient in feed ingredients could be effective for lowering the cost of feed. **OBJECTIVES:** This study was performed to evaluate the effect of pre-treatment of feed ingredients by commercial enzymes and different levels of pH on the release of phosphorus from phytate under in vitro condition. **METHODS:** Three solutions including Distilled water, HCl 0.5% and HCl 1% (with pH=5.5, 2.12 and 1.88 respectively) and three enzymes (None, Bio-phytase, Rovabio Excel AP, and Rovabio Max AP) were used to determine phytate content of corn and soybean meal. First, each sample was supplemented with the enzymes and pre-treated under the above mentioned solutions for 3 h at 25 and 40 ºC. **RESULTS:** The results indicated that pre-treatment of corn samples with Bio-phytase or Rovabio Max AP and different solutions (at 25 ºC and 40 ºC for 3 h) reduced phytate content significantly. The best results were obtained with corn samples supplemented with Rovabio Max AP and mixing by HCl 1% at 25 ºC, so that phytate content decreased up to 99.5% in comparison with control. The same results were also obtained for soybean samples. The highest reduction in phytate content (up to 47.4%) was observed by adding Rovabio Max AP and HCl 1% solution at 40 ºC. **CONCLUSIONS:** It could be concluded that pre-treating corn and soybean meal using various methods such as commercial enzymes including phytase and solutions with different pH were effective to reduce phytate content, which means increasing the bioavailability of phosphorous.

Introduction

Since the major part of costs in poultry production is related to feed, minimizing this part of the costs which depends on feed ingredients is very important. On the other hand, phosphorous is usually one of the expensive nutrients in poultry feed. Therefore, the amount of nutrients in feed ingredients, especially available phosphorus, has a very important role in lowering the cost of feed.

The main form of storage of phosphorus (P) in plant feedstuffs is phytate (myo-inositol-hexakis-phosphate or IP6-P) which contains approximately 60-80% of total phosphorus in plant feed ingredients (Dersjant-Li, 2015; Kishor Gupta, 2015; Besline Joshi, 2014; Esmaeilipour, 2012; Ravindran, 1995).

Monogastric animals including poultry birds produce endogenous phytase to certain extent. However, this enzyme has minimum effect on hydrolysis of dietary phytate in the intestine of poultry due to a number of micro-environmental factors such as pH of the site of action (intestine), presence of other dietary nutrients (divalent cations, amino acids) and low transit time of digesta. Phytate forms chelated complex with some mineral elements like calcium and magnesium and reduces their availability. Consequently, with reducing the digestibility of phytate, considerable quantities of P are excreted in the manure and lead to polluting the environment, poor absorption of mineral and protein and then high feed cost; unless plant or microbial phytases are added in the feed. Despite the low level of phytate content in feed ingredients, determining its quantity should be considered in order to supply the adequate and necessary phosphorus and also other bivalence like calcium and magnesium. Following the use phytase and its effect on phytate molecule in feed ingredients, some nutrients e.g. protein, starch, and minerals are released better, so they could be digested and absorbed more easily and quickly by the birds (Lamid, 2014; Esmaeilipour, 2012; Tahir, 2012; Woyengo, 2010).

The amount of phytic acid in feed ingredients is varied based on their type and the environment which they grow. Some researches show that the proportion of non-phytate P of total P in feed ingredients is approximately 33% but for corn is around 40% (Tahir, 2012; Ravindran, 1999). Data presented in Table 1 show the level of phytate in different ingredients (Tahir, 2012; Selle, 2007; Godoy, 2005).

Therefore, it seems that determining the amount of phytate in feed ingredients is necessary in order to balance the level of phosphorus and other elements in ration, precisely. It allows the nutritionist to formulate the feed efficiently, lower the feed cost and reduce the amount of P pollution in poultry excreta (Tahir, 2012; Woyengo, 2010; Cowieson, 2005; Common, 1940).

Exogenous enzymes are usually used to improve digestibility and nutritive value of rations including cereals, especially for poultry. There are several studies to describe the effects of exogenous enzyme on nutritional value of nutrients like energy and protein in diets while just a few researches pay attention to the effect of enzyme on nutritional value of ingredients, so it is necessary to determine the nutritional matrix of each ingredient. Therefore, some information about the effects of enzymes on nutrients and anti-nutrients availability of feed ingredients has been shown, permitting us to improve the diet formulation and making it more cost-effective (Beslin Joshi, 2014; Dourado, 2009; Olukosi, 2007; Cowieson, 2005).

Phytase is an enzyme which hydrolyzes phytate to inositol and inorganic phosphate. Some cereals like rye, triticale, and wheat and to a lower extent barley, have some phytase activity (Viveros, 2000) and also phytase exists at low level in the chicken gastro-intestinal tract but it is not enough to digest all P bounded phytate in diet even if diets are prepared directly on-farm, without any heat-treatment. Most diets are used as pellet form with heat treatment at temperature above 80 °C that deactivate the enzyme activity of cereals. Moreover, corn and soybean meal (SBM) which are the main ingredients used in poultry diet in our territory, have no enzyme activity. Therefore, it has been proven that supplementation of diets with exogenous phytase is effective for enhancing the P availability, reducing the requirement of inorganic P to the diet and hence, the amount of P excreted into the environment (Woyengo, 2013; Selle, 2000).

Recently, there are several studies on the effects of using the exogenous phytase along with combination of other enzymes, especially the cell wall degrading enzymes. These enzymes facilitate the access of phytase to phytate and also the release of phytate phosphorus but the results of these studies were vary (Woyengo, 2010; Kim, 2005).

Non-starch polysaccharide (NSPs) enzymes degrade the cell wall of cereals then the nutrients become more available for animals. In addition, NSPs enzymes reduce the intestinal viscosity so that digestion and absorption of the nutrients are accelerated, which leads to improved poultry performance. Some researchers explained that glycosidases are able to break the NSPs of the cell wall and thus accelerate the availability of phytase to the phytate which is imprisoned in the cell wall (Olukosi, 2007). Whilst if the phytase is used alone, its accessibility to phytate will be limited due to the substrate due to the substrate, which is imprisoned by NSP matrix (Olukosi, 2007). In addition, it has been shown that the effect of xylanase could be better when it is accompanied with other exogenous enzymes including protease, amylase and phytase (Dourado, 2009; Cowieson, 2005).

Since there is not enough time for digesta to reside in poultry gastrointestinal tract, enzymes are not enable to hydrolyze the ingredients completely. Therefore, benefiting from a method which increases contact time between enzymes and their substrate results in increased possibility of the positive effect of enzymes on nutrients, and also according to some researches, pre-treatment of feedstuffs or diets may have a beneficial effect on hydrolysis of phytate and also other anti-nutritional factors existed in feedstuffs. Consequently, pre-treatment would be a great way for using the vast quantity and variety of raw materials. Besides, it can be an added value to ration for improving the quality of diets.

Therefore, the objective of this research is to evaluate the effects of pre-treatment of feed ingredients by some factors like pH and exogenous enzymes (phytase and NSP enzyme) on content of phytic acid, in order to enhance the availability and utilization of phytate phosphorus in vitro conditions.

Materials and Methods

The influence of pre-treatment factors including pH and enzyme was evaluated on the bio-availability of phytate phosphorus in feed ingredients in two separate experiments. The samples of corn and soybean meal were supplemented with phytase and/or NSP enzymes. The design of trial for both ingredients was similar. Each trial was done at two temperatures (25 ° and 40 °C).

Experiment 1: the experiment had a completely randomized design with 3×4 factorial arrangements with three replicates for each treatment. For this purpose, the effect of three solutions with different pH (distilled water, HCl 0.5%, HCl 1%), and three commercial enzymes (None, RMAP = Rovabio Max AP, REAP = Rovabio Excel AP, Bio-phy = Bio-phytase) were studied after 3 h. Bio-phytase included (5,000 FYT U/g of CbS Canadian Bio-system company), and Rovabio AP (22000 U visco /g xylanase & 2000 U AGL/G B- gluconase of Adisseo company), and Rovabio Max AP (Phytase 10,000 FTU/g + 22000 of U visco /g xylanase + 2000 U AGL/G B- gluconase of Adisseo Company of France).

First, samples of corn were ground and randomly divided to three groups with 4 treatments in each group with 3 replications for each treatment. Then, samples of corn were supplemented with or without enzymes precisely. In the next step, 3 solutions with different pH (Distillated water, HCl 0.5% and HCl 1%) with pH=5.5, 2.12 and 1.88 respectively, were added to the mixture of corn samples and enzymes in room temperature, then were heated in oven 60°C or kept at room temperature (25 °C) for 3 h. Then all of the samples were kept at room temperature overnight in order to dry (with moisture not more than12%). The dried samples were prepared to measure their phytate contents. First, the samples were extracted with 0.2 normal HCl, then 0.5 ml of extract was transferred into a test tube. 1 ml of ferric solution was added to the tube and fitted with a ground-glass stopper. The tube was heated in a boiling water bath for 30 min. After cooling in ice water for 15 min. the solution was allowed to adjust to room temperature. Then 2 ml of 2, 2–Bipyridine solution was added and the contents of tube were mixed. Absorbance was measured after 0.5 min. The Bipyridine reacted with the iron phytate and the color of tube contents changed (Haug, 1983).

Experiment 2: In the second experiment, all of the above mentioned steps were conducted with SBM samples.

Statistical analysis: The experiment had a complete random design with a 3 × 4 factorial arrangement (ANOVA), R software (Version 3.0.0).The general linear model (GLM) was used to determine the main effects of factors of any possible interaction between factors using Bonferroni Postdoc test. Significance was accepted at the $P < 0.05$ level.

Table 1. Phytate phosphorus content of feed ingredients. Data derived from the study by Godoy et.al. (2005) & Sell, Ravindran et al (2007).

Feedstuff	Total P (g/kg)	Phytate P (g/kg)
Barley	2.73- 3.7	1.86- 2.2
Corn	2.3- 2.9	1.7- 2.2
Sorghum	2.6- 3.09	1.7- 2.46
Wheat	2.9- 4.09	1.8- 2.89
Canola meal	8.79- 11.5	4- 7.78
Cottonseed meal	6.4- 11.36	4.9- 9.11
Soybean meal	5.7- 6.94	3.54- 4.53

Results

Corn: The results presented in Table 2 indicated that the effects of enzymes and solutions (with different pH) on the lowering of phytate were significantly different at both temperatures (25 and 40 °C). At 25 °C, the effects of enzymes or solutions (different pH) alone, and also interaction effects of enzyme × solution on phytate content of corn samples were significant ($p<0.001$). According to the results presented in Table 3, adding NSP enzymes alone (REAP) to the corn samples and pre-treatment with different pH solutions for 3 h did not affect the content of phytate except with HCl 0.5%, in comparison with control. Pre-treated corn samples supplemented with phytase (Bio-phy) decreased phytate content ($p<0.001$). There were significant differences in phytate content of corn samples supplemented with phytase alone (Bio-phy) or in combination with phytase + NSP enzymes (RMAP) when compared with control and NSP enzymes alone (REAP) ($p<0.001$).

Table 2. Analysis of variance for treated corn samples with commercial enzymes and different solutions after 3 hours at 25 and 40 °C. [a] R Squared = .950 (Adjusted R Squared = .915). [b] R Squared = .980 (Adjusted R Squared = .966).

Source	25 °C			40 °C		
	df	F	P Value	df	F	P Value
Solution	2 [a]	8.44	.001	2 [b]	11.306	.000
Enzyme	3	156.34	.000	3	384.370	.000
Solution × Enzyme	6	8.715	.000	6	10.329	.000
Error	11			11		

Table 3. The mean of phytate content (± SD[1]) in corn samples treated with commercial enzymes and different solutions after 3 hours at 25 °C. [a-d] means within the same columns with common superscripts have no significant differences (p>0.05). [1]SD = Standard deviation, * = Increasing phytate content, ** = Decreasing phytate content. Bio-phy =Bio-phytase, REAP = Rovabio Excel AP, RMAP = Rovabio Max AP.

Enzyme	Distilled Water	Variation to control (%)	HCl 0.5%	Variation to control (%)	HCl 1%	Variation to control (%)
Without Enzyme	1.32±0.25^{ab}	0	1.31±0.08^{b}	0	1.60±0.22^{a}	0
REAP	1.43±0.14^{a}	*+ 8.3	1.78±0.40^{a}	+ 35.9	1.90±0.09^{a}	+ 18.8
Bio-phy	0.94±0.04^{bc}	**- 28.8	0.08±0.02^{c}	- 94.2	0.35±0.03^{b}	- 78.1
RMAP	0.62±0.57^{c}	- 53.0	0.21±0.08^{c}	- 84.0	0.01±0.00^{b}	- 99.4

Table 4. The mean of phytate content (± SD[1]) in corn samples treated with commercial enzymes and different solutions after 3 hours at 40 °C. [a-d] means within the same columns with common superscripts have no significant differences (p>0.05). [1] SD = Standard deviation, * = Increasing phytate content, ** = Decreasing phytate content. Bio-phy =Bio-phytase, REAP = Rovabio Excel AP, RMAP = Rovabio Max AP.

Enzyme	Distilled Water	Variation to control (%)	HCl 0.5%	Variation to control (%)	HCl 1%	Variation to control (%)
Without Enzyme	0.49±0.00b	0	1.27±0.08a	0	1.26±0.02a	0
REAP	1.15±0.04^{a}	**- 12.6	1.11±0.01^{a}	- 12.6	1.30±0.05^{a}	*+ 3.2
Bio-phy	0.29±0.19^{b}	- 40.8	0.16±0.07^{b}	- 87.4	0.14±0.10^{b}	- 88.9
RMAP	0.12±0.04^{b}	- 75.5	0.02±0.01^{b}	- 98.4	0.07±0.03^{b}	- 94.4

Table 5. Analysis of variance for treated soybean meal samples with different solutions, enzymes after 3 hours at 25 and 40 °C. [a] R Squared = .950 (Adjusted R Squared =.927). [b] R Squared = .969 (Adjusted R Squared = .947).

Source	25 °C			40 °C		
	df	F	P value	df	F	P value
Solution	2 [a]	74.379	.000	2	11.915	.000
Enzyme	3	28.202	.000	3	74.371	.000
Solution × Enzyme	6	6.993	.000	6	2.523	.041
Error	11			11		

Adding Bio-phy or RMAP and different pH solutions to corn samples caused a significant reduction of phytate content (p<0.001).

The results presented in Table 4 indicated that pre-treating corn samples supplemented with REAP and mixed with distilled water (pH=5.5) at 40 °C, increased phytate content in comparison with control while it had no significant effects with respect to 0.5 and 1% HCl. Adding Bio-phy or RMAP to corn samples and treatment with HCl 0.5 and 1% decreased phytate contents significantly (p<0.001) in comparison with control. The best results were obtained with corn samples by adding RMAP (Rovabio Max AP) and pre-treated with HCl 1% at 25 °C, that phytate content decreased up to 99.5% in comparison with control.

Table 6. The mean of phytate content (± SD[1]) in soybean meal samples treated corn samples with commercial enzymes and different solutions after 3 hours at 25 °C. [a-d] Means within the same columns with common superscripts have no significant differences (p>0.05). [1] SD = Standard deviation, * = Increasing phytate content, ** = Decreasing phytate content. Bio-phy =Bio-phytase, REAP = Rovabio Excel AP, RMAP = Rovabio Max AP.

Enzyme	Distilled Water	Variation to control (%)	HCL 0.5%	Variation to control (%)	HCL 1%	Variation to control (%)
Without Enzyme	3.55±0.54^{a}	0	2.05±0.16^{ab}	0	2.23±0.03^{a}	0
REAP	2.39±0.02^{b}	**- 32.7	2.18±0.03^{a}	*+ 6.3	1.95±0.60^{a}	- 12.6
Bio-phy	2.32±0.23^{b}	- 34.6	1.87±0.11^{ab}	- 8.78	1.94±0.12^{a}	- 13.0
RMAP	2.18±0.12^{b}	- 38.6	1.71±0.08^{b}	- 16.6	1.95±0.12^{a}	- 12.6

Table 7. The mean of phytate content (± SD[1]) in soybean meal samples treated corn samples with commercial enzymes and different solutions after 3 hours at 40 °C. [a-d] Means within the same columns with common superscripts have no significant differences (p>0.05). [1] SD=Standard deviation, * = Increasing phytate content, ** = Decreasing phytate content, Bio-phy =Bio-phytase, REAP = Rovabio Excel AP, RMAP = Rovabio Max AP.

Enzyme	Distilled Water	Variation to control (%)	HCL 0.5%	Variation to control (%)	HCL 1%	Variation to control (%)
Without Enzyme	3.46±0.00^{a}	0	3.65±0.00^{a}	0	3.4±0.04^{a}	0
REAP	3.55±0.00^{a}	**+ 2.6	3.76±0.00^{a}	+ 3.0	3.51±0.18^{a}	+ 3.2
Bio-phy	2.92±0.19^{b}	*- 15.6	2.39±0.15^{b}	- 34.5	2.41±0.01^{b}	- 29.1
RMAP	2.83±0.16^{b}	- 18.2	2.42±0.13^{b}	- 33.7	1.79±0.61^{b}	- 47.4

Soybean Meal: At two temperatures (25 and 40 °C), the effect of solutions and enzymes alone, and also interaction effect of solution with enzyme on phytate contents of soybean meal samples were significant (p<0.001, Table 5).

According to the results indicated in Table 6, adding all of the commercial enzymes to SBM samples and mixing with distilled water for 3 h at 25 °C reduced the content of phytate significantly (p<0.001) when compared with control, while no significant differences were observed for two other solutions (0.5 and 1% HCl) (p>0.05). A significant difference was observed between REAP and RAMP enzymes to reduce phytate content of soybean meal samples.

At 40 °C, supplementing soybean meals with REAP and different pH solutions did not affect phytate contents of samples after 3 h (p>0.05, Table 7). SBM samples with Bio-Phy or RMAP enzymes and mixing them with different pH solutions decreased phytate content. The highest reduction in phytate content (up to 47.4%) was observed by adding RMAP and treating with HCl 1% solution and at 40 °C.

Discussion

Chemical compositions of grains worldwide were measured during several studies. The results of those researches indicated some variations in composition of feed ingredients. For example, the amounts of phytate-P in different plants are very different. The reason of these variations could be due to different factors e.g. genetics, kind of plants, environmental conditions of growing plants, process, which are effective on availability of phosphorus in poultry. Similar results had been reported for chemical composition of feed ingredients which were used for preparation of poultry rations in Iran. For example, crude protein, calcium, and non-phytate phosphorus of corn samples could be in the range of 7.5 to 9.0, 0.1 to 0.2, and 0.8 to 1.2 gr/kg, respectively (Tahir, 2012; Liu, 2011; Steiner, 2007; Ravindran, 2006; Godoy, 2005; Kwanyuen, 2005; Lumpkins, 2005).

Corn and soybean meal are the two main ingredients in poultry rations. Phytic acid is generally aggregated in aleurone layer of monocotyledons like wheat, barley, rice, etc. Among the cereals, corn is different and the greatest proportion of phytic acid is found in germ (Tahir, 2012; Godoy, 2005).

Moreover, Zhou et al. (1992) declared that using the levels of Phosphorus as fertilizer is an important factor in determination of phytate-P content in feed ingredients. Significant regression is observed between phytate-P and total P in corn and soybean meal. It has been reported that phytate-P contents in corn samples were approximately 0.034% lower than the value in NRC, while for soybean meal samples they were approximately 0.151% higher (Tahir, 2012; Steiner, 2007; Cowieson, 2005).

Hidvegi et al. (2002) reported that cereals had a lower phytic acid content while its amount was higher in legume; so that maximum contents were 1.42g/100g and 1.75 g/100g, respectively. In addition, interaction between protein and phytic acid depends on pH and aggregation of protein (Rajendran, 1989; Schwenke, 1989), not the amount of phytic acid or this effect is very negligible (Hidvegi, 2002; Rajendran, 1989; Schwenke, 1989).

The results of present study indicated that the effect of solutions (with different pH) and commercial enzymes on the amount of non-phytate phosphorus released from phytate was significantly different at both temperatures (25 and 40 °C). According to some researches, in vitro pre-treatment of feedstuffs or diets may have beneficial effect on hydrolysis of phytate (Newkirk, 1998) and also other anti-nutritional factors existed in feedstuffs. Esmaeilipour et al. (2013) showed that soaking of broiler diet (in vitro conditions) improves phytate degradation, especially with increasing the time of soaking. Also, the result of present study indicates that pre-treating with HCl solutions had a better positive effect on decreasing the phytate content of corn and SBM sample when compared with distilled water. Other studies also determined the soaking of feed ingredients in citric acid was more effective in comparison with deionized water. Dephytinization or pre-treatment of feedstuffs with phytase could also be a good way, as soaking of feedstuffs prior to feeding might improve digestibility of P compared with dry feeding, because of providing a longer time for contact between phytate and phytase. Indeed, the dephytinization of individual feed ingredients has been shown to increase nutrients availability in chickens. However, the conditions of pre-treatment, like higher temperature and duration of incubation might affect the stability of enzyme (Esmaeilipour, 2012). On the other hand, Denstadli et al. (2006) reported that combination of low temperature and high moisture degraded the highest amount of phytate during incubation while moisture at high temperature had negative effect on enzyme stability.

The results of this study were consistent with the previous researches which showed that the effect of phytase along with soaking of feed ingredients on breaking of phytate phosphorus was dependent on the type of feedstuffs. Soaking of feed ingredients in water increased digestibility of P due to increasing contact time of phytate-P and exogenous phytase (Esmaeilipour, 2012; Blaabjerg, 2010). These findings are completely in agreement with the results of present study. According to the results of current experiment, combination of exogenous enzyme with HCl solutions had a better effect on decreasing phytate content of corn in comparison with SBM in the similar condition. Moreover, it has been demonstrated that interaction between phytase and soaking time (in water) had significant effects on breaking the phytae-P in SBM, while phytase with or without xylanase had no significant effect on degrading of phtate-P in wheat (Esmaeilipour, 2012; Blaabjerg, 2010).

In addition, it has been reported that cereals intrinsic phytases were stable at pH=3 - 5.5, while they were more sensitive to pH=8, so were degraded more easily. Increasing temperature reduced stability of intrinsic phytase of cereals. Incubation time of cereals in high temperatures was also a very important factor for stability of intrinsic phytase leading to decrease in the enzyme activity. Therefore, the availability of phosphorus in diets increased (Esmaeilipour, 2012). The results of present study are approved with Esmaeilipour et al. (2012), because the reaction of feed ingredients is generally different at various conditions. It could be due to several reasons including the location of phytate-P and phytase in grain and also their quantities.

Using the exogenous phytase along with the combination of other enzymes may facilitate the release of phytate phosphorus (Lu, 2013; Slominski, 2011). For example, phytate is concentrated in the aleurone layer of wheat (Ravindran, 1995) and xylanase may simplify availability of phytase to substrate in the aleurone. The combinations of phytase and various enzymes may be similarly advantageous for other feed ingredients (Cowieson, 2005). Researchers documented that combination of carbohydrase and phytase could facilitate the access of phytase to its substrate (Juanpere, 2005). In corn, phytic acid is located in the germ but in SBM is found in protein bodies of the seed. Solubility and accessibility of phytate salts and proteins from different feed ingredients and their effects on the extent of protein-phytate complex formation, coupled with variation in effectiveness of phytase in different diets (Selle, 2007). Thus using protease enzymes along with phytase may reduce the variability in phytase efficacy and maximize release of P from phytate.

However, the current research shows that the combination of phytase with NSPase enzyme had a better effect on decreasing the phytate content of corn and SBM but this difference was not significant. Supplementation of poultry diets with NSP-degrading enzymes and phytase might decrease the anti-nutritional effects of NSPs and phytic acid. NSPs can limit the accessibility of phytase to phytate (Kim, 2005). Therefore, NSP enzymes and phytase may act synergistically for improving nutrients utilization in poultry diets. NSP enzymes can hydrolyze NSPs to increase the availability of phytate for phytase. Cowieson et al. (2005) reported that using NSP enzymes like xylanase may hydrolyze the arabinoxylans in cell walls, so the release of encapsulated nutrients and their absorption will be increased (Olukosi, 2007; Cowieson, 2005). In addition, it seems that the lack of significant response to combination of phytase and NSPs enzymes (Xylanase, B-glucanase), might be due to low availability of substrate or inactivate of enzymes. It has been reported that glycosidases break down non-starch polysaccharides present in cell walls, then phytase would be able to access intrinsic phytate in cell wall. If phytase is used alone, accessibility to phytate will decrease, because it has been surrounded by NSP matrix. Besides, xylanase can hydrolyze the bond of soluble fiber. Then phosphorous and other minerals might be released and absorbed easily by animals (Olukosi, 2007; Coweison, 2005, 2010).

There are several reports that indicate adding the carbohydrases and phytase to ration increases the nutrients bioavailability and also performance of poultry (Adeola, 2010; Woyengo, 2010; Jia, 2008; Mori, 2007). Further, Juanpere et al. (2005) and Cowieson et al. (2010) declared that phytase along with β-glucanases decreased the excretion of calcium in the rations based on corn and barley. In addition, it may better to combine xylanase and glucanase in corn-soy based diets in broiler for maximizing the result of using NSP enzymes.

Dourado et al. (2009) determined that combination of phytase, xylanase, amylase and protease increased apparent metabolizable energy of corn but they were not effective on true metabolizable energy of SBM. Our result also shows that the effect of phytase and also phytase combined with NSPase decrease the phytate content in corn more than SBM.

Pre-treatment of corn in the solutions with different pH (including distilled water, and 0.5 or 1% HCl) at 25 and 40 °C could enhance the release of phosphorous from phytic acid and increase its bioavailability when supplemented with Bio-phytase (Bio-Phy) or Rovabio Max AP (RMAP).

With respect to SBM samples the highest bio-availability of phosphorous was observed by pre-treatment with HCl 1% solution at 40 °C and supplementing Rovabio Max AP.

According to the results of this study it could be concluded that pre-treating of feed ingredients (corn and SBM) of poultry diets using various methods such as using some commercial enzymatic products (including phytase) and solutions with different pH were effective to decrease the remaining phytate content in feed ingredients. It means that bioavailability of phosphorous increased.

Acknowledgments

This study was financially supported by Research Council of University of Tehran (Project No. 7509013/6/3).

References

Adeola, O., Jendza, J. A., Southern, L. L., Powell, S., Owusu-Asiedu, A. (2010) Contribution of exogenous dietary carbohydrases to the metabolizable energy value of corn distillers grains for broiler chickens. J Poult Sci. 89: 1947-1954.

Beslin Joshi, J. (2014) Phytase- A key to unlock phytate complex. Int J Pure Appl Biosci. 2: 304-313.

Blaabjerg, K., Carlsson, N.G., Hansen- Moller, J., Poulsen, H.D. (2010) Effect of heat-treatment, phytase, xylanase and soaking time on inositol phosphate degradation in vitro in Wheat, soybean meal and rapeseed cake. J Anim Feed Sci Technol. 162: 123-134.

Common, R.H. (1940) The phytic acid content of some poultry feeding stuffs. Analyst. 65: 79-83.

Cowieson, A.J., Bedford, M.R., Ravindran, V. (2010) Interactions between xylanase and glucanase in maize-soy-based diets for broilers. Br J Poult Sci. 51: 246-257.

Cowieson, A.J. (2005) Factors that affect the nutritional value of maize for broilers. J Anim

Feed Sci Technol. 119: 293- 305.

Cowieson, A.J., Adeola, O. (2005) Carbohydrase, Protease, and phytase have an additive beneficial effect in nutritionally marginal diets for broiler chicks. J Poult Sci. 84: 1860-1867.

Denstadli, V., Vestre, R., Svihus, B., Skrede, A., Storebakken, T. (2006) Phytate degradation in a mixture of ground wheat and ground defatted soybeans during feed processing: effects of temperature, moisture level, and retention time in small- and medium-scale incubation systems. J Agric Food Chem. 54: 5887–5893.

Dersjant-Li, Y., Awati, A., Schulze, H., Patridge, G. (2015) Phytase in non-ruminant animal nutrition: a critical review on phytase activities in the gastrointestinal tract and influencing factors. J Sci Food Agric. 95: 878-896.

Dourado, L.R.B., Sakomura, N.K., Barbosa, N. A.A., Bonato, M.A., Kawuauchi, I.M., Fernandes, J.B.K., Costa, F.G.P. (2009) Corn and soybean meal metabolizable energy with the addition of Exogenous Enzymes for poultry. Braz J Poult Sci. 11: 51- 55.

Esmaeilipour, O., Van Krimpen, M. M., Jongbloed, A. W., De Jonge, L. H., Bikker, P. (2013) The effects of temperature, moisture, duration of incubation time, calcium level, and soaking with water or citric acid on in vitro phytate degradation in a wheat–barley–rye–soybean meal-based diet. J Anim Feed Sci Technol. 183: 168-174.

Esmaeilipour, O., Van Krimpen, M. M., Jongbloed, A. W., De Jonge, L. H., Bikker, P. (2012) Effects of temperature, pH, incubation time and pepsin concentration on the in vitro stability of intrinsic phytase of wheat, barley and rye. Anim Feed Sci Technol. 175: 168-174.

Godoy, S., Chicco, C., Meschy, F., Requena, F. (2005) Phytic phosphorus and phytase activity of animal feed ingredients. Interciencia 30: 24-28.

Haug, W., Lantzsch, H. J. (1983) Sensitive Method for the Rapid Determination of Phytate in Cereals and Cereal Products. J Sci Food Agric. 34: 1423-1426.

Hidvegi, M., Radomir, L. (2002) Phytic Acid content of Cereal and Legumes and Interaction with Proteins. Period J Polytech Chem Eng. 46: 59-64.

Jia, W., Slominski, B.A., Guenter, W., Humphreys, A., Jones, O. (2008) The effect of enzyme supplementation on egg production parameters and omega-3 fatty acid deposition in laying hens fed flaxseed and canola seed. J Poult Sci. 87: 2005-2014.

Juanpere, J., Perez-Vendrell, A.M., Angulo, E., Brufau, J. (2005) Assessment of potential interactions between phytase and glycosidase enzyme supplementation on nutrient digestibility in broilers. J Poult Sci. 84: 571-580.

Kim, J.C., Simmins, P. H., Mullen, B. P., Pluske, J. R. (2005) Effect of wheat phosphorus content and supplemental enzymes on digestibility growth performance of weaner pigs. J Anim Feed Sci Technol. 118: 139-152.

Kishor Gupta, R., Singh Gangoliya, S., Kumar Singh, N. (2015) Reduction of phytic acid and enhancement of bioavailable micronutrients in food grains. J Food Sci Technol. 52: 676-684.

Kwanyuen, P., Burton, J. W., (2005) A simple and rapid procedure for phytate determination in soybeans and soy products. J Am Oil Chem Soc. 82: 81-85.

Lamid, M., Tri Puspaningsih, N.N., Asmarani, O. (2014) Potential of phytase enzymes as Biocatalysts for improved nutritional value of rice bran for broiler feed. J Appl Environ Biol Sci. 4: 377-380.

Liu, K., Han, J. (2011) Changes in mineral concentrations and phosphorus profile during dry-grind processing of corn into ethanol. J Bioresour Technol. 102: 3110–3118.

Lu, H., Adedokun, S.A., Preynat, A., Legrand-Defretin, V., Geraert, P.A., Adeola, O., Ajuwon, K.M. (2013) Impact of exogenous carbohydrases and phytase on growth performance and nutrient digestibility in broilers. Can J Anim Sci. 93: 243-249.

Lumpkins, B.S, Batal, A.B. (2005) The bioavailability of lysine and phosphorus in distillers dried grains with soluble. Poult Sci. 84: 581-586.

Newkirk, R. W., Classen, H. L. (1998) In vitro hydrolysis of phytate in canola meal with purified and crude sources of phytase. J Anim Feed Sci Technol. 72: 315-327.

Olukosi, O. A., Cowieson, A. J., Adeola, O. (2007) Age-related influence of a cocktail of xylanase, amylase, and protease or phytase individually or in combination in broiler. J Poult Sci. 86: 77-86.

Rajendran, S., Prakesh, V. (1989) Interaction of phytic acid with Alfa-Globulin from sesame seed (*Sesamus indicus* L.). In: Abhandlungen der Akademie der Wissenschaften der DDR. Schwenke, K.D., Raab, B. (eds.). Abteilung Mathematik, Naturwissenschaften, Technik Akademie Verlag Berlin. p. 247-251.

Ravindran, V, Bryden, W. L., Kornegay, E. T. (1995) Phytates: occurrence, bioavailability and implications in poultry nutrition. J Avian Poult Biol Rev. 6: 125-143.

Ravindran, V., Cabahug, S., Ravindran, G., Bryden, W. L. (1999) Influence of microbial phytase on apparent ileal amino acid digestibility in feedstuffs for broilers. J Poult Sci. 78: 699–706.

Ravindran, V., Morel, P. C., Partridge, G. G., Hruby, M. Sands, J. S. (2006) Influence of an *Escherichia coli*-derived phytase on nutrient utilization in broiler starters fed diets containing varying concentrations of phytic acid. J Poult Sci. 85: 82–89.

Schwenke, K. D., Mothes, R., Gast, K., Zirwer, D. (1989) Rapeseed protein- protein Interactions. In: Schwenke, K.D., Raab, B. (eds.). Abhandlungen der Akademie der Wissenschaften der DDR, Abteilung Mathematik, Naturwissenschaften, Technik Akademie Verlag Berlin. p. 105-114.

Selle, P. H., Ravindran,V. (2007) Microbial phytase in poultry nutrition. J Anim Feed Sci Technol. 135: 1–41.

Selle, P. H., Ravindran, V., Caldwell, A., Bryden, W. L. (2000) Phytate and phytase: consequences for protein utilization. Nutr Res Rev. 13: 255-278.

Slominski, B.A. (2011) Recent advances in enzymes for poultry diets. J Poult Sci. 90: 2013-2023.

Steiner, T., Mosenthin, R., Zimmermannb, B., Greiner, R., Roth, S. (2007) Distribution of phytase activity, total phosphorus and phytate phosphorus in legume seeds, cereals and cereal by-products as influenced by harvest year and cultivar. J Anim Feed Sci Technol. 133: 320-324.

Tahir, M., Shim, M. Y., Ward, N. E., Pesti, G. M. (2012) NIRS calibrations for total and phytate P in poultry feed ingredients. In proceedings: International Poultry Scientific Forum, Georgia World Congress Center, Atlanta, USA.

Tahir, M., Shim, M.Y., Ward, N.E., Smith, C., Foster, E., Guney A.C., Pesti, G.M. (2012) Phytate and other nutrient components of feed ingredients for poultry. J Poult Sci. 91: 928-935.

Viveros, A., Centeno, C., Brenes, A., Canales, A., Lozano, A. (2000) Phytase and acid phosphatase activities in plant feedstuffs. J Agric Food Chem. 48: 4009-4013.

Woyengo, T.A., Nyachoti C.M. (2013) Review: Anti-nutritional effects of phytic acid in diets for pigs and poultry-current knowledge and directions for future research. Can J Anim Sci. 93: 9-12.

Woyengo, T.A., Slominski, B.A., Jones, R.O. (2010) Growth performance and nutrient utilization of broiler chickens fed diets supplemented with phytase alone or in combination with citric acid and multicarbohydrase. J Poult Sci. 89: 2221- 2229.

Zhou, J.R., Fordyce, E.J., Raboy, V., Dickinson, D.B., Wong, M.S., Burns, R.A., Erdman, J.W. Jr. (1992) Reduction of phytic acid in soybean products improves zinc bioavailability in rats. Nutrition. 122: 2466-2473.

Investigation on mycoflora of poultry breeding houses' air and studying the efficacy of spraying and fumigation on inactivating the airspora

Shokri, H.*

Department of Pathobiology, Faculty of Veterinary Medicine, Amol University of Special Modern Technologies, Amol, Iran

Key words:
airspora, *Candida*, fumigation, mycoflora, poultry house

Correspondence
Shokri, H.
Department of Pathobiology, Faculty of Veterinary Medicine, Amol University of Special Modern Technologies, Amol, Iran

Email: hshokri@ausmt.ac.ir

Abstract:

BACKGROUND: A common concern of the poultry industry is the presence of fungal pathogens in the birds' environment, which may constitute a considerable health hazard to the birds, farmers, and those living in proximity of the farm. **OBJECTIVES:** The aims of this study were to assess the mycoflora in the indoor and outdoor environments of poultry breeding houses and studying the efficacy of disinfection methods, including spraying and fumigation, on reducing airspora concentration. **METHODS:** Indoor air of 12 poultry houses were sampled by exposing Petri dishes containing Sabouraud's glucose agar after removal of old litter, spraying with disinfectant solutions, and fumigation with formalin plus permanganate. The plates were incubated at 30 °C for seven days and fungi were counted and identified microscopically and macroscopically according to standard mycological methods. **RESULTS:** A total of 182 and 181 fungal colonies were recovered from indoor and outdoor air of poultry houses, respectively. *Candida* (30.2%) and *Aspergillus* (26.9%) species were the most common yeast and mold in the indoor, respectively, whereas *Alternaria* (37.6%) and *Candida* (19.3%) species were the most predominant fungi in the outdoor air of poultry houses. Disinfection of the poultry houses using spraying and fumigation methods led to a 38.1% and 75% reduction in airspora concentration ($p<0.05$), respectively. **CONCLUSIONS:** Based on the findings of the present study, *Candida* spp and *Alternaria* spp had the highest indoor and outdoor concentrations in poultry breeding houses' air, respectively, and fumigation was the most efficient method in reducing airspora.

Introduction

Intensive poultry production, implying large densities of animals in small areas, is a significant source of air pollution which may constitute a considerable health hazard to the birds, farmers, and those living in proximity of the farm (Lonc and Plewa, 2009). On the other hand, spread of bio aerosols outside of animal houses may result in local or even more extensive environmental pollution (Bakutis et al., 2004). The indoor air of poultry houses is usually contaminated with high concentrations of microorganisms (Jo et al., 2005). According to the existing studies, bacteria are the dominant microorganisms found in the poultry house bio aerosols, whose concentrations reach as much as 10^9 Colony Forming Unit (CFU)/m^3 (Radon et al., 2002), but fungi constitute a significant part of the airborne microflora in this sector as well. Their concentrations in stationary measurements usually range from 10^2 to 10^4 CFU/m^3 (Rimac et al, 2010), whereas in personal measurements for poultry farm workers- they are contained within 10^4-10^8 CFU/m^3 (Lee et al., 2006).

In general, outdoor atmosphere is dominated by representatives of the genera *Cladosporium*, *Penicillium*, *Aspergillus*, *Alternaria* and by yeasts and *Mycelia sterilia*. In relation to outdoor environments, indoor atmospheres typically display lower diversity (Araujo and Cabral, 2010). The fungal flora in the indoor air of breeding houses often contains molds from the genera: *Aspergillus*, *Penicillium*, *Cladosporium*, *Alternaria*, *Rhizopus*, *Scopulariopsis*, and *Trichophyton* (Lugauskas et al, 2004). Both viable forms of these fungi and their metabolites (mycotoxins) may cause a number of disorders in birds and poultry breeding workers, concerning mainly the respiratory tract (mucous membrane irritation, invasive mycoses of lungs, allergic rhinitis, allergic pulmonary alveolitis, asthma) and the skin (dermatomycoses and onychomycosis) (Dutkiewicz et al., 1999). Currently, fungal infections caused by *Microsporum gallinae* (Taghavi et al., 2014), A. fumigatus (Khosravi et al, 2007), and *Candida* species (Hashempour et al., 2014) are among the most frequent causes of fungal problems in poultry birds in Iran.

Poultry house sanitation plays a crucial role in controlling and preventing pathogenic infectious diseases. Removal of old litter, followed by cleaning and disinfecting poultry houses, can help reduce pathogen loads and break disease cycles. Methods for the application of disinfectants include spraying, misting, fogging, or fumigation (Eckman, 1994). A good sanitation program can benefit the grower by optimizing bird performance while lowering the incidence of contaminated flocks.

Mazandaran is a province in the North of Iran. It is located on the southern coast of the Caspian Sea. In the coastal plains - where we conducted our study - the humidity is high and the climate is temperate, which favors fungal growth; they are found through air. The present study was aimed to evaluate airspora concentration in the indoor and outdoor of poultry houses and studying the efficacy of disinfection methods including spraying and fumigation in inactivating a variety of common fungi in poultry houses.

Materials and Methods

Sampling sites: Twelve poultry breeding houses (broilers; Ross 308) were randomly selected from across the coastal plains of the Mazandaran province. Indoor and outdoor air samples were collected in the winter of 2014. The flock population in buildings was between 7000 and there were 35.000 birds. The rearing period was between 45 to 56 days for birds.

Air sampling: Indoor air samples for determining concentrations of fungi were collected by exposing Petri dishes containing Sabouraud's glucose agar (Merck Co., Darmastadt, Germany) in three steps as follows: Step 1: after the removal of old litter; Step 2: after spraying with disinfectant solutions (dispatag, chloracid 2000, nanosil, savlon, and formalin); Step 3: after fumigation using formalin along with permanganate. Petri dishes were placed at the height of 1.5 meters above the floor. Sampling took 30 minutes. During indoor mycoflora sampling at the same point, outdoor air sampling was performed as well (Shokri et al., 2010).

Laboratory analysis: Samples were incubated at 30 °C for seven days, after which the resulting colonies were counted as Colony Forming Units (CFU/plate/30 min). The culture plates were discarded after 4 weeks if no signs of fungal growth were seen. At least one colony of each apparently different types of colonies from indoor and outdoor air samples was selected for subculture and identification. The isolated fungi were identified to the genus level on the basis of colonial morphology on diagnostic media and on microscopic morphology by keys to identification and also using biochemical tests with API 20C AUX kit (bioMerieux-Vitek, Inc., Hazelwood, USA) (Pitt, 2000; Larone, 2002; Samson et al., 2004).

Statistics: For statistical analysis, a chi-square test was performed to reveal the differences among different poultry breeding houses; with respect to the concentration of isolated airborne fungi. A p value less than 0.05 was considered statistically significant.

Results

Forty-eight plates were collected, of which 36 were indoor air samples and 12 outdoor. Thirty-eight plates turned out positive. The types and concentrations of airborne culturable fungi determined in poultry breeding houses and outside of those houses were presented in Table 1. The analysis of airspora showed that the indoor concentration of fungi (no. 182 CFU) was to some extent higher than that of outdoor concentration (no. 181 CFU) at a distance of 20 meters from the poultry houses. No significant differences were observed between airspora in the indoor and outdoor air of poultry breeding houses.

In this study, a total of 13 genera of fungi from the indoor air samples were identified from poultry houses. As shown in Table 2, the most predominant yeasts were *Candida* spp (30.2%), *Trichosporon* spp (6%), *Rhodotorula* spp (1.6%), and *Geotrichum* spp (0.5%), as well as nine genera of molds which were identified as follows: *Aspergillus* spp (26.9%), *Alternaria* spp (11.5%), *Mycelia sterilia* (9.9%), *Penicillium* spp (8.8%), *Chrysosporium* spp (1%), *Mucor* spp (1%), *Cladosporium* spp (1%), *Rhizopus* spp (0.5%), and *Dematiaceous fungi* (0.5%). There was a statistically significant difference between the concentrations of molds (61.5%) and yeasts (38.5%) ($p<0.05$) (Fig. 1). A total of 11 fungal genera were identified from the outdoor air samples of poultry houses. As shown in Table 2, *Alternaria* spp were the most frequent organisms and formed about 37.6% of the total fungal community.

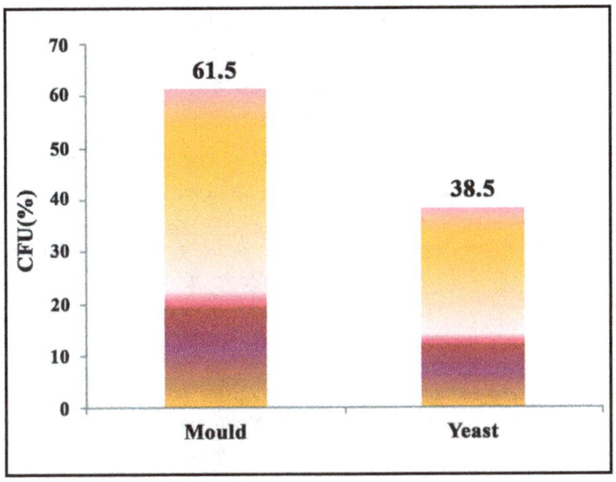

Figure 1. Comparison of the concentrations of moulds and yeasts in the inside air of poultry breeding houses (CFU/plate/30 min).

Table 1. Concentrations of airspora in the indoor and outdoor environments of the poultry breeding houses (CFU/plate/30 min). (*) Step 1: After removal of old litter; Step 2: After spraying with disinfectant solutions (dispatag, chloracid 2000, nanosil, savlon and formalin); Step 3: After fumigation using formalin along with permanganate.

	Indoor air (CFU)			Outdoor air (CFU)
	Step 1	Step 2	Step 3	
Poultry house 1	54	4	9	44
Poultry house 2	6	17	2	12
Poultry house 3	23	18	0	33
Poultry house 4	5	5	0	6
Poultry house 5	10	4	0	12
Poultry house 6	47	0	0	17
Poultry house 7	6	11	10	3
Poultry house 8	4	0	0	5
Poultry house 9	6	32	0	1
Poultry house 10	5	7	7	20
Poultry house 11	6	5	0	6
Poultry house 12	9	9	0	22

Table 2. The composition of fungal genera in outside and inside air of poultry breeding houses (CFU/plate/30 min). (*) Step 1: After removal of old litter; Step 2: After spraying with disinfectant solutions (dispatag, chloracid 2000, nanosil, savlon and formalin); Step 3: After fumigation using formalin along with permanganate.

Poultry houses	Indoor air (CFU)			Outdoor air (CFU)
	Step 1	Step 2	Step 3	
Poultry house 1	*Aspergillus* (5), *Penicillium* (1), *Alternaria* (4), *Mycelia sterilia* (1), *Candida* (30), *Rhodotorula* (1), *Geotrichum* (1), *Trichosporon beigelii* (11)	*Cladosporium* (2), *Trichosporon beigelii* (2)	*Alternaria* (1), *Cladosporium* (1), *Mycelia sterilia* (7)	*Aspergillus* (1), *Penicillium* (7), *Alternaria* (2), *Mycelia sterilia* (13), *Candida* (21)
Poultry house 2	*Alternaria* (2), *Mycelia sterilia* (2), *Chrysosporium* (2)	*Drechslera* (1), *Aspergillus* (1), *Penicillium* (3), *Fusarium* (1), *Alternaria* (4), *Cladosporium* (1), *Mycelia sterilia* (4), *Rhodotorula* (1), *Candida* (1)	*Rhizopus* (1), *Mucor* (1)	*Alternaria* (3), *Mycelia sterilia* (1), *Chrysosporium* (2), *Penicillium* (4), *Candida* (2)
Poultry house 3	*Aspergillus* (17), *Penicillium* (5), *Candida* (1)	*Aspergillus* (1), *Cladosporium* (1), *Alternaria* (7), *Rhodotorula* (1), *Candida* (8)	0	*Aspergillus* (2), *Penicillium* (1), *Alternaria* (30)
Poultry house 4	*Aspergillus* (2), *Alternaria* (3)	*Mycelia sterilia* (1), *Candida* (1)	0	*Fusarium* (3), *Mycelia sterilia* (1), *Alternaria* (1), *Candida* (1)
Poultry house 5	*Aspergillus* (5), *Penicillium* (3), *Rhizopus* (1), *Alternaria* (1)	*Penicillium* (1), *Mycelia sterilia* (3)	0	*Penicillium* (1), *Mycelia sterilia* (1), *Alternaria* (4), *Dematiaceous fungi* (3), *Rhodotorula* (3)
Poultry house 6	*Aspergillus* (20), *Penicillium* (4), *Alternaria* (3), *Candida* (20),	-	0	*Penicillium* (1), *Mycelia sterilia* (3), *Alternaria* (5), *Fusarium* (1), *Candida* (7)
Poultry house 7	*Alternaria* (2), *Mucor* (1), *Mycelia sterilia* (3)	*Cladosporium* (8), *Alternaria* (2), *Trichosporon beigelii* (1)	*Cladosporium* (8), *Alternaria* (1), *Penicillium* (1)	*Aspergillus* (1), *Alternaria* (1), *Mycelia sterilia* (1)
Poultry house 8	*Alternaria* (1), *Mucor* (1), *Penicillium* (2)	-	0	*Aspergillus* (1), *Alternaria* (1), *Penicillium* (3)
Poultry house 9	*Mycelia sterilia* (6)	*Cladosporium* (10), *Alternaria* (1), *Mycelia sterilia* (1), *Rhodotorula* (20)	0	*Mucor* (1)
Poultry house 10	*Mycelia sterilia* (2), *Cladosporium* (1), *Dematiaceous fungi* (1), *Rhodotorula* (1)	*Alternaria* (3), *Cladosporium* (3), *Penicillium* (1)	*Stemphylium* (1), *Cladosporium* (2), *Alternaria* (1), *Penicillium* (2), *Mycelia sterilia* (1)	*Aspergillus* (7), *Cladosporium* (2), *Alternaria* (3), *Penicillium* (2), *Mycelia sterilia* (2), *Candida* (4)
Poultry house 11	*Cladosporium* (1), *Alternaria* (1), *Penicillium* (1), *Mycelia sterilia* (2), *Rhodotorula* (1)	*Cladosporium* (3), *Dematiaceous fungi* (1), *Rhodotorula* (1)	0	*Mycelia sterilia* (3), *Cladosporium* (1), *Dematiaceous fungi* (1), *Alternaria* (1)
Poultry house 12	*Alternaria* (4), *Mycelia sterilia* (2), *Candida* (3)	*Cladosporium* (8), *Mucor* (1),	0	*Alternaria* (20), *Mucor* (1), *Rhodotorula* (1)

Results of this study indicated that disinfection by spraying method of the poultry houses led to a 38.1% reduction in airspora concentration, while the application of fumigation, especially formaldehyde along with potassium permanganate, led to a 75% reduction in airspora concentration in the indoor air of poultry breeding houses, representing significant efficacy of fumigation method in reducing the airspora concentration ($p<0.05$).

Discussion

The presence of fungi in the indoor air of poultry house is a natural phenomenon. Microorganisms are constituents of saprophytic and pathogenic fungi, which were found in the poultry houses air. Aerial count of fungal elements in the indoor air of poultry house and monitoring of its emission from this building to the adjacent environment are important parameters for the assessment of the influence of poultry houses on the animals' health and environmental pollution (Lonc and Plewa, 2009). In the present study, fungal contamination in the indoor air was determined at 12 poultry breeding houses in Mazandaran province, Iran.

In the current study, a total of 48 impacted plates were collected, of which 36 were indoor air samples and 12 outdoor. Thirty-eight plates turned out positive. As shown in Table 1, the indoor concentration of fungi (no. 182 CFU) was to some extent higher than that of outdoor concentration (no. 181 CFU) at a distance of 20 meters from the poultry houses. No significant differences were observed between airspora in the indoor and outdoor air of poultry breeding houses. Baykov and Stoyanov (1999) also reported higher fungal levels inside poultry houses than in nearby areas and the average values were similar to our results.

The present study indicated 13 genera of fungi from the indoor air samples of poultry houses. The most predominant yeasts were *Candida* spp (30.2%), *Trichosporon* spp (6%), *Rhodotorula* spp (1.6%), and *Geotrichum* spp (0.5%), as well as nine genera of molds which were identified as follows: *Aspergillus* spp (26.9%), *Alternaria* spp (11.5%), *Mycelia sterilia* (9.9%), *Penicillium* spp (8.8%), *Chrysosporium* spp (1%), *Mucor* spp (1%), *Cladosporium* spp (1%), *Rhizopus* spp (0.5%), and *Dematiaceous fungi* (0.5%). While the share of yeasts in the entire pool of the determined fungi reached only 38.5%, molds constituted 61.5% in that pool, representing significant difference between molds and yeasts ($p<0.05$; Fig. 1). The fungal mycoflora isolated in these houses was largely diversified. A similar diversity was observed by other researchers, who surveyed poultry houses (Radon et al., 2002; Lugauskas et al., 2004; Karwowska, 2005). Furthermore, consistent with the data presented in their studies, the molds' population prevailed in the indoor air of breeding houses. According to the data obtained by Soliman et al. (2009), fungi, e.g. *Candida albicans*, *A. niger*, *A. nidulans*, *Penicilium* spp, and *Mucor* spp were prevalent in poultry farms in Egypt. However, Romanowska-Słomka and Mirosławski (2009) described the occurrence of the molds and yeasts such as, *Aspergillus*, *Penicillium*, *Candida* and *Cryptococcus* species, in the poultry houses.

Other investigators (Gigli et al., 2005; Nieguitsila et al., 2011) isolated and identified many fungal strains, including *Cladosporium* spp, *Aspergillus* spp, *Penicillium* spp, *Scopulariopsis* spp, *Fusarium* spp, *Epicoccum* spp, *Mucor* spp, *Trichophyton* spp, *Alternaria* spp, *Ulocladium* spp, *Basidiospores* spp, *Acremonium* spp, *Aureobasidium* spp, *Drechslera* spp, *Pithomyces* spp, *Chrysosporium* spp, *Geomyces* spp, and *Rhizomucor* spp from breeding houses. The presence of such fungi in poultry houses was proved by the results of our study.

The present study exhibited *Aspergillus* and *Candida* species as the predominant genera in the indoor air of poultry breeding houses, comprising over 50% of all the determined genera with a significant difference with other fungi ($p<0.05$). The high prevalence of these fungi could be related to humid environment of Mazandaran province. These results are in consistent with most studies, which mentioned *Aspergillus* species as the dominant mycoflora in the poultry house air (Jo et al., 2005; Vučemilo et al., 2007). This genus comprises many saprophytic species, as well as pathogens. *Aspergillus* species may induce aspergillosis and allergic symptoms in both human and birds (Flannigan et al., 2001; Libudzisz et al., 2007). According to the literature, *Candida* species were also isolated from the indoor air of poultry houses, but they do not always make the dominant fungal mycoflora (Radon et al., 2002; Lonc and Plewa, 2009; Rimac et al., 2010). Yeasts of genus *Candida* are ranked among opportunistic pathogens, which only in specific conditions (e.g. deficient immunity system) may induce various types of candidiasis in birds (Larone, 2002).

A total of 11 fungal genera were identified from the outdoor air samples of poultry houses. As shown in Table 2, *Alternaria* spp were the most frequent organisms with the frequency of 37.6% of the total fungal community. *Alternaria* spp are one of the most common fungi associated with asthma. Not only the presence of asthma, but also the persistence and severity of asthma is strongly associated with sensitization and exposure to *Alternaria* spp (Salo et al., 2006). In this study, other commonly occurring fungi from outdoor air were associated with *Candida* (19.3%), *Mycelia sterilia* (13.8%), *Penicillium* (10.5%), and *Aspergillus* (6.6%) species. In a study conducted by Shokri et al. (2010), *Alternaria*, *Cladophialophora*, and *Mucor* species were the most predominant fungi isolated from the air of different locations of Mazandaran province, Iran.

A good sanitation program of poultry breeding houses is the removal of old litter, cleaning, washing, and disinfecting, which are very important in controlling the accumulation and spread of disease-causing microorganisms (Lugauskas et al., 2004). This study was continued to determine whether different disinfection methods including spraying and fumigation are effective in reducing fungal populations. Results of this study indicated that disinfection by spraying method of the poultry houses led to a 38.1% reduction in airspora concentration, while the application of fumigation, especially formaldehyde along with potassium permanganate, led to a 75% reduction in airspora concentration in the indoor air of poultry breeding houses, representing significant efficacy of fumigation method in reducing the airspora concentration ($p<0.05$).

Finally, our study indicated that fumigation appears to be more effective for the inactivation of airspora as compared to routine chemical disinfectant solutions. A total of 100% reduction in the concentration of airspora was achieved in poultry breeding houses 3, 4, 5, 6, 8, 9, 11, and 12 after 48 hours of fumigation. In addition, an 83.3% and 66.7% reduction in airspora concentration was observed in poultry houses 1 and 2, respectively (Table 1). In contrast, airspora concentration increased in poultry houses 7 and 10 after disinfection by spraying and fumigation methods. Poultry houses 7 and 10 were disinfected only using one disinfectant solution (dispatag), while other houses used dispatag along with one or two other antiseptic solutions (chloracid 2000, nanosil, savlon, and formalin). Another probable explanation for this may be the fact that, in the houses 7 and 10, the litter bed system was not correctly removed. In fact, if disinfectants are used without properly cleaning the house prior to application, then the effectiveness of the disinfectants may be compromised. Many disinfectants are ineffective in the presence of organic matter, such as soil or litter (Witkowska et al, 2010). The application of disinfectants, level of organic charge, synergy, temperature, dilution rate, and examination methods influence the antimicrobial activity of disinfectants (Russel, 2003). The mechanisms of action of antiseptics and disinfectants on microorganisms include examination of uptake, lysis, and leakage of intracellular constituents, perturbation of cell homeostasis, effects on model membranes, and inhibition of enzymes, electron transport, and oxidative phosphorylation (McDonnell and Russell, 1999; Christopher et al., 2007). Previous studies demonstrated that any number of best management practices, treatments, or disinfectants can comprise a sanitation program. However, if used improperly, sanitation procedures can adversely affect disease prevention, thus, lowering bird performance (Davies et al., 1995). For this reason, it is important to routinely reevaluate the effectiveness of poultry house sanitation programs.

In summary, the dominant fungal mycoflora in the air of poultry breeding houses were molds (61.5%), with the most abundant *Aspergillus* genus. Yeasts constituted another 38.5% of fungal aerosol and were mainly represented by *Candida* spp. In addition, this research has demonstrated the potential for fumigation method to achieve a large percentage reduction in viable spore counts in the indoor air of poultry houses. Results of this study indicated that variables, such as application rate, disinfectant type, and the presence or absence of organic matter, are all important considerations when including a chemical disinfectant application into a sanitation program.

Acknowledgments

This study was funded by Research Council of Faculty of Veterinary Medicine, Amol University of Special Modern Technologies, Amol, Iran.

References

1. Araujo, R., Cabral, J.P. (2010) Fungal air quality in medical protected environments. In: Air Quality. Ashok, K. (ed.). (1st ed.) Sciyo Publisher. Sciyo, India. p. 357- 382.
2. Bakutis, B., Monsteviliene, E., Januskeviciene, G. (2004) Analyses of airborne contamination with bacteria, endotoxins and dust in livestock barns and poultry houses. Acta Vet Brno. 73: 283-289.
3. Baykov, B., Stoyanov, M. (1999) Microbial air pollution caused by intensive broiler chicken breeding. Microbiol Ecol. 29: 389-392.
4. Christopher, J.I., Geoff, W.H., Stephen, P.D. (2007) Action of disinfectant quaternary ammonium compounds against *Staphylococcus aureus*. Antimicrob Agents Chemother. 51: 296-306.
5. Davies, R.H., Wray, C. (1995) Observations on disinfection regimens used on *Salmonella enteritidis* infected poultry units. Poult Sci. 74: 638-647.
6. Dutkiewicz, J., Śpiewak, R., Jabłoński, L. (1999) Classification of occupational biohazards and exposed worker groups. Inst Med Wsi. 3: 143-148.
7. Eckman, M.K. (1994) Chemicals used by the poultry industry. Poult Sci. 73: 1429-1432.
8. Flannigan, B., Samson, R.A., Miller, J.D. (2001) Microorganisms in Home and Indoor Work Environments. CRC Press LLC. Boca Raton, USA.
9. Gigli, A.C.S., Baracho, M.S., Naas, I.A., Silva, R.A., Zago, R., Dall'Anese, F.P. (2005) Diagnosis and evaluation of fungi presence in the air of two different ventilation systems for broiler houses. Braz J Poult Sci. 7: 205-208.
10. Hashempour, A., Sadeghi Zali, M.H., Seyedgholizadeh, S., Malekan, M., Yahyapour, H. (2014) Prevalence of subclinical candidiasis in broiler flocks in Urmia, Iran. Sch J Agric Vet Sci. 1: 153-155.
11. Jo, W.K., Kang, J.H. (2005) Exposure levels of airborne bacteria and fungi in Korean swine and poultry sheds. Arch Environ Health. 60: 140-146.

12. Karwowska, E. (2005) Microbiological air contamination in farming environment. Polish J Environ Stud. 14: 445-449.
13. Khosravi, A.R., Bozorgmehrifard, M.H., Yahyaraeyat, R., Shokri, H. (2007) Identification of isolated fungi from different lesions of birds with aspergillosis referred to mycology research center, Faculty of Veterinary Medicine, University of Tehran. J Vet Res. 62: 243-246.
14. Larone, D.H. (2002) Medically Important Fungi. A Guide To Identification. (4th ed.) ASM Press. Washington D.C., USA.
15. Lee, S.A., Adhikari, A., Grinshpun, S.A., McKay, R., Shukla, R., Reponen, T. (2006) Personal exposure to airborne dust and microorganisms in agricultural environments. J Occup Environ Hyg. 3: 118-130.
16. Libudzisz, Z., Kowal, K., Żakowska, Z. (2007) Technical Microbiology. Wydawnictwo Naukowe PWN, Warszawa. Poland.
17. Lonc, E., Plewa, K. (2009) Microbiological air contamination in poultry houses. Polish J Environ Stud. 14: 445-449.
18. Lugauskas, A., Krikstaponis, A., Sveistyte, L. (2004) Airborne fungi in industrial environments- potential agents of respiratory diseases. Ann Agric Environ Med. 11: 19-25.
19. McDonnell, G., Russell, A.D. (1999) Antiseptics and disinfectants: activity, action, and resistance. Clin Microbiol Rev. 12: 147-179.
20. Nieguitsila, A., Arn´e, P., Durand, B. (2011) Relative efficiencies of two air sampling methods and three culture conditions for the assessment of airborne culturable fungi in a poultry farmhouse in France. Environ Res. 111: 248-253.
21. Pitt, J.I. (2000) A laboratory guide common *Penicillium* species. (3rd ed.) Food Science Australia Press. North Ryde, Australia.
22. Radon, K., Danuser, B., Iversen, M., Monso, E., Weber, C., Hartung, J. (2002) Air contaminants in different European farming environments. Ann Agric Environ Med. 9: 41-48.
23. Rimac, D., Macan, J., Varnai, V.M., Vučemilo, M., Matković, K., Prester, L. (2010) Exposure to poultry dust and health effects in poultry workers: impact of mould and mite allergens. Int Arch Occup Environ Health. 83: 9-19.
24. Romanowska-Słomka, I., Mirosławski, J. (2009) Biological hazards in an industrial poultry farm- research results. Bezpieczeństwo Pracy. 7: 16-19.
25. Russell, A.D. (2003) Biocide use and antibiotic resistance: the relevance of laboratory findings to clinical and environmental situations. Lancet Infect Dis. 3: 794-803.
26. Salo, P., Arbes, S., Sever, M., Jaramillo, R., Cohn, R., London, S., Zeldin, D. (2006) Exposure to *Alternaria alternata* in US homes is associated with asthma symptoms. J Allergy Clin Immunol. 118: 892-898.
27. Samson, R.A., Hoekstra, E.S., Frisvad, J.C. (2004) Introduction to Food- and Airborne Fungi. (7th ed.) Centraalbureau Voor Schim-Melcultures, Utrecht, The Netherlands.
28. Shokri, H., Khosravi, A.R., Naseri, A., Ghiasi, M., Ziapour, S.P. (2010) Common environmental allergenic fungi causing respiratory allergy in North of Iran. Int J Vet Res. 4: 169-172.
29. Soliman, S., Sobeih, M., Hussein, M., Abdel-Latiff, H., Moneim, A. (2009) Seasonal epidemiological surveillance on bacterial and fungal pathogens in broiler farms in Egypt. Int J Poult Sci. 8: 720-727.
30. Taghavi, M., Ghorbani-Choboghlo, H., Khosravi, A.R., Erfanmanesh, A., Balal, A. (2014) Fungal flora of the combs and wattles of Iranian native chickens. Iran J Microbiol. 6: 46-50.
31. Vučemilo, M., Matković, K., Vinković, B., Jakšić, S., Granić, K., Mas, N. (2007) The effect of animal age on air pollutant concentration in a broiler house. Czech J Anim Sci. 52: 170-174.
32. Witkowska, D., Chorąży, L., Mituniewicz, T., Makowski, W. (2010) Microbiological contamination of litter and air during rearing of broiler chickens [in Polish]. Water Environ Rural Areas. 10: 201-210.

Comparison of *Leptospira interrogans* infection in the goats and sheep

Rezaei, S.[1], Haji Hajikolaei, M.R.[1*], Ghadrdan Mashhadi, A.R.[1], Ghorbanpour, M.[2], Abdollahpour, G.[3]

[1]*Department of Clinical Sciences, Faculty of Veterinary Medicine, Shahid Chamran University of Ahvaz, Ahvaz, Iran*

[2]*Department of Pathobiology, Faculty of Veterinary Medicine, Shahid Chamran University of Ahvaz, Ahvaz, Iran*

[3]*Department of Internal Medicine, Faculty of Veterinary Medicine, University of Tehran, Tehran, Iran*

Key words:
goat, leptospirosis, seroprevalence, sheep,

Correspondence
Haji Hajikolaei, M.R.
Department of Clinical Sciences, Faculty of Veterinary Medicine, Shahid Chamran University of Ahvaz, Ahvaz, Iran

Email: mhajih@scu.ac.ir

Abstract:

BACKGROUND: Most leptospiral infections in sheep and goat are asymptomatic but may result in high fever, abortion, stillbirth, agalactiae. There is a different foraging behavior between sheep and goat that may cause the different prevalence of Leptospira interrogans infection in sheep and goats. **OBJECTIVES:** The purpose of the present study was to compare the prevalence of *L. interrogans* antibodies in sheep and goats. **METHODS:** Blood samples were taken from 246 sheep and 210 goats in 12 herds from 8 areas of Ahvaz where the animals were kept together. Sera were initially screened at dilution of 1:100 against 8 live serovars of *L. intrrogans*: pomana, canicola, hardjo, ballom, ictrohaemorrhagiae, grippotyphosa, tarasovi and australis using the microscopic agglutination test (MAT). **RESULTS:** The prevalence of leptospiral infection was 8.53% in sheep and 10.95% in goats. The highest reacting leptospira in both species was *L.i.* Pomona with a reactor rate of 68.18% in sheep and 56% in goats, followed in descending order by ictrohaemorrhagiae (18.8%), canicula, hardjo and grippotyphosa (each of them 4.54%), in sheep and ictrohaemorrhagiae (28%), canicula (16%) in goats. Statistical analysis showed that were no significant differences between sheep and goat (P=0.428). There were no significant differences among age groups in sheep (p=0.301) and goats (p= 0.363), but there was a tendency in adults sheep and goats (≥3years) to be more seropositive than young sheep and goats. Seroprevalence of leptospiral infection among various areas in sheep (p= 0.464) and goats (p= 0.710) was also not significantly different. **CONCLUSIONS:** It is concluded that there is no difference between sheep and goats in terms of leptospiral infection when they are kept together in the same herd and husbandry condition.

Introduction

Leptospirosis is a reemerging zoonotic disease of human and animals worldwide. It is presumed to be the most widespread zoonosis in the world. The disease is caused by pathogenic species of spirochetes of the genus leptospira (Samir et al., 2015). Among sheep and goats, most of the outbreak goes unnoticed due to lack of proper clinical signs and they usually react asymptomatically to the infection (OIE, 2000). The clinical manifestation of leptospires ranges from mild to severe life threatening disease with jaundice, renal failure or abortion during pregnancy (Shivaraj et al. 2009). Unfortunately, a definitive diagnosis of leptospirosis is difficult to make. Most diagnostic laboratories do not try to isolate leptospires because of their fragile nature, cost and complexity of the isolation media, and prolonged incubation period. Therefore, recognition of leptospiral infection has generally been based on serological evidence. Two tests have a role in veterinary diagnosis: the Microscopic Agglutination Test (MAT) and the Enzyme Linked Immunosorbent Assay (ELISA) (OIE, 2000)

Previous serological surveys of leptospiral infection in Ahvaz were carried out on cattle, horse and donkey (Hajikolaei et al., 2006, 2005a, 2005b) and two studies have been conducted to determine seroprevalence of leptospiral infection in goats and sheep, separately (Hajikolaei et al., 2007a, 2007b). A big different between sheep and goats is their foraging behavior and diet selection. Goats are natural browsers, preferring to eat leaves, twigs, vines and shrubs. They are very agile and will stand on their hind legs to reach vegetation. Goats like to eat the tops of plants. Sheep are grazers, preferring to eat short, tender grasses and clover. Their dietary preference is forbs and they like to graze close to the soil surface. These differences between sheep and goats may be responsible for the difference in prevalence of leptospiral infection in sheep and goats (Bojkovski et al., 2014). As there has been no study on comparison of leptospiral infection in sheep and goats in similar region, this study was undertaken to compare the prevalence of *L. interrogans* antibodies in sheep and goats in different areas of Ahvaz, the center of Khouzestan province in the southwest of Iran.

Materials and Methods

Blood samples were taken from 246 sheep and 210 goats from 8 areas of Ahvaz, in the southwest of Iran, during May to July of 2015. None of these animals had been vaccinated against leptospires and there was no history of leptospirosis-related symptoms or sign of the disease at the time of sampling. According to dental formula, these goats and sheep were divided into 5 ages groups (≤ 1, 1, 2, 3 and ≥4 years old). The number of samples of goats from area A to H were 40(A), 40(B), 40(C), 24(D), 14(E), 13(F), 16(G), 20(H) and those numbers of sheep were 40(A), 40(B), 40(C), 40(D), 20(E), 14(F), 21(G), 30(H), respectively.

The blood samples were allowed to clot and were centrifuged for 8 min at 3000g. After centrifugation, the sera were removed and stored at -20 °C until ready for test. The sera were tested for antibodies to 8 live antigens of *leptospira interrogans* (*L.introgans* serovars pomona, canicola, hardjo, ballum, ictrohemorrhagiae, grippotyphosa, tarasovi, australis) using the microscopic agglutination Test (MAT), in leptospiral research laboratory in faculty of veterinary medicine, university of Tehran. According to the methods of OIE, sera were initially screened at a dilution of 1:100 against these antigens. At first, serum dilution of 1:50 was performed and a volume of each serovar, equal to the diluted serum volume, was added to each well of microtitrations plates, making the final serum dilution 1:100. The microtitrations plates were incubated at 29 °C for 2h. The plates were examined by dark-field microscopy. Results were considered positive when 50% or more of agglutination of leptospires was found (OIE, 2000). Sera with positive result were titrated against reacting antigens in serial two-fold dilution from 1:100 to 1:800.

Statistical analysis was achieved using Chi-Square and Fisher's exact test which aimed to

Table 1. The Results of MAT on sheep and goats in some areas of Ahvaz-Iran.

Animals	No. positive (%)	No. negative (%)	No. exam
Sheep	21 (8.53)	225(91.47)	246
Goats	23 (10.95)	187(89.05)	210

detect differences between all variables.

Results

Out of 246 sheep and 210 goats tested, 21 (8.53%) and 23 (10.95%), were seropositive and antibodies against one or more serovars were detected (Table 1). One goat (4.76%) and two sheep (8.69%) were positive for more than one serovar. Significant difference (p= 0.428) between the sheep and goats as reactors to leptospires were not found. The highest number of reactors in sheep (68.2%) and goats (56%) was due to *L.introgans* serovar pomona, followed in descending order by icterohaemorrhagiae (18.2%), hardjo (4.5%), canicola (4.5%), and grypothyphosa (4.5%) in sheep and icterohaemorrhagiae (28%), and canicola (16%), in goats (Table 2). With the exception of one sample that had a titer level of 200, the other samples had a titer level of 100.

There was no significant difference among age groups in sheep (p=0.301) and goats (p= 0.363), but there was a tendency in adult sheep and goats (≥3years) to be more seropositive than the younger animals (Table 3 and 4). Distribution of leptospiral infection in sheep (p= 0.464) and goats (p= 0.710) among various areas was also not significantly different (Table 5 and 6). In area F, none of the examined sheep and goats have shown antibodies against various serovars of *L.interrogans* (Table 5, 6).

Discussion

Leptospirosis is an infectious zoonotic disease caused by different serotypes of the leptospires in any geographical area and information about the serotypes in one region may help the epidemiology and pathogenesis of this bacteria. Cattle are maintenance host for many serotypes of this bacteria. Sheep and goats are not naturally maintenance hosts for some of the serotypes such as pomona or hardjo and are likely to have infection of relatively short duration and produce severe pathologic effects. However, persistent leptospiruria and high seroprevalence rates of infection in sheep and goat where no contact with cattle have occurred suggest that sheep and goat may be a maintenance host for some serovars. This could complicate control of the infection in cattle, sheep and goat. Infected sheep and goat are a potential zoonotic risk to humans such as abattoir workers, sheep and goat farmers and shearers which previously had not been considered (Radostits et al., 2007). Long-term survival of pathogenic leptospires outside the host requires a warm, moist environment with a near natural pH (Miller et al., 1991). According to different foraging behavior in sheep and goats it is suspected that leptospiral infection in these animals has substantial differences but in this study there were no significant differences of the seroprevalence infection between sheep and goats in similar regions and situations. However, it may be due to the fact that neither of them like to get their feet wet and both prefer upland grazing to lowland that results in less exposure to leptospires (Bojkovski et al., 2014). We found that the seroprevaalence of leptospiral infection in goat and sheep in Ahvaz was 10.95% and 8.53%, respectively. The prevalence of leptospiral infection in goats and sheep from other countries based on serological survey has been reported to be 1.2%, 12.3%, 13.1, 14.3%, 16.8%, 32%, 40%, 42%, 42.1%, 55.2% and 70% in France, Italy, Nigeria, Bolivia, Greece, Croix, Belize, Australia, Egypt, India and New Zealand (Agunloye, 2002; Ciceroni et al., 1997; Flint et al., 1988; Maronpot and Barsoum, 1972; Sratnam, 1992; Trap and Gaumont, 1983) and

Table 2. The Prevalence of leptospiral antibody titer to different serovars in sheep and goats in some areas of Ahvaz-Iran. G-grypothyphosa, P-ponnona, I-icterohaemorrhagiae, C-canicola, H-hardjo, B-ballum, T- tarasovi, A-australis.

Animals	G	P	I	C	H	B	T	A
Sheep	1 (4.5%)	15 (68.2%)	4 (18.2%)	1 (4.5%)	1 (4.5%)	0 (0%)	0 (0%)	0 (0%)
Goats	0 (0%)	14 (56%)	7 (28%)	4(16%)	0 (0%)	0 (0%)	0 (0%)	0 (0%)

Table 3. Age distribution in leptospiral seroprevalence of sheep in some areas of Ahvaz-Iran.

Age (year)	No. positive (%)	No. negative (%)	Total (%)
<2	0 (0)	10 (100)	10 (4.06)
2	1 (2.7)	36 (97.29)	37 (15.04)
3	8 (13.33)	52 (86.66)	60 (24.39)
≥4	12 (8.63)	127 (91.37)	139 (56.50)
Total	21 (8.53)	225 (91.47)	246

Table 4. Age distribution in leptospiral seroprevalence of goat in some areas of Ahvaz-Iran.

Age (year)	No. positive (%)	No .negative (%)	Total(%)
<2	3 (5.36)	56 (94.64)	59 (28.09)
2	3 (13.04)	20 (86.96)	23 (10.95)
3	5 (13.51)	32 (86.49)	37 (17.61)
≥4	12 (13.18)	79 (86.82)	91 (43.33)
Total	23 (10.95)	187 (89.04)	210

14.3%, 19.7%, 4.2%, 60.4%, 6.1% and 16.8% in Bolivia, Argentina, Egypt, India, Italy and Greece, respectively (Ciceroni et al., 1997; Draghi et al., 1984; Maronpot and Barsonm, 1972; Stratname et al., 1992; Ciceroni et al., 2000 and Burriel et al., 2002).

There are some reports of leptospiral infection in goat and sheep from Iran (Hajikolaei et al., 2007a; 2007b; Hassanpour et al., 2012; Zainali et al., 1997; Ramin, AG and Azizzadeh, F., 2013). According to these reports, the seroprevalence of leptospiral infection in goat was 27.5%, 10.46% and 13.3% in Ahvaz, Uremia and Khoy, respectively and in sheep 14.9% and 19.3% respectively in Ahvaz and Uremia. The results of these reports confirm that prevalence of leptospiral infection in goat and sheep is different from region to region or country to country. These differences may be the consequence of environmental factors and control efforts (Maleki et al., 2014 and Milller et al., 1991). The results of this study showed that the serological infection rate in goat and sheep in Ahvaz is relatively high and consequently the preventive methods must be applied to stop the spread of disease and its transmission to the human and other farm animals and the important role of goat and sheep on the epidemiology of the infection must be emphasized. The predominant leptospire serovars in serological reaction varies somewhat among countries. For example, *L. interrogans* serovars poi and pommona in Bolivia (Ciceroni et al., 1997), wollfi, pomona and ballum in Argentina (Draghi et al, 1984), pomona in India (Manickavel et al., 1991), autumnalis in Egypt (Maronpot and Baarsoum, 1972) and pomona in Malaysia (Bahaman et al., 1987) were the predominant serovars in sheep and automnalis, pomona, automnalis, poi, bratislava and ictrohemorrhagiae were the common serovars in goats in Egypt, Nigeria, India, Bolivia, Italy and France, respectively (Agunloye, 2002; Cerri, 2003; Ciceroni et al., 1997; Maronpot and Barsoum, 1972 and Trap and Gaumont, 1983).

In this study, *L. interrogans* serovars pomona and icterohaemorrhagiae were detected as the

Table 5. Distribution of leptospiral infection in sheep from various areas of Ahvaz-Iran.

Area	No. positive (%)	No. negative (%)	Total
A	2 (5)	38 (95)	40
B	6 (15)	34 (85)	40
C	3 (7.5)	37 (92.5)	40
D	3 (7.5)	37 (92.5)	40
E	1 (5)	19 (95)	20
F	0 (0)	14 (100)	14
G	2 (9.09)	20 (90.9)	22
H	4 (13.33)	26 (86.67)	30
Total	21	225	246

Table 6. Distribution of leptospiral infection in goats from various areas of Ahvaz-Iran.

Area	No. positive (%)	No. negative (%)	Total
A	4 (10)	36 (90)	40
B	7 (17.5)	33 (82.5)	40
C	3 (7.5)	37 (92.5)	40
D	4 (16.66)	20 (83.33)	24
E	1 (6.66)	14 (93.33)	15
F	0 (0)	14 (100)	14
G	2 (11.76)	15 (88.23)	17
H	2 (10)	18 (90)	20
Total	23	187	210

most prevalent serovars with 68.18%, 18.8% and 56%, 28% in sheep and goats, respectively. In previous studies in Tehran, Tabriz, Ahvaz and Khorramabad, the predominant serovars in cattle were Pomona; Pomona; grippotyphosa and Pomona; canicola and grippotyphosa, respectively, respectively (Hajikolaei et al., 2007; Hassanpour et al., 2012; Maleki et al., 2013). It is probable that this serovar may be adapted to and maintained by these farm animals in Ahvaz. There is a need for futher investigation on clinical cases of leptospirosis to determine whether this serovar is the main cause of leptospirosis in this region.

Percentage of seropositive for more than one serovar was 8.6% and 4.76% in seropositive goats and sheep, respectively. In serological tests for leptospirosis such as MAT, the results often indicate infection with more than one serovar (Egan and Yearly, 1989; Hajikolaei et al, 2005, Hataway et al., 1981). This may be the result of mixed serovar infection but the existence of cross reactivity in the MAT among the serovars is well known and can be excluded from this interpretation. The high prevalence of infection and dominant titre of 1:100 reveal that leptospiral infection in goats and sheep in Ahvaz (in the southwest of Iran) is endemic and occurs mostly in subclinical form. There were no significant differences among the ages and areas groups in sheep and goats, but there was a tendency in adult sheep and goats (≥3 years) to be more seropositive than young sheep and goats that is in agreement with the other studies (Hassanpour et al., 2008 and 2012 and Maleki et al., 2014).

These results confirm that leptospiral infection may exist in the goat and sheep population in Ahvaz area and the presence of antibodies in the absence of infection indicates the exposure to the organism and must be acknowledged. In addition, these results confirm that the majority of leptospiral infections is asymptomatic. Because of the importance of leptospira interrogans as an abortifacient agent in goat and sheep, it will be considered as one of the possible causes of abortion in goat and sheep in Ahvaz, southwestern Iran.

Acknowlegments

The authors would like to acknowledge the research vice chancellor of Shahid Chamran University of Ahvaz for financial support.

References

1. Agunloye, C.A. (2002) Leptospiral agglutination antibodies in sheep and goat in southwest Nigeria. Israel Vet Med Assoc. 57: 2.
2. Bahaman, A.R., Ibrahim, A.L., Adam, H. (1987) Serological prevalence of leptospiral infection in domestic animals in west Malaysia. Epidemiol Infect. 99: 379-392.
3. Bojkovski, D., Stuhee, I., Kompan, D., Zupan, M. (2014) The behavior of sheep and goats co-grazing on pasture with defferent types of vegetation in the karst region. J Anim Sci. 92: 2752-278.
4. Burriel, A.R., Vougiouka, D.M., Butsini, S., Nomikou, K., Patakakis, M. (2002) A serological investigation of some causes of reproductive failure among small ruminants in Greece. Online J Vet Res. 6: 57-63.
5. Cerri, D., Ebani, V.V., Fratini, F., Pinzauti, P., Andreani, E. (2003) Epidemiology of leptospirosis: observation on serological data obtained by a diagnostic laboratory for leptospirosis from 1995 to 2001. New Microbiol. 26: 383-389.
6. Ciceroni, L., Bartoloni, A., Pinto, A., Guglielmetti, P., Vasquez, C.V. (1997) Serological survey of leptospiral infection in sheep, goats and dogs in Cordillera province, Bolivia. New Microbiol. 20: 77-81.
7. Ciceroni, L., Lombordo, D., Pinto, A., Ciarrocchi, S., Simeoni, J. (2000) Prevalence of antibodies to leptospira serovars in sheep and goats in Alto Adige-South Tyrol. J Vet Med. 47: 217-223.
8. Draghi de Benitez, M.G., Zubriggen, M.A., Vanzini, V.R. (1984) Serological survey for ovine leptospirosis in Correentes province, Argentina. Vet Argent. 1: 336-340.
9. Egan, J., Yearley, D.A. (1989) Serological survey of leptospiral infection in Republic of Irland. Vet Rec. 119: 306.
10. Flint, S.H., Corner, R.J., Marshall, R.B. (1988). Leptospirosis in farmed goats. New-Zealand. Vet J. 36: 156-158.
11. Haji Hajikolaei, M.R., Ghorbanpour, M., Keshavarzi-Yangabadi, M., Abdollapour, G.R. (2007a) Seroprevalence of leptospiral infection in goats of Ahvaz. Iran J Vet Res. 4: 93-96.
12. Haji Hajikolaei, M.R., Ghorbanpour, M., Gharibi, D., Abdollapour, G.R. (2007b) Serologic study on leptospiral infection in sheep of Ahvaz, southwestern Iran. J Vet Res. 8: 333-336.
13. Haji Hajikolaei, M.R., Ghorbanpour, M., Abdollapour, G.R. (2005a) Serological study of leptospirosis in cattle in Ahvaz. J Vet Res (University of Tehran). 60: 7-14.
14. Haji Hajikolaei, M.R., Ghorbanpour, M., Haidari, M., Abdollapour, G.R (2005b) Comparison of leptospiral infection in the horse and donkey. Bull Vet Inst Pulawy. 49: 175-178.
15. Hasanpor, A., Asgarloo, S., Imandar, M., Mashayekhi, M., Abdollhapour, G.R., Safarmashaei, S. (2012) Seroepidemiologic study of Goats leptospirosis in Khoy-Iran. J Anim Vet Adv. 11: 229-233.
16. Maleki, S.H., Abdollapour, G.R., Bahonar, A.R. (2013) Serological and bacteriological study of leptospirosis in dairy herds and feedlot in Tehran areas. Iran J Vet Med. 7: 177-183.
17. Maleki, S.H. (2014) Serological study on leptospiral infection in goats in Khorramabad. Bull Georg Natl Acad Sci. 8: 553-558.
18. Manickavel, K., Kalyanasundaram, C.K., Venkataraman, K.S., Rao, V.N.A., Thanagavelu, S. (1991) Reports on leptospirosis in sheep in Tamil Nadu. Indian Vet J. 68: 503-505.
19. Maronpot, R.R., Barsoum, I.S. (1972) Lepto-

spiral Microscopic agglutination antibodies in sera of man and domestic animals in Egypt. Am J Tropic Clinic Microbiol. 30: 2219-2224.

20. Miller, D.A., Wilson, M.A., Beran, G.W. (1991) Relationship between prevalence of *Leptospira introgans* in cattle and regional climatic and seasonal factors. Am J Vet Res. 52: 1761-1768.
21. O.I.E. (2000) Manual of standards of diagnostic tests and vaccines, leptospirosis, part 2, section 22: chapter 2.2.4., Paris, France.
22. Radostits, O.M., Gay, C.C., Hinchcliff, K.W., Constable, P.D. (2007) Veterinary Medicine: A Textbook of the Disease of Cattle, Horses, Sheep, Pigs and Goats. (10th ed.) Saunders Elsevier, Philadelphia, PA, USA.
23. Ramin, A.G., Azizzadeh, F. (2013) Seroepidemiological detection of antibodies against leptospiral spp using microscopic agglutination test in uremia cows and sheep. Acta Vet. 63: 53-61.
24. Saglama, Y.S., Yenerb, Z., Temurc, A., Yalcinc, E. (2007) Immonohistochemical detection of leptospiral antigens in cases of naturally occurring abortion in sheep. Small Rumin Res. 74: 119-122.
25. Samir, A., Soliman, R., El-Hariri, M., Abdel-Moein, K.H., Hatem, M.E. (2015) Leptospirosis in animal and human contacts in Egypt: broad range surviilance. Rev Soc Bras Med Trop. 48: 272-727.
26. Shivaraj, M.D., Venkatesha, Rajkumari, S., Sripad, K., Sanjeevkumar, B., Chandranaik, M., Renukapraasad, C. (2009) Leptopriosis in sheep and its diagnosis. Vet World. 2: 263-264.
27. Sratnam, K.L. (1992) Leptospiral antibodies among sheep and goat. Indian J Anim Sci. 62: 1041-1043.
28. Zainali, A., Vand-yousefi, J., Ahoraei, P. (1997) The survey of leptospiral infection in Uremia. J Pajouhesh Va Sazandegi (In Persian). 37: 76-78.

Isolation, phenotypic and molecular characterization of motile *Aeromonas* species, the cause of bacterial hemorrhagic septice-mia in affected farmed carp in Iran

Soltani, M.[1*], Moghimi, S.M.[1], Ebrahimzade Mousavi, H.[1], Abdi, K.[2], Soltani, E.[3]

[1]*Department of Aquatic Animal Health, Faculty of Veterinary Medicine, University of Tehran, Tehran, Iran*
[2]*Aquatic Animal Health Expert, Office of Health and Control of Aquatic Animal Diseases, Iranian Veterinary Organization, Tehran, Iran*
[3]*Department of Microbiology, Faculty of Science, University of Tehran, Tehran, Iran*

Key words:
Farmed carp, Motile *Aeromonas* septicemia, 16S rRNA gene

Correspondence
Soltani, M.
Department of Aquatic Animal Health, Faculty of Veterinary Medicine, University of Tehran, Tehran, Iran

Email: msoltani@ut.ac.ir

Abstract:

BACKGROUND: Motile *Aeromonas* species cause heavy mortalities in carp farms during spring and summer in Iran. **OBJECTIVES:** The aim of this study was to detect phenotypic and genotypic characterization of motile *Aeromonas* species isolated from diseased carps in some northern and southern provinces of Iran. **METHODS:** A number of 40 samples from 22 fish farms were collected. The identified motile *Aeromonas* species were sequenced and phylogenetic tree was drawn by MEGA6 using UPGMA analysis. **RESULTS:** A number of 19 bacterial isolates were identified as motile *Aeromonas* sp. by biochemical tests, and the DNA segments of 16S rRNA gene of all these strains gave 1200 bp after running on 1% agarose electrophorus gel. Also, the sequencing results showed that the bacterial samples were determined as *A. hydrophila* and *A. veronii* biovar veronii. **CONCLUSIONS:** Phylogenetic analysis revealed that motile *Aeromonas* strains in this study were separated in two clusters and four genogroups with high similarities.

Introduction

Aeromonas hydrophila and other motile *Aeromonas* species which cause motile *Aeromonas* septicemia are known as the most common bacterial infections in freshwater aquaculture worldwide (Borrell et al., 1997; Leblanc, et al., 1981; Woo et al., 2011; Henebry et al., 1988). The species of *A. hydrophila, A. sobria, A. caviae* and *A. veronii* are the cause of carp mortalities (Popoff and VéEron, 1976; Garrity et al., 2004). Motile *Aeromonas* species cause some pathologic conditions including acute, chronic and latent infections with different clinical signs (Soltani, 2002). The disease occurrence is common in spring and summer in farmed carp that is related to high temperature, fish metabolism and organic loading rate (Soltani, 2002). According to the Iranian veterinary organization, the most epizootics occur in the north and south regions of Iran where the carp aquaculture is located (Iranian Veterinary Organization, unpublished data, 2011). So far, some epizootics of the disease have occurred in various species of carp in the north and south provinces (Peyghan and Esmaili, 1997; Soltani et al., 1998; Alishahi et al., 2009). Although the morphological and biochemical approaches have been applied to identify the genus *Aeromonas* in Iran, there is no adequate data on the phylogenetic position of the *Aeromonas* species involved in morbidity and mortality of carps. Therefore, the aim of this study was to isolate and characterize the motile *Aeromonas* species involved in carp mortality in the north and south regions of the country. Such data are useful for prevention and control criteria of disease and outbreaks.

Materials and Methods

Collection of bacterial isolates and phenotypic identification: After collecting 40 samples from different carp ponds, a total of 19 *Aeromonas* strains were isolated from common carp (*Cyprinus carpio*) and silver carp (*Hypophthalmichthys molitrix*) with clinical symptoms of bacterial infection such as hemorrhages in skin and gill, exophthalmia and dropsy. The samples were collected from three different geographical locations in Iran during a two-year period (2014 - 2015): 10 samples from Mazandaran province, 14 samples from Gilan province and 16 samples from Khuzestan province. The samples were isolated from kidney, cultivated on blood agar and incubated at 30°C for 72 h. First, the morphological characteristics of the colonies were identified by Gram staining which confirmed the bacterial colonies were Gram negative. Biochemical tests were carried out in all strains including SIM (Sulfide, Indole, and Motility), gelatin and esculin hydrolysis, lysine and ornothine decarboxylase, nitrate reduction, fermentation and gas production of glucose, maltose and inositol, triple sugar iron agar (TSI), methyl red and voges-proskauer (MRVP) tests.

DNA extraction: The DNA Biospin Bacteria Genomic Extraction Kit, Bioflux Co. (Gapan) was used to extract the genomic DNA. Briefly, a volume of 10 ml of culture was collected by centrifugation for 1min at 14000 g and resuspended in 100 µl of EL buffer incubated at 37°C for 40 min. Then RS buffer and PK solution were added, respectively and incubated at 56°C for 15 min. 200 µl of GA buffer was then added and centrifuged at 12,000 x g for 1 min and the supernatant was transferred to a new 1.5ml tube. An aliquot of 400 µl of BA buffer was then added and centrifuged at 10,000 x g for 1 min. A volume of, 500 µl of G binding buffer was then added into the spin column and centrifuged at 10,000 x g for 1 min. A volume of 500 µl of washing buffer was added to the spin column and centrifuged at 10,000 x g for 1 min two times. After transferring the spine column to a sterile 1.5ml micro centrifuge tube, 100 µl of elution buffer was added and the mixture was incubated at room temperature for 1 min, centrifuged at 12,000 x g for 1 min. The spin column was removed with the buffer in the micro centrifuge tube containing the DNA. The analysis of DNA concentration and quality were based on the 260 /280 nm and absorbance ratio using the spectrophotometer (Biophotometer Eppendorf) according to manufacturer's instructions. The solution was kept at -20°C when stored.

Polymerase chain reaction: The polymerase chain reaction was used to detect the presence of the 16S rRNA gene in all isolates. Briefly, the 25 µl PCR mix consisted of 2.5µl 10x reaction buffer, Fermentas Co. (Lithuania), 0.2U Taq polymerase, 1µl of the two primer solutions (forward: 5′-AGA GTT TGA TCA TGG CTC AG -3′; reverse: 5′-GGT TAC CTT GTT ACG ACT T-3′), 4µl mix dNTP (2.5mM each) and 1µl of DNA sample. PCR was carried out on the thermocycler Bio-Rad Co. (USA) performed the following cycles of denaturation at 94°C for 3 min followed by 35 cycles at 94°C for 1 min, annealing at 45°C for 1 min and extension at 72°C for 1/5 min and an extension cycle at 72°C was allowed for 10 min. Negative controls with no template DNA were included. Also, PCR products were electrophoresed in 1% agarose gel in TBE buffer. The gel was stained with GenDireX (Biohelix-USA) and photographed on a UV transilluminator XR-plus, Bio-Rad Co. (USA). The identified *Aeromonas* strains by 16S rRNA PCR analysis on 1% agarose gel electrophoresis were then sequenced directly by

Table 1. Biochemical characteristics of *A. hydrophila* isolates in this study.

Tests	M1	M2	M3	M4	G1	G2	G3	G4	G5	K1	K3	K4	K5	K7	K9
Indole	+	+	+	+	+	+	+	+	+	+	+	+	+	+	+
Motility	+	+	+	+	+	+	+	+	+	+	+	+	+	+	+
H2S	+	-	+	+	+	+	+	+	+	+	+	+	+	+	+
Gelatin hydrolysis	-	-	+	+	+	+	+	+	+	-	+	-	+	+	+
Ornithine decarboxylase	-	-	-	-	-	-	-	-	-	-	-	-	-	-	-
Nitrate reduction	+	+	+	+	+	+	+	+	+	+	+	+	+	+	+
MR	+	+	+	+	+	+	+	+	+	+	+	+	+	+	+
VP	+	+	+	+	+	+	+	+	+	+	+	+	+	+	+
TSI	-/+	-/-	-/-	-/-	-/-	-/+	+/+ Gas	+/+ Gas	+/+ Gas	+/+	+/+ Gas	+/+ Gas	+/+	+/+	+/+ Gas
Lysine decarboxilase	+	+	+	+	+	+	+	+	+	+	+	+	-	-	+
Esculin hydrolysis	+	+	-	-	+	+	+	+	+	+	+	+	+	+	+
Inositol fermentation	-	-	-	-	-	-	-	-	-	-	-	-	-	-	-
Maltose fermentation	+	+	+	+	+	+	+	+	+	-	-	-	-	-	-
Glucose fermentation	+	+	+	+	+	+	+	+	+	+	+	+	+	+	+
Gas production of glucose	+	-	-	-	+	+	-	-	-	-	-	-	-	-	-

Table 2. Biochemical characteristics of *A. veronii* isolates in this study.

Tests	K2	K6	K8	K10
Indole	+	+	+	+
Motility	+	+	+	+
H2S	+	+	+	+
Gelatin hydrolysis	-	+	+	+
Ornithine decarboxylase	-	-	-	-
Nitrate reduction	+	+	+	+
MR	+	+	+	+
VP	+	+	+	+
TSI	+/+	+/-	+/+	+/+
Lysine decarboxilase	+	+	+	+
Esculin hydrolysis	-	-	-	-
Inositol fermentation	-	-	-	-
Maltose fermentation	-	-	-	-
Glucose fermentation	-	+	+	+
Gas production of glucose	-	-	-	-

Takapouzist Co. (Tehran, Iran). The results were aligned by the Finch TV software and then compared with available sequences in GeneBank using BLAST service. The phylogenetic tree was drawn by MEGA6 using UPGMA analysis.

Results

Clinical signs and gross pathology: Fish samples collected from 22 farms showed distinct clinical signs of lethargy, anorexia, loss of balance, exophthalmia, ulcers, hemorrhages in skin and gill and abdominal distention (Figs. 1 and 2). Internally, the spleen was enlarged and hemorrhagic. Petechial hemorrhages were observed on the surface of kidney, intestines and many tissues. Also, accumulation of ascetic fluid was observed in almost all the diseased fish.

Biochemical tests: In primary phenotypic tests, grown colonies were gram negative, cocobacilli shaped, motile and oxidase positive which are supposed to be in genus *Aeromonas*. The results of the biochemical tests were compared with the key table in Bergey's manual systematic bacteriology to determine the species. The results are shown in Tables 1and 2.

Analysis of 16S rRNA gene PCR: The results of PCR amplification of DNA from bacterial strains showed the expected amplicons of 1200 bp (Fig. 3).

Sequencing and phylogenetic analysis: The sequencing of the PCR products resulted in detection of KT378601, KT378602, KT378603, KT378604, KU201534,

Table 3. The Aeromonas strains isolated from carp ponds (sampling region, number of fish samples, number of isolated strains of motile Aeromonas, laboratory code and accession number).

Region	Number of fish samples	Number of isolates identified as Aeromonas sp.	Laboratory Code	Accession Number
Khuzestan State	16	10	K1, K2, K3,K4, K5,K6, K7, K8, K9, K10	KU201536, KU201537, KU201538, KU201539, KU201540, KU216160, KU216161, KU216162, KU216163, KU216164
Gilan State	14	5	G1, G2, G3 G4, G5	KT378601, KT378602, KU201534, KU201535, KU257639
Mazandaran State	10	4	M1, M2, M3, M4	KT378603, KT378604, KU257637, KU257638

KU201535, KU201536, KU201537, KU201538, KU216160, KU216161, KU216164, KU257637, KU257638 and KU257639 as *A. hydrophila* and KU201539, KU201540, KU216162 and KU216163 as *A. veronii* biovar veronii (Table 3). The MEGA 6 software has been applied to show the phylogenetic relationship between all isolates in this study (Fig. 4). According to the phylogenetic tree, high similarities were observed among motile *Aeromonas* species isolated from carps in Iran. The strains were classified in two clusters, A and B with 1.6% variations. There were two genogroups in cluster A, genogroup A1 and A1. In genogroup A1, the similarity between the strain, KU216163 and the other strains including KU216162, KU257637 and KU201154 was 99.4%. Also, the cluster A was divided to two genogroups, B1 and B2 with 99.3% similarity. In genogroup B1, the similarity between the two strains, KU216160 and KU216164 and the strains, KU216161, KU257637, KU 257638 and KU257639 was 99.5%. Also, the strains in genogroup B2 showed high similarities so that the similarity between the strain, KU201537 and the others strains was 99.5%.

Discussion

Recently, there have been many reports of heavy mortalities in carps during spring and summer in Iran. Although motile *Aeromonas* species are usually known as secondary opportunistic pathogens, they can be as primary pathogens in some conditions. So, there are no effective approaches for control and treatment of disease in carp farms since Aeromons infection is related to the environmental conditions and physicochemical parameters of water. Therefore, isolation and identification of the bacteria would be useful for control and prevention of disease. Today, molecular techniques are used widely since they provide a relatively rapid and highly sensitive method for the detection of bacterial pathogens (Chu and Lu, 2005). In this regard the most commonly used gene for taxonomic and phylogenetic purposes in bacteria is the 16S rRNA which is the most conserved gene in bacteria (Clarridge, 2004; Roy et al., 2013). In the present study, various biochemical tests have been applied to identify 40 clinical isolates of motile *Aeromonas* sp. Also, 19 isolates have been characterized as motile *Aeromonas* sp. by PCR analysis of 16S rRNA gene. Most results from both approaches have shown similarities, however, some discrepancies have been observed. Four strains, KT378602, KU257637, KU257638 and KT378603 that were characterized as *A. veronii* biochemically (esculin hydrolysis negative), were identified by PCR and DNA sequencing as *A. hydrophila*. Also, the gelatin hydrolysis test was negative in five

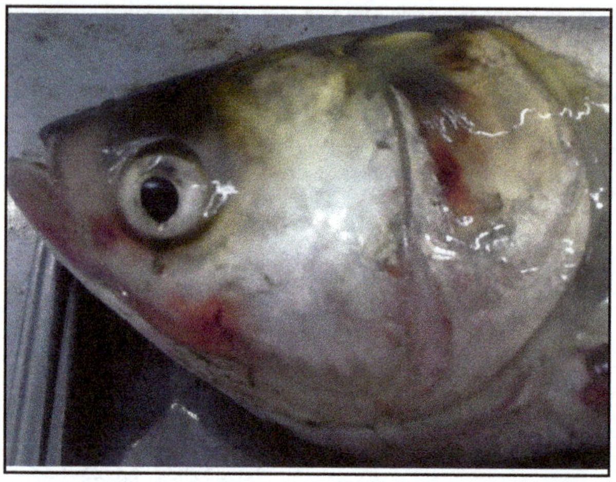

Figure 1. Skin hemorrhage and exophthalmia of silver carp (H. molitrix).

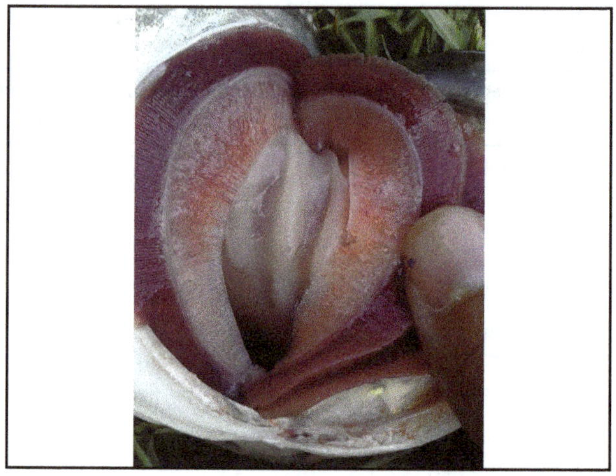

Figure 2. Hemorrhage in gill filaments of silver carp (H. molitrix).

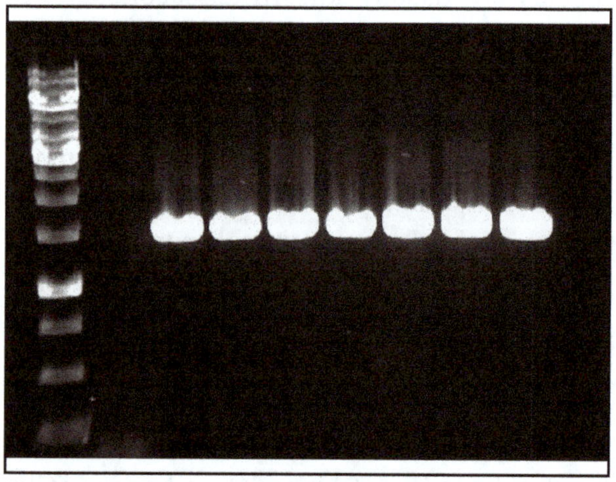

Figure 3. PCR detection of 16S rRNA genes in several Aeromonas recovered from diseased carp in Iran. Lane M= 1 kbp DNA ladder, Lane 1= negative control, Lane 2= positive control (*Aeromonas hydrophila* - IRTCC1032), Lane 3 to 8= several test samples.

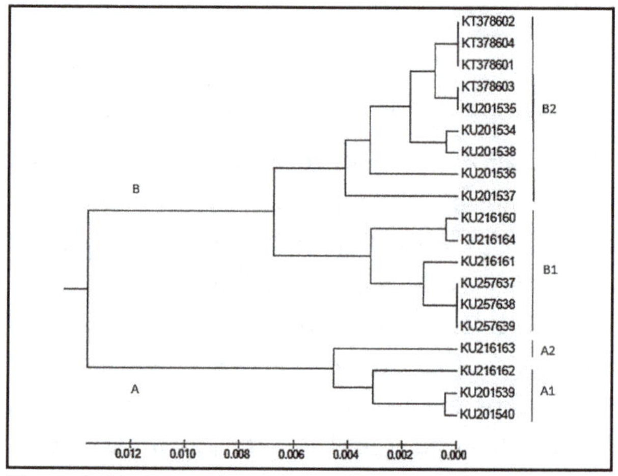

Figure 4. Phylogenetic analysis of Aeromonas strains based on the 16S rRNA sequences using UPGMA method.

strains, KT378601, KT378602, KU216160 and KU201537 and KU201439. But they identified phylogenetically as *A. hydrophila* and *A. veronii*. These results were confirmed by repeating the tests. Such discrepancies may result from the fact that biochemical tests are not reliable for identification of *Aeromonas* sp.. Other strains showed the same results in both biochemical and molecular tests. The phylogenetic tree of 19 bacterial isolates of this study showed 97.2-100% similarity based on the analysis of 16S rRNA gene. Such similarities among the isolates of the country can be applied to promote some prevention methods like vaccination.

Alzahrani (2015) used the 16S rRNA gene to identify and characterize *Aeromonas* species in drinking water since this gene is known as a specific molecular marker for bacterial identification and is useful for the bacterial molecular taxonomy. The results showed that all bacterial samples were *A. veronii* or a new species. Moreover, classical tests as well as molecular studies on the 16S rRNA gene have been applied by Sarkar et al. (2012) for classification of the phylogenetic relationships among *Aeromonas* species isolated from various sources. The biochemical and molecular results were similar to those of the present study and the isolates registered in GeneBank were used for comparison with the isolates of this study by using MEGA6 software. The results showed similarities in 16S rRNA sequences of the strains even though the samples have been collected from different sources. Arora et al. (2006) applied several methods to identify *Aeromonas* species and concluded that both indirect ELISA and duplex-PCR are reliable methods to detect *Aeromonas* species in foods of animal origin due to their specificity and duplex-PCR is the best method among others used in the study on account of its rapidity, sensitivity and specificity. Borrel et al. (1997) used the same gene to identify *Aeromonas* species from different clinical samples such as blood, soft tissue infection and urine. Most results from the biochemical tests and RFLP method were similar but some discrepancies were seen. For instance, some species detected biochemically as *A. veronii* were characterized as *A. hydrophila* and *A. caviae* by RFLP analysis. In conclusion, the RFLP method is proposed as a rapid and reliable method without the need for sequencing to identify *Aeromonas* species. In addition to the 16S rRNA gene, many virulence genes have been detected to identify *Aeromonas* species (Sechi et al., 2002; Yogananth et al., 2009; Uma et al., 2010; Cagatay and Şen, 2014; Hussain et al., 2014). Among the virulence factors of motile *Aeromonas* species, antigen-O, the presence of capsule, S layer, exotoxins such as hemolysins and enterotoxins, exoenzymes such as lipase, amylase and protease and the type III secretion system are well known (Oliveira et al., 2012). Hussain et al. (2014) studied the ahh1, asa1 and 16S rRNA genes by using multiplex PCR to detect the hemolytic strains of *Aeromonas* isolated from fish and fishery products. The results proved the presence of 16S rRNA and asa1 genes in *A. sobria*, 16S rRNA and ahh1 genes in *A. hydrophila* and 16S rRNA gene in *A. liquifaciencs* and provided reliable data to detect the hemolytic strains of *Aeromonas*. In the study of Cagatay and Şen (2014) on the virulence genes of *A. hydrophila* regarding the cause of bacterial hemorrhagic septicemia in rainbow trout, the AHCYTOEN, Hly and OmpTS genes have been detected. All these genes were detected in the *Aeromonas* strains and are known as specific virulence determinants and genetic markers to identify the bacteria before the disease spread. Biochemical tests as well as PCR for detecting the aerolysin and hemolysin genes of *Aeromonas* strains have been carried out by Yoganath et al. (2009) in which seven strains of 15 strains have been identified as *A. hydrophila*. The PCR assay applied in this study was known as a useful tool to detect the aerolysin and hemolysin genes which can be the genetic virulence markers. A similar study has been done by Uma et al. (2010) that indicated the aerolysin and hemolysin genes are a better indicator of the potential health risk since the pathogenicity of *Aeromonas* strains is associated with such virulence factors. Besides the molecular and biochemical tests, the LD50 determination can be used to identify the virulent *Aeromonas* strains, as Alishahi et al. (2009) applied this method to detect the pathogenic motile *Aeromonas* species. The results showed the presence of *A. hydrophila* (%11), *A. veronii* (%4) and *A. sobria* (%2.7) from a total of 300 samples. Also, *Aeromonas* species were known as the secondary pathogens since they have not presented enough virulence needs for mortalities.

Furthermore, motile *Aeromonas* infection is related to the physicochemical parameters of water quality which can exacerbate the disease outbreaks. In the present study, water temperature was higher than the standard levels and the acidity of water was in the maximum range. Other parameters including dissolved oxygen, carbon dioxide, total hardness as calcium carbonate, nitrite, nitrate and total dissolved solids were in the normal ranges. According to previous studies on detecting *Aeromonas* sp. in carp ponds, this bacteria was known as a secondary pathogen and the disease can occur at stress conditions (Alishahi et al., 2009). Recently, the motile *Aeromonas* species have been isolated from warm water fish in Iran and numerous factors can be associated with the incidence of the disease. Some of these factors were mentioned in the following: The temperature in summer is more than 40 °C as a result of climate change and the ammonia level and the acidity of water occasionally increase in warm weather. Also, the atmospheric pressure decreases in summer and as a result the water capacity to keep oxygen reduces. Another reason of reducing the dissolved oxygen level is toxins produced by algae which increase the organic loading range in water. Further, unsuitable structure of fish ponds leads to an inadequate water exchange and prevent refilling water. Waste water is periodically used for filling the ponds. The organic loading rate increases by the use of animal-based fertilizer in feeding fish. Besides, the owners do not pay attention to the rules and regulations defined by the responsible organizations about the control and prevention of the disease in summer. In this regard, several methods are suggested to prevent the disease such as systematically preparing the ponds before new larva and fish are put into the ponds, water filtration, quarantine process and collecting the dead fish on a daily basis and reporting the mortality rate to the veterinary organization.

In addition, the carp species are sensitive to some viral diseases such as Spring Viremia of Carp (SVC) and Koi Herpes Virus (KHV). Recently, several fresh water ornamental fishes were imported to the country for research aims and experimental studies. SVCV and KHV were detected in the imported ornamental fishes (Soltani, unpublished data, 2012; Zamani et al., 2014). So occurrence of the viral diseases in carp pond is possible and needs further studies.

Acknowledgments

This work was financially supported by Iranian Veterinary Organization, Center of Excellence of Aquatic Animal Health and Research Council of University of Tehran.

References

1. Alishahi, M., Soltani, M., Zargar, A. (2009) Study of the mortality of grass carp (*Ctenopharyngodon idella*) in Khuzestan province. Iran Vet J. 4: 25-34.
2. Borrell, N., Acinas, S.G., Figueras, M.J., Martinez-Murcia, A.J. (1997) Identification of Aeromonas clinical isolates by restriction fragment length polymorphism of PCR-amplified 16S rRNA genes. J Clin Microbiol. 35: 1671-1674.
3. Brenner, D.J., Krieg, N.R., Staley, J.T. (2005) Bergey's Manual of Sustematic Bacteriology (2nd ed.). Baltimore, USA.
4. Cagatay, I.T., Sen, E.B. (2014) Detection of pathogenic *Aeromonas hydrophila* from rainbow trout (*Oncorhynchus mykiss*) farms in Turkey. Intl J Agric Biol. 16: 435-438.
5. Chu, W.H., Lu, C.P. (2005) Multiplex PCR assay for the detection of pathogenic *Aeromonas hydrophila*. J Fish Dis. 28: 437-441.
6. Clarridge, J.E. (2004) Impact of 16S rRNA gene sequence analysis for identification of bacteria on clinical microbiology and infectious diseases. Clin Microbiol Rev. 17: 840-862.
7. Garrity, G.M., Bell, J.A., Lilburn, T.G. (2004) Taxonomic Outline of the Prokaryotes. Bergey's Nanual of Systematic Bacteriology. (2nd ed.). New York, USA.
8. Henebry, M.S., Gorden, R.W., Buck, D.H. (1988) Bacterial populations in the gut of the silver carp (*Hypophthalmichthys molitrix*). Prog Fish Cult. 50: 86-92.
9. Hussain, I., Jeyasekaran, G., Shakila, R.J., Raj, K., Jeevithan, E. (2014) Detection of hemolytic strains of *Aeromonas hydrophila* and *A. sobria* along with other *Aeromonas* spp. from fish and fishery products by multiplex PCR. J Food Sci Technol. 51: 401-407.
10. Leblanc, D., Mittal, K., Olivier, G., Lallier, R. (1981) Serogrouping of motile Aeromonas species isolated from healthy and moribund fish. Appl Environ Microb. 42: 56-60.

11. Oliveira, S.T., Veneroni-Gouveia, G., Costa, M.M. (2012) Molecular characterization of virulence factors in *Aeromonas hydrophila* obtained from fish. Pesquisa Vet Brasil. 32: 701-706.
12. Peyghan, R., Esmaili, F. (1997) Infection of the grass carp with the motile Aeromonas like microrganism. J Fish. 6: 1-8.
13. Popoff, M., VéEron, M. (1976) A taxonomic study of the *Aeromonas hydrophila-Aeromonas punctata* group. J Gen Microbiol. 94: 11-22.
14. Roy, R.P., Bahadur, M., Barat, S. (2013) Isolation, identification and Antibiotic resistance of *Aeromonas* spp. and *Salmonella* spp. from the fresh water loach, *Lepidocephalichthys guntea* and water of Terai River Lotchka, West Bengal, India. Zool Pol. 58: 5-17.
15. Sarkar, A., Saha, M., Roy, P. (2012) Identification and typing of *Aeromonas Hydrophila* through 16S rDNA-PCR finger printing. J Aquacult Res Dev. 3: 1-5.
16. Sechi, L.A., Deriu, A., Falchi, M.P., Fadda, G., Zanetti, S. (2002) Distribution of virulence genes in *Aeromonas* spp. isolated from Sardinian waters and from patients with diarrhoea. J Appl Microbiol. 92: 221-227.
17. Soltani, M. (2002) Fish bacterial diseases. (1st ed.). Published by Iranian Veterinary Oraganization Press, Tehran, Iran.
18. Soltani, M., Mirzargar, S.S., Ebrahimzadeh Maboud, H. (1998) Occurrence of the *Aeromonas septicemia* in the ornamental fish, oscar (*Astronotus ocellatus*), isolation, characterization and pathogenicity. Iran J Vet Med. 53: 62-65.
19. Uma, A., Rebecca, G., Meena, S., Saravanabava, K. (2010) PCR detection of putative aerolysin and hemolysin genes in an *Aeromonas hydrophila* isolate from infected Koi carp (Cyprinus carpio). Tamil J Vet Anim Sci. 6: 31-33.
20. Woo, P.T.K., Leatherland, J.F., Bruno, D.W. (2011). Fish Diseases and Disorders (2nd ed.). Cambridge, UK.
21. Yogananth, N., Bhakyaraj, R., Chanthuru, A., Anbalagan, T., Nila, K.M. (2009) Detection of virulence gene in *Aeromonas hydrophila* isolated from fish samples using PCR technique. Global J Biotech Biochem. 4: 51-53.
22. Zamani, H., Ghasemi, M., Hosseini, S., Karsidani, S.H. (2014) Experimental susceptibility of Caspian white fish, *Rutilus frisii kutum* to Spring viraemia of carp virus. Virus Dis. 25: 57-62.

Molecular evaluation of M2 protein of Iranian avian influenza viruses of H9N2 subtype in order to find mutations of adamantane drug resistance

Malekan, M.[1], Vasfi Marandi, M.[1*], Barin, A.[2], Mokhtari Azad, T.[3], Ranjbar, M.M.[3], Bashashati, M.[1]

[1]*Department of Avian Medicine, Faculty of Veterinary Medicine, University of Tehran, Tehran, Iran*
[2]*Department of Microbiology, Faculty of Veterinary Medicine, University of Tehran, Tehran, Iran*
[3]*Department of Virology, School of Public Health, Tehran University of Medical Sciences, Tehran, Iran*

Key words:
adamantane drug resistance, avian influenza virus, H9N2, M2 protein, poultry

Correspondence
Vasfi Marandi, M.
Department of Avian Medicine, Faculty of Veterinary Medicine, University of Tehran, Tehran, Iran

Email: mvmarand@ut.ac.ir

Abstract:

BACKGROUND: The H9N2 subtype of influenza A viruses is considered to be widespread in poultry industry. Adamantane is a group of antiviral agents which is effective both in prevention and treatment of influenza A virus infections. These drugs inhibit M2 protein ion channel which has role on viral replication. **OBJECTIVES:** The main objective of this study is to evaluate M gene of avian influenza viruses (AIVs) of H9N2 subtype in order to find adamantane drug resistance mutations. **METHODS:** Over 100 suspected samples were collected from different geographical regions of Iran during 2012-2013. Samples were injected via allantoic sac of 9-11 day-old chicken embryos. A total of 11 out of 100 were AIV. The H9N2 subtype was confirmed by specific RT-PCR. The RT-PCR was conducted for full length M gene. PCR amplified products were purified and then conducted for commercial direct sequencing. Finally, sequences were checked for possible sites of adamantane resistance mutations. **RESULTS:** Overall, 8 out of 11 viruses harbored the adamantane resistance-associated mutations. Of which, four viruses were isolated in 2013 and four viruses in 2012. Two different resistance-associated mutations were observed during different years. **CONCLUSIONS:** The present study provided clear evidence concerning resistance AIVs of H9N2 subtype that were circulating in Iranian poultry sector. This concern is always present as M segment might be introduced into human influenza viruses by reassortment phenomenon.

Introduction

Disease of poultry caused by type A influenza viruses in the family Orthomyxoviridae has been recognized since the late 19th century, causing mainly sporadic but serious outbreaks in poultry industry (Swayne et al. 2013). These viruses are divided into two subtypes based on their two surface glycoproteins including hemagglutinin (HA) and neuraminidase (NA) (Zambon, 1999). Sixteen HA subtypes (H1-16) and nine NA subtypes (N1-9) are recognized among avian influenza viruses (AIVs) (Swayne et al. 2013). From late on, H9N2 subtype of influenza A viruses have been considered to be widespread in poultry industry (Peiris et al. 1999). The H9N2 subtype is known to be a cause of subclinical and clinical diseases with mild to severe manifestations in respiratory system associated with egg decline, diarrhea and renal disorders (Swayne et al. 2013; Davison et al., 1999; Shalaby et al., 1994).

First isolation and characterization of H9N2 subtype of influenza A in Iran was conducted by Vasfi Marandi and Bozorgmehri Fard in 1998 (Vasfi Marandi et al., 2002). Nowadays, several researchers are working on different aspects of H9N2 subtype because of its importance both in public health and poultry sector (Bashashati et al., 2013; Emadi Chashmi et al., 2013; Nili and Asasi, 2003; Homayounimehr et al., 2010; Karimi et al., 2004).

Type A viruses consist of 8 segmented negative strand genome (Lamb et al. 2001; Swayne et al. 2013). Both matrix and membrane proteins encode by M gene of 7th segment. This gene has 1027 bp in which nucleotide positions of 26-784 encode M1 and positions of 26-51 and 740-1007 encode M2 protein. The M2 is a tetramer membrane protein where locates intra the viral envelope and projects from the surface of the virus. The M2 protein comprises 3 parts of extracellular, transmembrane and cytoplasmic domain (97 amino acids) (Furuse et al., 2009). Transmembrane domain of M2 is a proton channel which balances pH of viral membrane during cell entry and also during viral maturation, and equilibrates pH across the trans-Golgi membrane of infected cells.

Adamantane is a group of antiviral agents which is effective both in prevention and in treatment of influenza A virus infections (Saito et al., 2002). During early stage of infection, these drugs inhibit virus replication by blocking proton flow through M2 ion channel and suppressing viral ribonucleoprotein complex release into cytoplasm of infected cells (Iwahashi et al., 2001; Kitahori et al., 2006). In general they prevent virus replication within the infected cell.

Mutation which causes substitution of Aspargine to Serine at position 31in M2 protein is responsible for all resistant viruses (Iwahashi et al., 2001; Bright et al. 2006). Furthermore, single amino acid substitution of residue 26, 27, 30, 31, 34 or 38 over helical turns of M2 transmembrane domain lead to drug resistance (Lee et al. 2008; Ilyushina et al., 2005; Schnell et al., 2008; Saito et al., 2007; Shiraishi et al., 2003).

The objective of present study was evaluation of AIVs of H9N2 subtype isolated from Iranian poultry sector during 2012 and 2013 to identify single amino acid mutations responsible for adamantane drug resistance.

Material and Methods

Virus isolation: Over one-hundred tissue samples were collected from different geographical regions of Iran during 2012-2013 and stored at -70°C. These samples include of trachea, lung and cecal tonsil of susceptible birds to avian influenza.

Samples were prepared by procedure described by Swayne, et al.'s 2008 method. Four 9-11 days-old chicken embryos were used for each sample. Samples were injected via allantoic sac. Inoculated embryos were incubated at 35-37°C for 5 days. Eggs were candled daily and died embryos were collected. After 5 days all live embryos were killed by chilling up to 4°C. Amnioallantoic fluids of dead embryos were collected for hemagglutinating activity (HA) test. The HA positive samples were confirmed by

Hemagglutinin and Nuaraminidase specific primers of H9 and N2 subtypes with RT-PCR (Lee et al., 2001; Qiu et al., 2009). A total of eleven positive AIVs of H9N2 Subtype samples were detected for further tests.

Viral RNA extraction and cDNA synthesis: Viral RNA was extracted by RNX-PlusTM solution (Cinaclon® ,Iran) as indicated on manufacturer's instructions. cDNA was prepared with the following method: 10 μl of prepared RNA was mixed with 2 μl of 20 pmol oligonucleotide influenza universal primer,Uni12 (5′-AGCRAAAGCAGG-3′). The mixture was incubated at 65°C for 5 min. Then, mixture was put on ice and 2 μl Reaction buffer 10X, 1 μl ribonuclease inhibitor (Fermantase®, Canada), 2 μl dNTP 10 mM and 1 μl M-MULV reverse transcriptase enzyme (Fermantase®, Canada) were added. The reaction was carried at 42°C for 60 min and was terminated by heating at 70°C for 5 min.

Polymerase chaise reaction (PCR) amplification: Amplification of M gene was performed by universal primers as follows: Bm-M-1F: 5′- TATTCGTCTCAGGGAGCAAAAGCAGGTAG-3′ and Bm-M-1027 R: 3′-ATATCGTCTCGTATTAGTAGAAACAAGGTAGTTTTT-5′. Mentioned primers amplified complete M gene segment of avian influenza with length of 1027 bp (Hoffmann et al., 2001).

A 50 μl total volume of master mix contained: 5 μl PCR buffer 10X, 20 pmol of each forward and reverse primer (2 μl), 2 μl dNTP 10 mM, 4 μl MgCl2 50 mM, 0.5 μl Pfu DNA polymerase (Fermentase, Canada) and 2 μl cDNA samples. The amplification protocol was: one step denaturation at 95°C for 3 min, 35 cycle of 94°C for 15 sec, 58°C for 30 Sec, 72°C for 1 min and final extension at 72°C for 5 min (Hoffmann et al.,

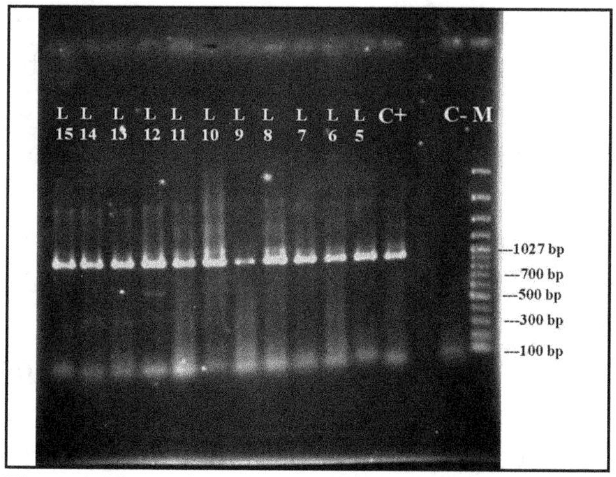

Figure 1. Illustration of gel electrophoresis result of amplified M gene fragments of Iranian avian influenza H9N2 subtype isolates . M=Marker (Ladder) 100bp, L=Lanes, C=Control.

2001). A volume of 10μ of PCR products were electrophoresed on 1% agarose gel in 1x TBE buffer near 100bp Marker, and visualized by ethidium bromide staining. After ethidium bromide staining, the gels were photographed under UV light with a Gel Doc system (VilberLourmat Inc. Cedex, France).

The DNA sequencing: PCR amplified products were purified by QIA quick Gel Extraction Kit (Qiagen, Valencia, CA, USA) and then conducted for commercial direct sequencing service by Takapouzist Co. (Bioneer, Republic of Korea).

Bioinformatics analysis: The obtained sequences were analyzed and trimmed by FinchTV software (http://www.geospiza.com/finchtv) and then registered in NCBI. Nucleotide sequences were translated to protein sequences, comparatively aligned and their variations evaluated by taking advantage of Bioedit version 7.7.9 software. Finally, sequences were checked for possible sites of adamantane resistance mutations including L26F, A30T, A30S, A30V,S31N, G34E and L38F.

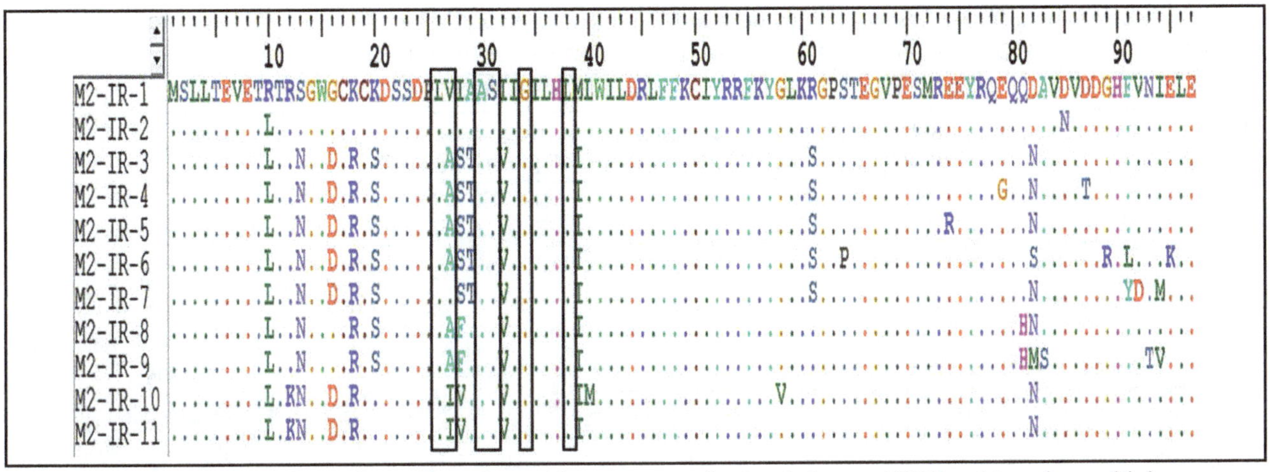

Figure 2. Demonstration of complete M2 amino acid sequences of avian influenza H9N2 subtype by multiple sequence alignment (MSA). Results are illustrated and edited by Bioedit 7.7.9 . Conserve, semi-conserved and variable regions along M2 protein could be seen in this figure. All residues that are identical to the top sequences in an alignment as a dot ('.') used. Rectangular shape showing sequences with possible sites of adamantane resistance mutations.

Results

RT-PCR analysis and sequencing results: Complete M gene was amplified by PCR and electrophoresis results depicted in Fig. 1. The RT-PCR products of H9N2 isolates showed the same length (approximately 1027bp) at electrophoresis. Briefly, lane M is Molecular weight marker (100 bp) and lanes 5-15 are specific molecular sized 1027 bp amplicons representing M gene obtained from Iranian avian influenza H9N2 subtype.

Alignment and comparison of sequencing results: After sequencing, M gene sequences chromatograms were analyzed by FintchTV software for quality checking and editing. Nucleotide sequences of complete M2 gene were translated to protein sequences, and comparatively aligned. Results (Fig.2) revealed limited variations of M2 gene of Iranian avian influenza H9N2 subtype and these limited variations are due to the conserve nature of M gene.

Then, analysis across 6 possible mutation sites related to adamantane resistance were shown by rectangular shape/marking. Details will be described later in Table 1.

Adamantane resistance mutations analysis: The M2 sequence of 11avian influenza (H9N2) isolates collected during 2012-2013 in Iran were obtained. A total of 6 out of 11 (54.5%) harbored the adamantane resistance-associated V27A mutation and 2 (18.2%) harbored V27I. Of these, 4 (66.6%) viruses showed V27A were isolated in 2013 and 2 (40%) viruses of V27A in 2012. All mutation V27I belonged to 2012 isolates . No mutations were observed in all other adamantine resistance associated sites including L26F, A30T, A30S, A30V,S31N, G34E and L38F (Fig. 2 and Table 1). Also, there were significant variations in amino acid 28 and 82 (Table 2).

Discussion

Current study aimed to evaluate M2 protein of Iranian avian influenza H9N2 subtype in order to find mutation of adamantane drug resistance. Under field conditions, sequenced isolates caused considerable complexities in affected poultry farms such as significant respiratory complications.

Sequence analysis of the M gene of these

Table 1. Observed Adamantane Resistance Mutations in M2 protein of Iranian avian influenza H9N2 subtype during 2012 and 2013. 1- L26F; 2- [a]V27A, [b]V27I; 3- A30T, A30S, A30V; 4- S31N; 5- G34E; 6- L38F.

Year	2013							2012				
Isolated Virus	M2-IR-1	M2-IR-2	M2-IR-3	M2-IR-4	M2-IR-5	M2-IR-6	M2-IR-7	M2-IR-8	M2-IR-9	M2-IR-10	M2-IR-11	Reference
AA Code												
26 1	-	-	-	-	-	-	-	-	-	-	-	Iwahashi et al., 2001; Shiraishi et al., 2003; Saito et al., 2007; Ilyushina et al., 2005; Lee et al., 2008; Schmidke et al., 2006
27 2	-	-	+a	+ a	+ a	+ a	-	+ a	+ a	+ b	+ b	Iwahashi et al., 2001; Shiraishi et al., 2003; Saito et al., 2007; Ilyushina et al., 2005; Lee et al., 2008; Schmidke et al., 2006; Cheung et al., 2006
30 3	-	-	-	-	-	-	-	-	-	-	-	Iwahashi et al., 2001; Shiraishi et al., 2003; Saito et al., 2007; Ilyushina et al., 2005; Lee et al., 2008; Schmidke et al., 2006
31 4	-	-	-	-	-	-	-	-	-	-	-	Iwahashi et al., 2001; Shiraishi et al., 2003; Saito et al., 2007; Ilyushina et al., 2005; Lee et al., 2008; Schmidke et al., 2006
34 5	-	-	-	-	-	-	-	-	-	-	-	Iwahashi et al., 2001; Ilyushina et al., 2005; Lee et al., 2008; Schmidke et al., 2006
38 6	-	-	-	-	-	-	-	-	-	-	-	Lee et al., 2008; Schmidke et al., 2006

Table 2. Amino acid variation at different sites of M2 protein in H9N2 subtype viruses isolated in 2012-2013.

Site Number	Amino acid Variation
16	Glycine, Aspartic acid
20	Serine, Lysine
28	Isoleusine, Serine, Phenyalanine, Valine
29	Alanine, Threonine
61	Serine, Argenine
82	Aspartic acid, Aspargine, Methionine, Serine

viruses revealed that six out of eleven isolates harbored the adamantane resistance associated V27A and two harbored V27I mutations. Also, there were significant variations in amino acids 28 and 82 among analyzed sequences.

Yavarian et al., in two different studies in 2009 and 2010, reported an increase in amantadine resistance, due to a S31N mutation in the M2 protein, among influenza A H3N2 isolates circulating in Iran during 2005-2007 and 2005-2008 (Yavarian et al., 2009 and 2010). Ilyushina et al., 2005 by analysis of north America and Asian isolates showed diversity of adamantane resistant mutants among AIVs in different positions of V27A, A30S, S31N (Ilyushina et al., 2005). Saito et al., 2003 found that the overall frequencies of amantadine-resistant strains were 29.6% (24 of 81) during the 1999-2000 influenza season and 23.3% (7 of 30) during the 2000-2001 influenza season. They also found dominant amino acid substitution residues differ significantly with the subtype: namely, V27A in H1N1 strains and S31N in H3N2 strains (Saito, et al., 2003). Barr et al., 2007 investigated 102 (H3) and 37 (H1) influenza viruses isolated at WHO Reference Research Center of Influenza in Melbourne. 43% of H3 and 0% of H1 subtypes showed S31N resistance mutation. They concluded, despite the introduction of neuraminidase inhibitors, amantadine and rimantadine continue to be used for the treatment or prevention of influenza A, mainly due to their low cost (Barr et al., 2007). Higgins et al., 2009 found that from 49 H3N2 subtype isolates 46 carried a point mutation in the M gene coding for the M2 protein which would be associated with amantadine resistance (S31N and V27A) (Higgins et al., 2009). Schmidke et al., 2005 reported a total 3 of 12 isolates show S31N and V27A major substitution in resistant isolates of H1N1, H1N2 and H3N2 subtypes (Schmidke et al., 2006).

Antiviral resistance analysis of M2 protein sequences of H9N2 subtype from United Arab Emirates from 2000 to 2003 revealed that 6 viruses carried a V27A substitution at position 27 and only one virus possessed S31N at position 31. Then, testing resistance against amantadine quantitatively, by using serially increasing concentrations of the drug showed all the Dubai isolates had a high level of resistance to amantadine in cell culture (Aamir et al., 2007).

Therefore, the main substitution position of adamantane resistance of Iranian viruses circulating between 2012 and 2013 in present study is similar to that observed among H9N2 isolates reported before from the United Arab Emirates.

Kitahori et al., 2006 isolated H3N2 and reported 3.4% of isolates revealed adamantane resistance mutations at position 31 (S31N), 26 (L26F) and 27 (V27I) (Kitahori et al., 2006). Pabbaraju et al., 2008 conducted a study to find adamantane resistance in circulating human influenza from 1970 to 2003 in Canada. A total of 73 (23%) of the 317 influenza A H3 subtype viruses tested contained one or two amino acid substitutions in the M2 protein known to cause resistance to adamantanes. Most of the resistant isolates showed S31N mutation and few of them showed V27I substitution. No resistance was observed in the influenza A H1 subtype viruses tested. Their results showed a significant increase in adamantane resistance levels in circulating influenza A H3 viruses from December 2005 to March 2006 (Pabbaraju et al., 2006). Tang et al., 2008 reported overall 58 out of 281 H3N2 subtype isolates collected during 1997-2006 in Hong Kong harbored the adamantane resistance-associated S31N mutation. One of these S31N-containing isolates also harbored the V27I mutation (Tang et al., 2008). Here, in our results two isolates showed mutation on V27I which is compatible with their results.

In conclusion, the present study provided clear evidence that resistant AIVs of H9N2 subtype were circulating in Iranian poultry sector. We suggest adamantane resistance may arise due to selection pressure of illegal drug usage. A high frequency of adamantane drug resistance may cause a problem in environment and human health care system. This concern is always present as M segment may be introduced to human influenza virus by reassortment. This fact may cause special concern with regard to pandemic highly pathogenic influenza viruses.

Furthermore, results of present study help to make us awareness about resistance to adamantane drugs in Iranian poultry farms and to avoid the arbitrary use of adamantane to treat and prevent infections from avian influenza. Finally, it seems practical tests of the drug influence in-vivo and in-vitro, can ensure effective use of the drugs and their probable resistance.

Acknowledgments

Current study was supported by grant No 12/6/7508001 of Research Council of Tehran University. We are glad to acknowledge Mrs. Yazdani and Mr.Soleimani for their kind cooperation.

References

1. Amir, U.B., Wernery, U., Ilyushina, N., Webster, R.G. (2007) Characterization of avian H9N2 influenza viruses from United Arab Emirates 2000 to 2003. Virology. 361: 45-55.
2. Barr, I.G., Hurt, A.C., Iannello, P., Tomasov, C., Deed, N., Komadina, N. (2007) Increased adamantane resistance in influenza A (H3) viruses in Australia and neighboring countries in 2005. Antiviral Res. 73: 112-117.
3. Bashashati, M., Vasfi Marandi, M., Bozorgmehri Fard, M.H., Hematzadeh, F., Sabouri, F. (2013) Genetic and phylogenetic analysis of the ribonucleoprotein complex genes of H9N2 avian influenza viruses isolated from commercial poultry in Iran. Iranian Journal of Veterinary Medicine. 7: 159-168.
4. Bright, R.A., Shay, D.K., Shu, B., Cox, N.J., Klimov, A.I. (2006) Adamantane resistance among influenza A viruses isolated early during the 2005-2006 influenza season in the United States. J Am Med Assoc. 295: 891-894.
5. Cheung, C.L., Rayner, J.M., Smith G.J., Wang, P., Naipospos, T.S.P., Zhang, J., Yuen, K.Y., Webster, R.G., Peiris, J.S.M., Guan, Y., Chen, H. (2006) Distibution of amantadine resistant H5N1 avian variant in Asia. J Infect Dis. 193: 1626-1629.
6. Davison, S., Benson, C.E., Ziegler, A.F., Eckroade, R.J. (1999) Evaluation of disinfectants with the addition of anti-freezing compounds against nonpathogenic H7N2 avian influenza virus. Avian Dis. 43: 533-537.
7. Emadi Chashmi, H., Vasfi Marandi, M., Bozorgmehri Fard, M.H., Bashashati, M., Barin, A. (2013) Molecular characterization of non-structural gene of H9N2 subtype of avian influenza viruses isolated from broiler chickens in Iran. Iranian Journal of Veterinary Medicine. 7: 23-34.
8. Furuse, Y., Suzuki, A., Kamigaki, T., Oshitani, H. (2009) Evolution of the M gene of the influenza A virus in different host species: large-scale sequence analysis. Virol J. 6: 67.
9. Higgins, R.R., Eshaghi, A., Burton, L., Mazzulli, T., Drews, S.J. (2009) Differential patterns of amantadine-resistance in influenza A (H3N2) and (H1N1) isolates in Toronto, Canada. J Clin Virol. 44: 91-93.
10. Homayounimehr, A.R., Dadras, H., Shoushtari, A., Pourbakhsh, A.A. (2010) Sequence and phylogenetic analysis of the haemagglutinin genes of H9N2 avian influenza viruses isolated from commercial chickens in Iran. Trop Anim Health Prod. 42: 1291-1297.
11. Ilyushina, N.A., Govorkova, E.A., Webster, R.G. (2005) Detection of amantadine-resistant variants among avian influenza viruses isolated in North America and Asia. Virology. 341: 102-106.
12. Iwahashi, J., Tsuji, K., Ishibashi, T., Kajiwara, J., Imamura, Y., Mori, R., Hara, K., Kashiwagi, T., Ohtsu, Y., Hamada, N., Maeda, H., Toyoda, M., Toyoda, T. (2001) Isolation of amantadine-resistant influenza A viruses (H3N2) from patients following administration of amantadine in japan. J Clin Microbiol. 39: 1652-1653.
13. Karimi, V., Bozorgmehri Fard, M.H., Shabazzadeh, D., Esmaeilzaded, M., Pourbakhsh, S.A. (2004) Sequence analysis and phyloge-

netic study of hemagglutinin gene of H9N2 subtype of Avian influenza virus isolated during 1998-2002 In Iran. Iran Biomed J. 8: 167-172.

14. Kitahori, Y., Nakano, M., Inoue, Y. (2006) Frequency of amantadine-resistanat influenza A virus isolated from 2001-02 to 2004-05 in Nara Prefecture. Jpn J Infect Dis. 59: 197-199.
15. Lamb, R.A., Krug, R.M. (2001) Orthomyxoviridae: the viruses and their replication. In: Fields Virology. Fieldds, B.N., Knipe, D.M., Howley, P.M., Chanock, R.M., Melick, J.L., Momath, T.P., Roizman, B. (eds.). (4th ed.) Lippincott-Raven. Philadelphia. PA, USA. p. 1487-1531.
16. Lee, J., Song, Y.J., Park, J.H., Lee, J.H., Baek, Y.H., Song, M.S., Oh, T.K., Han, H.S., Pascua, P.N., Choi, Y.K. (2008) Emergence of amantadine-resistant H3N2 avian Influenza A virus in south korea. J Clin Microbiol. 46: 3788-3790.
17. Lee, M.S., Chang, P.C., Shein, J.H., Cheng, M. C., Shieh, H. K. (2001) Identification and subtyping of avian influenza viruses by reverse transcription-PCR. J Virol Methods. 97: 13-22.
18. Nili, H., Asasi, K. (2003) Avian Influenza (H9N2) Outbreak in Iran. Avian Dis. 47: 828-831.
19. Pabbaraju, K., Ho., K.C., Wong, S., Shokoples, S., Pang, X., Fonseca, K., Fox, J.D. (2008) Adamantane resistance in circulating human influenza A viruses from Alberta, Canada (1970-2007). Antiviral Res. 79: 81-86.
20. Peiris, M., Yam, W.C., Chan, K.H., Ghose, P. Shortridge, K.F. (1999) Influenza A H9N2: Aspects of laboratory diagnosis. J Clin Microbiol. 37: 3426-3427.
21. Qiu, B.F., Liu, W.J., Peng, D.X., Hu, S.L., Tang, Y.H., Liu, X.F. (2009) A reverse transcription-PCR for subtyping of the neuraminidase of avian influenza viruses, J Virol Methods. 155: 193-198.
22. Saito, R., Li, D., Suzuki, Y., Sato, I., Masaki, H., Nishimura, H., Kawashima, T., Shirahige, Y., Shimomura, C., Asoh, N., Degawa, S., Ishikawa, H., Sato, M., Shobugawa, Y., Suzuki, H. (2007) High prevalence of amantadine-resistance influenza A (H3N2) in six prefectures, Japan, in the 2005-2006. J Med Virol. 79: 1569-1576.
23. Saito, R., Oshitani, H., Masuda, H., Suzuki, H. (2002) Detection of amantadine-resistant influenza A virus strains in nursing homes by PCR-restriction fragment length polymorphism analysis with nasopharyngeal swabs. J Clin Microbiol. 40: 84-88.
24. Schmidke, M., Zell, R., Bauer, K., Krumbholx, A., Schreder, C., Suess, J., Wutzler, P. (2006) Amantadine resistance among porcine H1N1, H1N2 and H3N2 influenza A viruses isolated Germany between 1981 and 2001. Interviro. 49: 286-293.
25. Schnell, J.R., Chou, J.J. (2008) Structure and mechanism of the M2 proton channel of influenza A virus. Nature. 451: 591-595.
26. Shalaby, A.A., Slemons, R.D., Swayne D.E. (1994) Pathological studies of A/chicken/Alabama/7395/75 (H4N8) influenza virus in specificpathogen-free laying hens. Avian Dis. 38: 22-32.
27. Shiraishi, K., Mitamura, K., Sakai-Tagawa, Y., Goto, H., Sugaya, N., Kawoaka, Y. (2003) High frequency of resistant viruses harboring different mutations in amantadine-treated children with influenza. J Infect Dis. 188: 57-61.
28. Swayne, D.E., Suarez, D.L., Sims, L.D. (2013) Influenza. In: Disease of Poultry. Swayne, D.E., Glisson, J.R., McDougald, L.R., Nolan, L.K., Suarez, D.L., Nair, V. (eds.). (13th ed.) Wiely-Blackwell. Iowa. USA. p. 181-218.

29. Swayne, D.E., Senne, D.A., Suarez, D.L. (2008) A laboratory manual for the isolation, identification and characterization of avian pathogens. Dufour-Zavala, L., Swayne, D.E., Glisson, J.R., Pearson, J.E., Reed, W.M., Jackwood, M.W., Woolcock, P.R. (eds.). (15th ed.) Am Assoc Avian Pathologists, USA. p. 128-133.
30. Tang, J.W., Ngai, K.L., Wong, J.C., Lam, W.Y., Chan, P.K. (2008) Emergence of adamantane-resistanat influenza A (H3N2) Viruses in Hong Kong between 1997 and 2006. J Med Virol. 80: 895-901.
31. VasfiMarandi, M., Bozorgmehri Fard, M.H. (2002) Isolation of H9N2 Subtype of Avian Influenza Viruses during an Outbreak in Chickens in Iran. Iran Biomed J. 6: 13-17.
32. Yavarian, J., Mokhtari Azad, T., Zheng, X., Gregory, V., Lin, P., Hay, A. (2010) Amantadine resistance in relation to the evolution of influenza A(H3N2) viruses in Iran. Antiviral Res. 88: 193-196.
33. Yavarian, J., Mokhtari Azad, T., Jandaghi, N.Z., Nategh, R. (2009) Amantadine-resistant influenza A (H3N2) viruses in Iran. Acta Virol. 53: 135-138.
34. Zambon, M.C. (1999) Epidemiology and pathogenesis of influenza. J Antimicrobiol Chemother. 44: 3-9.

Investigating the effect of progestrone (Cue-Mate™) administration on ovulation induction in photostimulated anestrus mares

Ghasemzadeh Nava, H.*, Kaveh Baghbadorani, M., Gharavi, J., Ghahremani, N., Gharagozloo, F.

Department of Theriogenology, Faculty of Veterinary Medicine, University of Tehran, Tehran, Iran

Key words:
anestrus, mare, ovulation, photostimulation, progestrone

Correspondence
Ghasemzadeh Nava, H.
Department of Theriogenology, Faculty of Veterinary Medicine, University of Tehran, Tehran, Iran

Email: Hghasem@ut.ac.ir

Abstract:

BACKGROUND: In mare, different methods of earlier cyclicity induction and hastening first ovulation of the year have been reported. **OBJECTIVES:** The goal of present study was to investigate the effect of progesterone (Cue-mate®) on synchronization and acceleration of the first ovulation of the year in winter anestrous mares under artificial lighting system. **METHODS:** After detection of anestrus mares, artificial lighting regimen of 16h light was conducted from early December for both treatment and control groups mares. After detecting of 25 mm follicle in the ovary, treatment group mares received Cue-Mate and examined were through rectal ultrasound until follicle reached the size of 35mm, when cue-mate was removed. Daily ultrasound examination and teasing were done until detection of ovulation. **RESULTS:** Based on our results, no significant difference in rate of ovulation (66% vs 60%) and size of ovulatory follicle existed between treatment and control group. In addition, despite of decreasing time interval of follicular growth from 25 mm to 35 mm (8.33±0.88 vs 10.75±2.28 in treatment and control groups respectively) and from each of these sizes to ovulation size, no significant difference existed between treatment and control groups. **CONCLUSIONS:** This was the first preliminary report of investigating the effect of progesterone plus artificial lighting on hastening first ovulation of the year in early winter anestrous. It seems more studies considering the greater number of mares in different ages are needed.

Introduction

The mare is seasonally polyestrous with regular ovulatory cycles occurring in response to increasing day length (Donadeu and Watson, 2007). In mares that have entered a seasonal anestrous phase during the winter of temperate latitudes, ovulatory cycles do not normally commence until April or early May (October or early November in the Southern Hemisphere) (Ginther, 1974). Most breeder associations use a single date, January 1st for registering all foals born in a calendar year, however, from an economic standpoint production of foals early in the year is essential for performance in the show ring and maximizing prices obtained for yearlings (Squires, 2008). Getting mares pregnant around February 15th is essential and various hormonal and non-hormonal methods have been described for advancing first ovulatory cycle of mares in both anestrus and transitional phase. Non-hormonal method which is based on photo-stimulation can be implemented by using various artificial lighting procedures including: Indoor conventional and modified light therapy which requires mares to be kept in stalls during lighting period or mobile light therapy which allows outdoor maintenance of mares by using blue light emitting diode (LED; 468nm) mask (Murphy, et al. 2014). Conventional lighting regimen can be done by 14.5 to 16h daily light (8-9.5h darkness) beginning from December in deep anestrus mares. Modified light regimens use photosensitive phases of the mare's circadian clocks including that of post dusk therapy which uses 2.5h additional light after sunset or skeletal lighting which works based on night interruption through 1 -2 h. lighting, 9.5-10.5 hours after beginning of darkness. Lighting regimens are successful, albeit variable in response time between individuals, but must be started many weeks before ovulation (McKinnon, et al. 2011).

Hormonal treatment methods for induction or hastening earlier cyclicity can be classified into two categories: treatments for inducing onset of cyclicity in anestrus mares including administration of GnRH osmotic pump or implant and recombinant LH and FSH or those whose efficacy has been mainly proved for hastening cyclicity among mares in transition phase like using ovulation inducing agents (GnRH agonists and hCG), dopamine D2-receptor antagonists for increasing prolactin secretion (Panzani, et al. 2011) and progesterone or progestin treatment to suppress GnRH release allowing a surge after cessation of treatment (Squires, 2008). Efficacy of reFSH in stimulating follicular development and advancing the first ovulation of the year in deep anestrous mares maintained under ambient lights was determined. The results of this study indicated that reFSH was effective in stimulating the development of ovarian follicles and advancing the first ovulation of the year in seasonally anestrous mares under ambient lights but was not successful in inducing continued cyclicity (Meyers-Browna, et al. 2013). Diastral level of progesterone inhibit ovulation and cause follicular regress in ruminants, while in equids they just prevent showing of estrus behavior and with regards to the possibility of continuing diastral follicles' development, ovulation is presumable. In one study, short-term preovulatory progestogen (CIDR or altrenogest) treatment in mares could not delay ovulation. Also, treatments had no effect on follicular growth rate or the size of the ovulatory follicle immediately preceding ovulation (Caniso, et al. 2013).

We hypothesized that progesterone supplementation increase efficiency of lighting therapy and results in earlier ovulation induction compared with control group.

The goal of present study was to investigate the effect of progesterone on synchronization and acceleration of the first ovulation of the year in winter anestrous mares under artificial lighting system.

Material and Methods

Animals: Crossbred and mixed bred barren mares (n=10), aged from 5 to 10 years old, body weight averaged of 500 Kg and good body condition were used in this study.) in research and training hospital of Faculty of Veterinary Medicine, University of Tehran-Iran located in Mohammad Abad (in Alborz province-Iran). They were fed with hay, alfalfa and cereals concentrate in standard rations. Because of stallion exposure effect on hastening onset of cyclicity, we were careful not to be allowed the mares to have contacted with stallions. Mares were weekly examined by rectal palpation and ultrasonography from late November of 2014. Mares with signs of anestrus condition, were characterized by inconclusive or no estrous behavior, a relatively relaxed cervical canal, little or no uterine tone, absence of ultrasonically visible endometrial edema or a corpus luteum, and usually follicles of less than 20 mm. They were examined at least 2 weeks apart and were divided randomly in two groups (each group = 5 mares).

Treatments: All of enrolled mares were exposed daily to artificial lighting regimens of 16h light (8h darkness) from early December by using incandescent 200 W bulb and daily programmed analog time switcher (theben Co.). The status of mares' reproductive system in terms of follicular growth and uterine edema was evaluated by ultrasonography examination, twice a week. Unfortunately, 2 mares in treatment group were eliminated from the study after about one month due to some problems. So, we continued with 3 and 5 mares in study and control group respectively. Treatment group mares also received Cue-mate (Bayer Animal Health, New zealand), which is a type of progesterone releasing intravaginal device (PRID) containing Progesterone 1.56g within two silicone pods attached to a flexible 'wishbone' for insertion into the vagina (Fig. 1). The device was originally designed for use in cattle to induce and synchronize estrus. In the mare, sufficient progesterone is absorbed through the vaginal wall to give peripheral plasma concentrations above 10.5 nm/l for the first 4 days. Concentrations diminish to about 7 nm/l by the 8 day and to 5.3 nm/l or lower by day 16.

Study design: If the follicle with a diameter of 25 mm was observed, mares were divided randomly into two groups:

Treatment group: Mares treated by insertion of a Cue-Mate in vaginal region. They were re-examined ultrasonographically about 6 days after insertion of the Cue-Mate and then daily according to the level of follicular activity found. When a follicle of 35 mm or greater had developed, the Cue-Mate was removed. If such a follicle had not developed after 12 to 16 days, the Cue-Mate was also removed. Daily teasing began on the day after Cue-Mate removal until estrus was detected. Then, reproductive examination for detection of reproductive signs of estrus and ovulation was done by ultrasonography.

Control group: Mares were not treated using insertion of a Cue-Mate, but they were re-examined daily according to the level of follicular activity. When a follicle with ≥35 mm diameter had developed, teasing and ultrasonography was performed daily until ovulation.

Statistical analysis: The obtained data such as rate of estrous, rate of ovulation, and rate of antral hemorrhagic follicles occurrence were analyzed by Chi-square statistical test. The numerical data included time interval from size of deviation (≈ 20 mm diameter) to becoming inducible follicle (≈ 35 mm), time interval from gaining capability of ovulation (≈ 35 mm) to ovulation, and diameter of follicles at ovulation and day of ovulation following photostimulation program were tested by T-test. All of the data were analyzed by SAS statistical software version 9.2 through PROC FREQ and PROC T-TEST, respectively.

Results

Mares in treatment group were treated by Cue-Mate for a mean of 11.6±0.6 days. During the treatment period, none of the intravaginal devices (Cue-Mate) was expelled. Mild vaginitis was seen in just one mare and resolved spontaneously after Cue-Mate removal. One of the mares in control group did not respond to lighting regimen and her ovaries remained inactive during the study. All mares in both groups ovulated after Cue-Mate removal except one in treatment group.

In spite of shortened duration observed in follicular growth from ≈25 mm to ≈35 mm (8.33±0.88 days vs 10.75±2.28 days in treatment and control groups respectively) and from each of these sizes to ovulatory size, no significant difference existed between treatment and control groups (Table 1). It was found that mean diameter of follicles at the time of ovulation (44.7 ± 3.3 mm and 43.1 ± 3.3 mm in treatment and control groups respectively) did not show any difference between two groups (Table 2). Also, there was no significant difference in time interval from the beginning of lighting program to ovulation (Table 2). No significant difference was found in ovulation rate and proportion of mares showing estrus between treatment and control group (Figure 2).

Discussion

Various types of progesterone therapy, including long act injectable (Lopez-Bayghen, et al. 2008) or orally administered progestins (Squires, et al. 1983) and intravaginal releasing progesterone (Handler, et al. 2007) has been used for synchronizing and hastening of ovulation in the mares. Intravaginal route offers a relatively cheap and convenient method of delivering progesterone to mares which does not require daily administration. Treatment of transitional mares with an intravaginal progesterone containing device specifically designed for mares (Cue-Mare) for 10 days, resulted in follicular growth and ovulation within 4 days of device removal and it was associated with minimal discomfort and vaginitis (Grimmett, et al. 2002). Induction of ovulation of mare using hormonal methods did not receive as much attention in the past as dairy cattle and sheep (Squires, 2008, Talebkhan Garoussi, and Golzar, 2012a). It was associated with earlier pregnancy

Table 1. Comparison mean time interval from Cue-mate administration (≈ 20 mm) to ovulation capacity (≈ 35mm), from this time to ovulation and from beginning of treatment to ovulation between treatment and control groups.

Variable (Mean±SEM)	Control	Treatment	P-value
Time interval to ovulation capacity (day)	10.75±2.28	8.33±0.88	0.4
Time interval of inducible follicle ovulation (day)	8±1.78	5±2	0.3
Time interval to ovulation from 25mm (day)	18.2±6.7	12±2.82	0.1

Table 2. Comparison mean diameter of follicles at the time of ovulation and time interval from the beginning of lighting program to ovulation between treatment and control groups.

Variable (Mean±SEM)	Control	Treatment	P-value
Diameter of follicle at ovulation (mm)	3.3 ± 44.7	3.3 ± 43.1	0.9
Day of ovulation following lightening (day)	8.8 ± 58.3	6.2 ± 53.3	0.6

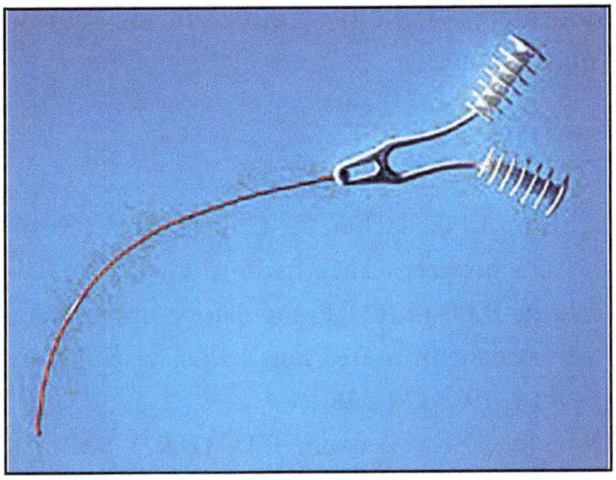

Figure 1. Cue-Mate.

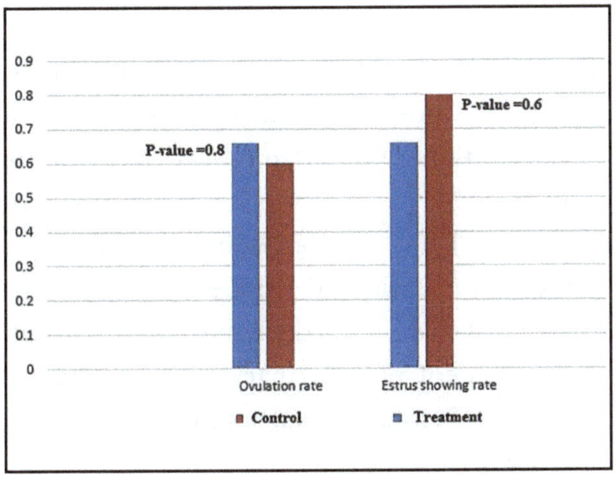

Figure 2. Comparison of proportion of mares ovulated or showed estrus behavior between treatment and control group.

during breeding season and increased risk of pregnancy at the end of it (Hanlon and Firth, 2012). Moreover, intravaginal devices designed for cattle, including CIDR (1.38 g P4), PRID (1.55 g P4) and cue-mate (1.56g P4) have been used off-label in mares and are effective in stimulating follicle growth in transitional mares (Klug and Jochle 2001). Regardless of shape and a little difference in amount of progesterone content, all of these devices have a silicone layer which slowly releases progesterone and maintains its plasma level over 1 ng/ml during 7 to 10 days of treatment period (Klug and Jochle 2001).

Even though artificial photoperiod has been shown to be quite effective in hastening the first ovulation of the year, mares still experience a transition period from winter anestrus to normal cyclicity. Conversely, administration of PRID to anestrus mares without sufficient pre-treatment artificial lighting has limited value and generally results in the follicular growth without ovulation, hence combination of artificial photoperiod for approximately 30 to 60 days and then 12 to 15 day exposure to exogenous progesterone after some follicular development on the ovary can be used to synchronize and accelerate the first ovulation of the year, resembling applied procedure during vernal transition period (Squires, et al. 1979).

Most experiments about the use of PRID are confined to vernal transition mares. It has been reported that using PRID together with ovulation inducing agents (GnRH analogs and hCG) enhanced efficacy of both treatments in comparison with administration of each of them alone (Newcombe, et al. 2002). It should be mentioned that we did not use any ovulation agent in this study. Newcombe (2002) reported that PRID administration to photostimulated anestrus mares resulted in ovulation in 92% of mares, 6.6 days after PRID removal, our finding about ovulation of 66% of mares, 5±2 days after removal is comparable with this result. Although positive effect of PRID for induction of estrus in transition mares has been reported (Hanlon and Firth, 2012, Kumar, 2011), based on our finding no significant difference in rate of showing of estrus existed between treatment and control group. Sufficient effect of lighting therapy for induction of follicular growth in control group mares can justify our results. Lack of difference in time interval to ovulation from beginning of lighting therapy in treatment and control groups mares also imply this point.

Regarding the size of ovulatory follicles, it has been reported that administration of CIDR in transitional mares stimulates follicular growth (Handler, et al. 2006), possibly due to mimicking changes of luteal phase progesterone level and enhancing LH concentration after day 6 of its insertion (Hanlon, et al. 2010). However, our results did not show significant differences in size of ovulatory follicles between treatment and control groups. The good results may arise from different study designs and time of transition phase in which treatment has been applied.

It has been reported that priming the follicles by progesterone decreased time interval of 20 mm follicle to 35 mm follicle (Staempfli, et al. 2011) and 35 mm follicle to ovulation (Newcombe, et al. 2002). According to our results, time interval from beginning of treatment at the time of follicular growth to 35mm, from 35 mm follicle to ovulation and from beginning of treatment to ovulation, were all lower in treatment group mares compared with control group. Lack of significance is probably due to low number of mares in the experiment. It seems that additional studies are needed to evaluate the effect of progesterone and lighting on induction of ovulation and hastening the first ovulation of the year in early winter anestrous. Also, ovulation induction agents such as hCG can also be applied in a discrete group to evaluate their effect on these criteria.

Acknowledgments

This study was supported by Faculty of Veterinary Medicine, University of Tehran, Tehran, Iran.

References

Caniso, I.F., Gallacher, K., Gilbert, M-A., Korn, A., Schweizer, C.M., Bedford-Guaus, S., Gilbert, R.O. (2013) Preovulatory progestagen treatment in mares fails to delay ovulation. Vet J. 197: 324-328

Donadeu, F.X., Watson, E.D. (2007) Seasonal changes in ovarian activity: Lessons learnt from the horse. Anim Reprod Sci. 100: 225-242.

Ginther, O.J. (1974) Occurence of anoestrus, oestrus, dioestrus and ovulation over a 12-month period in mares. Am J Vet Res. 35: 1173-1179.

Ginther, O.J. (1979) Reproductive Biology of the Mare: Basic and Applied Aspects. Ginther, O.J. (ed.). (1st ed.) Published by author. Department of Veterinary Science, University of Wisconsin, Madison, Chapters 6 and 7, USA.

Grimmett, J.B., Hanlon, D.W, Duris, G.F., Jochle, W. (2002) A new intravaginal progesterone-releasing device (Cue-Mare (TM)) for controlling the estrous cycle in mares. Theriogenology. 58: 585-587

Handler, J., Schönlieb, S., Hoppen, H.O., Aurich, C. (2006) Seasonal effects on attempts to synchronize estrus and ovulation by intravaginal application of progesterone-releasing device (PRID TM) in mares. Theriogenology. 65: 1145-1158.

Handler, J., Schönlieb, S., Hoppen, H.O., Aurich, C. (2007) Influence of reproductive stage at PRID TM insertion on synchronization of estrus and ovulation in mares. Anim Reprod Sci. 97: 382-393.

Hanlon, D.W., Evans, M.J., Firth, E.C. (2010) Effects of intravaginal progesterone on follicular dynamics and FSH, LH, and progesterone concentrations in transitional mares. Anim Reprod Sci. 121: 32-34.

Hanlon, D.W., Firth, E.C. (2012) The reproductive performance of Thoroughbred mares treated with intravaginal progesterone at the start of the breeding season. Theriogenology. 77: 952-958.

Klug, E., Jochle, W. (2001) Advances in synchronizing estrus and ovulations in the mare: A mini review. J Equine Vet Sci. 21: 474-479.

Kumar, R., Phogat, J.B., Mann, J.S., Singh, U., Sharma, A.K. (2011) Estrus induction and fertility response in anestrus mares with exogenous progesterone releasing device (CIDR-B) during late breeding season. Biol Med. 3: 359-364.

Lopez-Bayghen, C., Zozaya, H., Ocampo, L., Brumbaugh, G.W., Sumano, H. (2008) Melengestrol acetate as a tool for inducing early ovulation in transitional mares. Acta Vet Hung. 56: 125-131.

McKinnon, A.O., Squires, E., Vaala, W.E., Varner, D.D. (2011) Equine Reprod. (2nd ed.). Wiley-Blackwell, UK.

Murphy, B.A., Walsh, C.M., Woodward, C.M, Prendergast, R.L., Ryle, J.P., Fallon, L.H., Troedsson, M.H. (2014) Blue light from individual light masks directed at a single eye advances the breeding season in mares. Equine Vet J. 46: 601-5.

Meyers-Browna, G.A., McCue, P.M., Troedsson, M.H.T., Klein, C., Zent, W., Ferris, R.A., Lindholm, A.R., Scofield, D.B., Claes, A.N., Morganti, M., Colgin, M.A., Wetzel, R.L., Peters. (2013) Induction of ovulation in seasonally anestrous mares under ambient lights using recombinant equine FSH (reFSH). Theriogenology. 80: 456-462.

Newcombe, J.R., Handler, J., Klug, E., Meyers, P.J., Jöchle, W. (2002) Treatment of transition phase mares with progesterone intravaginally and with deslorelin or hCG to assist ovulations. Vet Rev. 22: 57-64.

Newcombe, J.R. (2002) Field observation on the use of a progesterone-releasing intravaginal device to induce estrus and ovulation in seasonally anestrus mares. J Equine Vet Sci. 22: 378-382.

Panzani, D., Zicchino, I., Taras, A., Marmorini, P., Crisci, A., Rota, A., Camillo, F. (2011) Clinical use of dopamine antagonist sulpiride to advance first ovulation in transitional mares. Theriogenology. 75: 138-43.

Staempfli, S.A., Clavier, S., Thompson, D.L., Burns, P.J., Lyle, S.K., McKinnon, A.O. (2011) Effect of a single injection of long-acting progesterone on the first ovulation in early and late spring transitional mares. J Equine Vet Sci. 31: 744-748.

Squires, E.L., Stevens, W.B., McGlothlin, D.E., Pickett, B.W. (1979) Effect of an oral progestin on the estrous cycle and fertility of mares. J Anim Sci. 49: 729-735.

Squires, E.L., Heesemann, C.P., Webel, S.K., Shideler, R.K., Voss, J.L. (1983) Relationship of altrenogest to ovarian activity, hormone concentrations and fertility of mares. J Anim Sci. 56: 901-910.

Squires, E.L. (2008) Hormonal Manipulation of the Mare: A Review. J Equine Vet Sci. 28: 627-634.

Talebkhan Garoussi, M., Golzar, E. (2012a). Survey of clinical effects of norgestomet implant and estradiol valerate on conception rate of subfertile high yielding Holstein dairy cows. Iranian Journal of Veterinary Clinical Sciences. 6: 71-78.

Talebkhan Garoussi, M. Gallehdar, E., Farzaneh, N., Mohri, M. (2012b). The effect of Norgestomet on the reproductive performance of out of breeding season of ewes with or without PMSG. Trop Anim Health Prod. 44: 965-968.

PERMISSIONS

All chapters in this book were first published in IJVM, by Faculty of Veterinary Medicine of University of Tehran; hereby published with permission under the Creative Commons Attribution License or equivalent. Every chapter published in this book has been scrutinized by our experts. Their significance has been extensively debated. The topics covered herein carry significant findings which will fuel the growth of the discipline. They may even be implemented as practical applications or may be referred to as a beginning point for another development.

The contributors of this book come from diverse backgrounds, making this book a truly international effort. This book will bring forth new frontiers with its revolutionizing research information and detailed analysis of the nascent developments around the world.

We would like to thank all the contributing authors for lending their expertise to make the book truly unique. They have played a crucial role in the development of this book. Without their invaluable contributions this book wouldn't have been possible. They have made vital efforts to compile up to date information on the varied aspects of this subject to make this book a valuable addition to the collection of many professionals and students.

This book was conceptualized with the vision of imparting up-to-date information and advanced data in this field. To ensure the same, a matchless editorial board was set up. Every individual on the board went through rigorous rounds of assessment to prove their worth. After which they invested a large part of their time researching and compiling the most relevant data for our readers.

The editorial board has been involved in producing this book since its inception. They have spent rigorous hours researching and exploring the diverse topics which have resulted in the successful publishing of this book. They have passed on their knowledge of decades through this book. To expedite this challenging task, the publisher supported the team at every step. A small team of assistant editors was also appointed to further simplify the editing procedure and attain best results for the readers.

Apart from the editorial board, the designing team has also invested a significant amount of their time in understanding the subject and creating the most relevant covers. They scrutinized every image to scout for the most suitable representation of the subject and create an appropriate cover for the book.

The publishing team has been an ardent support to the editorial, designing and production team. Their endless efforts to recruit the best for this project, has resulted in the accomplishment of this book. They are a veteran in the field of academics and their pool of knowledge is as vast as their experience in printing. Their expertise and guidance has proved useful at every step. Their uncompromising quality standards have made this book an exceptional effort. Their encouragement from time to time has been an inspiration for everyone.

The publisher and the editorial board hope that this book will prove to be a valuable piece of knowledge for researchers, students, practitioners and scholars across the globe.

LIST OF CONTRIBUTORS

Urzúa, N., Errecalde, C., Prieto and G. Paula Tonini M.
Department of Pharmacology, Faculty of Agriculture and Veterinary, National University of Río Cuarto, Río Cuarto, Argentina

Lüders, C.
School of Veterinary Medicine, Catholic University of Temuco, Temuco, Chile

Picco, E.
Department of Pharmacology, Faculty of Veterinary Sciences, National University of the Litoral, Esperanza, Argentina

Dehghan, M. M.
Department of Surgery and Radiology, Faculty of Veterinary Medicine, University of Tehran, Tehran, Iran

Sookhtehzari, A.
Department of Clinical Sciences, School of Veterinary Medicine, Lorestan University, Khorramabad, Iran

Alirezaei, M.
Division of Biochemistry, School of Veterinary Medicine, Lorestan University, Khorramabad, Iran

Fakour, Sh.
Department of Clinical Sciences, Faculty of Veterinary Medicine, Sanandaj Branch of Islamic Azad University, Sanandaj, Iran

Hajizadeh, P.
Graduated from the Faculty of Veterinary Medicine, Sanandaj Branch of Islamic Azad University, Sanandaj, Iran

Habibian Dehkordi, S., Esmaeili, M. and Kabutari J.
Department of Pharmacology, School of Veterinary Medicine, Shahrekord University, Shahrekord, Iran

Arab, H. A.
Department of Pharmacology, Faculty of Veterinary Medicine, University of Tehran, Tehran, Iran

Shahbazfar, A. A.
Department of Pathobiology, School of Veterinary Medicine, University of Tabriz, Tabriz, Iran

Ghand Foroushan, M., Zendehdel, M. and Babapour, V.
Department of Basic Sciences, Faculty of Veterinary Medicine, University of Tehran, Tehran, Iran

Chalmeh, A. and Hajimohammadi, A.
Department of Clinical Sciences, School of Veterinary Medicine, Shiraz University, Shiraz, Iran

Mohamadi R.
Graduated Student of Animal Physiology, College of Agriculture and Natural Resources, University of Gonbad Kavous, Gonbad Kavous, Iran

Rahchamani, R., Ghanbari, F. and Farivar, F.
Department of Animal Sciences, College of Agriculture and Natural Resources, University of Gonbad Kavous, Gonbad Kavous, Iran

Taheriyan, M. R., Baghbanzadeh, A. and Zendehdel, M.
Department of Basic Sciences, Faculty of Veterinary Medicine, University of Tehran, Tehran, Iran

Hassanzadeh, M. and Moghimi Niaki, A. A.
Department of Avian Diseases, Faculty of Veterinary Medicine, University of Tehran, Tehran, Iran

Babapour, V.
Department of Basic Sciences, Faculty of Veterinary Medicine, University of Tehran, Tehran, Iran

Mohit, A.
Department of Animal Sciences, Faculty of Agriculture, University of Guillan, Rasht, Iran

Mirzaie, S.
Institute for Agricultural Research of Iranian Organization for Sciences and Technology, Tehran, Iran

Tolouei, T., Hassanzadeh, M. and Rezaei Far, A.
Department of Avian Diseases, Faculty of Veterinary Medicine, University of Tehran, Tehran, Iran

Chalmeh, A., Hajimohammadi, A., Asadollahpour, S. and Mazrouei Sebdani, M.
Department of Clinical Sciences, School of Veterinary Medicine, Shiraz University, Shiraz, Iran

Nikbakht, Gh. and Alkaragoly, H.
Department of Microbiology and Immunology, Faculty of Veterinary Medicine, University of Tehran, Tehran, Iran

Ghahri, H.
Department of Poultry Sciences, Faculty of Veterinary Medicine, Islamic Azad University, Urmia Branch, Urmia, Iran

Rassoli, A. and Fatouraee, N.
Biological Fluid Dynamics Laboratory, Biomechanics Department, Biomedical Engineering Faculty, Amirkabir University of Technology, Tehran, Iran

Mirderikvandi, M., Kiani, A. and Khaldari, M.
Animal Sciences Group, Faculty of Agriculture, Lorestan University, Khorram Abad, Iran

Alirezaei, M.
Division of Biochemistry, School of Veterinary Medicine, Lorestan University, Khorram Abad, Iran

Mehrparvar, M., Mazhari, M. and Esmaeilipour, O.
Department of Animal Sciences, Faculty of Agriculture, University of Jiroft, Kerman, Iran

Sami, M.
Department of Food Hygiene, Faculty of Veterinary Medicine, Shahid Bahonar University, Kerman, Iran

Mokhber Dezfouli, M. R., Tavanaeimanesh, H. and Sadeghian Chaleshtori, S.
Department of Internal Medicine, Faculty of Veterinary Medicine, University of Tehran, Tehran, Iran
Institute of Biomedical Research, Faculty of Veterinary Medicine, University of Tehran, Tehran, Iran

Hayati, F.
Department of Surgery and Radiology, Faculty of Veterinary Medicine, University of Tehran, Tehran, Iran

Dehghan, M. M.
Department of Surgery and Radiology, Faculty of Veterinary Medicine, University of Tehran, Tehran, Iran
Institute of Biomedical Research, Faculty of Veterinary Medicine, University of Tehran, Tehran, Iran

Akbarein, H.
Department of Food Hygiene and Quality Control, Faculty of Veterinary Medicine, University of Tehran, Tehran, Iran

Pournaghi, P.
Department of Biology, Payame Noor University, Tehran, Iran

Fakour, Sh.
Department of Clinical Sciences, Faculty of Veterinary Medicine, Sanandaj Branch of Islamic Azad University, Sanandaj, Iran

Alimohammadzadeh, P.
Young Research and Elite Club, Sanandaj Branch Islamic Azad University, Sanandaj, Iran

Vaziry, A.
Department of Clinical Sciences, Faculty of Agriculture, University of Kurdistan, Sanandaj, Iran

Sasani, F., Khaki, F. and Gharagouzloo, M. J.
Department of Pathology, Faculty of Veterinary Medicine, University of Tehran, Tehran, Iran

Nouri Gharajalar, S. and Zare, P.
Department of Pathobiology, Faculty of Veterinary Medicine, Tabriz University, Tabriz, Iran

Raoofi, A.
Department of Internal Medicine, Faculty of Veterinary Medicine, University of Tehran, Tehran, Iran

Yourdkhani, S.
Department of Clinical Sciences, Faculty of Veterinary Medicine, Garmsar Branch, Islamic Azad University, Garmsar, Iran

Bokaie, S.
Division of Epidemiology and Zoonoses, Department of Food Hygiene and Quality Control, Faculty of Veterinary Medicine, University of Tehran, Tehran, Iran

Ghasemifard, M., Rahchamani, R., Ghanbari, F. and Mostafalo, Y.
Department of Animal Sciences, College of Agriculture and Natural Resources, University of Gonbad Kavous, Gonbad Kavous, Iran

Rahimi, Z. S., Modirsanei, M., Mansoori, B., Rezaeian, M., Farkhoy, M. and Honarzad, J.
Department of Animal and Poultry Health and Nutrition, Faculty of Veterinary Medicine, University of Tehran, Tehran, Iran

Shokri, H.
Department of Pathobiology, Faculty of Veterinary Medicine, Amol University of Special Modern Technologies, Amol, Iran

Ghasemzadeh Nava, H., Kaveh Baghbadorani, M., Gharavi, J., Ghahremani, N. and Gharagozloo, F.
Department of Pathobiology, Faculty of Veterinary Medicine, Amol University of Special Modern Technologies, Amol, Iran

Index

R

S

T

www.ingramcontent.com/pod-product-compliance
Lightning Source LLC
LaVergne TN
LVHW060518210926
848485LV00005B/1105
* 9 7 8 1 6 3 9 8 7 2 2 3 7 *